Skin Changes and Diseases in Pregnancy

BASIC AND CLINICAL DERMATOLOGY

Series Editors

Alan R. Shalita, M.D.

Professor and Chairman
Department of Dermatology
State University of New York
Health Science Center at Brooklyn
Brooklyn, New York

David A. Norris, M.D.

Director of Research
Professor of Dermatology
The University of Colorado
Health Sciences Center
Denver, Colorado

1. Cutaneous Investigation in Health and Disease: Noninvasive Methods and Instrumentation, *edited by Jean-Luc Lévêque*
2. Irritant Contact Dermatitis, *edited by Edward M. Jackson and Ronald Goldner*
3. Fundamentals of Dermatology: A Study Guide, *Franklin S. Glickman and Alan R. Shalita*
4. Aging Skin: Properties and Functional Changes, *edited by Jean-Luc Lévêque and Pierre G. Agache*
5. Retinoids: Progress in Research and Clinical Applications, *edited by Maria A. Livrea and Lester Packer*
6. Clinical Photomedicine, *edited by Henry W. Lim and Nicholas A. Soter*
7. Cutaneous Antifungal Agents: Selected Compounds in Clinical Practice and Development, *edited by John W. Rippon and Robert A. Fromtling*
8. Oxidative Stress in Dermatology, *edited by Jürgen Fuchs and Lester Packer*
9. Connective Tissue Diseases of the Skin, *edited by Charles M. Lapière and Thomas Krieg*
10. Epidermal Growth Factors and Cytokines, *edited by Thomas A. Luger and Thomas Schwarz*
11. Skin Changes and Diseases in Pregnancy, *edited by Marwali Harahap and Robert C. Wallach*

ADDITIONAL VOLUMES IN PREPARATION

Biomedical Mycology, *edited by Paul H. Jacobs and Lexie Nall*

Skin Changes and Diseases in Pregnancy

edited by
Marwali Harahap
University of North Sumatra Medical School
Medan, Indonesia

Robert C. Wallach
New York University School of Medicine
New York, New York

Marcel Dekker, Inc. New York • Basel • Hong Kong

Library of Congress Cataloging-in-Publication Data

Skin changes and diseases in pregnancy / edited by Marwali Harahap,
Robert C. Wallach.
p. cm. — (Basic and clinical dermatology ; 11)
Includes index.
ISBN 0-8247-9401-X (hardcover : alk. paper)
1. Skin diseases in pregnancy. I. Harahap, Marwali.
II. Wallach, Robert C. III. Series.
[DNLM: 1. Skin Diseases—in pregnancy. 2. Skin Diseases—therapy.
3. Genital Diseases, Female—in pregnancy. 4. Pregnancy
Complications. W1 CL69L v.11 1996 / WR 140 S6274 1996]
RG580.S54S55 1996
618.3—dc20
DNLM/DLC
for Library of Congress 95-40122
CIP

The publisher offers discounts on this book when ordered in bulk quantities. For more information, write to Special Sales/Professional Marketing at the address below.

This book is printed on acid-free paper.

Marcel Dekker, Inc.
270 Madison Avenue, New York, New York 10016

Current printing (last digit):
10 9 8 7 6 5 4 3 2 1

PRINTED IN THE UNITED STATES OF AMERICA

Preface

No book or monograph has yet been written that is sufficiently detailed to provide a comprehensive guide to the diagnosis and management of skin changes and diseases in pregnancy. The relevant literature is scattered throughout numerous journals. Contradictory advice and opinion are rife, terminology is inconsistently used, and the burden of sorting fact from fiction is a daunting prospect. Given this situation, the utility of a thorough treatment of the topic is self-evident.

Skin Changes and Diseases in Pregnancy provides the reader with an authoritative and timely review of advances in the diagnosis and management of skin diseases in pregnancy. It also serves as a comprehensive source of current information on skin diseases that may have impact on the outcome of pregnancy. It is a useful reference for the diagnosis and management of perinatal genital infections. This book is also essential for all those who require basic guidance through the mass of drug information emanating from sources of varying authenticity. Full coverage is given to current knowledge of the risk and benefit of dermatological therapy during pregnancy and lactation. This book will be invaluable for dermatologists and obstetricians, as well as for general physicians and other medical practitioners.

Contributors were selected because of their expertise and special interest in the subject they cover. This volume is the end product of the coordinated efforts of two editors and fifteen authors from seven countries, and is designed to summarize the best in thought and research on skin changes and diseases in pregnancy.

Marwali Harahap
Robert C. Wallach

Contents

Contributors

Ingrun Anton-Lamprecht Professor and Director, Institute for Ultrastructure Research of the Skin, Department of Dermatology, Ruprecht-Karls University Heidelberg, Heidelberg, Germany

Betty Bellman, M.D. Department of Dermatology and Cutaneous Surgery, University of Miami School of Medicine, Miami, Florida

Brian Berman, M.D., Ph.D. Professor, Department of Dermatology and Cutaneous Surgery, University of Miami School of Medicine, Miami, Florida

Robert Charles-Holmes, M.D., F.R.C.P. Department of Dermatology, Warwick Hospital, Warwickshire, England

Susan M. Forster, B.Sc., M.B., B.S., M.R.C.P. Department of Genito-Urinary Medicine, Hinchingbrooke Hospital, Huntingdon, Cambridgeshire, England

Marwali Harahap, M.D. Professor, Department of Dermatology, University of North Sumatra Medical School, Medan, Indonesia

Michael John Hare, M.A., M.D., F.R.C.O.G. Department of Obstetrics and Gynecology, Hinchingbrooke Hospital, Huntingdon, Cambridgeshire, England

Wolfgang Jurecka, M.D. Professor, Division of General Dermatology, Department of Dermatology, University of Vienna, Vienna, Austria

Marek Lewandowski, M.D. Department of Human Anatomy, University of Bydgoszcz Medical Academy and City Hospital, Bydgoszcz, Poland and Visting Professor, Department of Cell Biology, Neurobiology, and Anatomy, The Ohio State University, Columbus, Ohio

Douglas J. Perkins Department of Cell Biology, Neurobiology, and Anatomy, Laboratory of Perinatal Research, Department of Obstetrics and Gynecology, The Ohio State University, Columbus, Ohio

Denis Sasseville, M.D., F.R.C.P.C., D.A.B.D. Assistant Professor, Department of Medicine (Dermatology), McGill University, Montreal, Quebec, Canada

Stephen T. Sonis, D.M.D., D.M.Sc. Chief, Division of Oral Medicine, Oral and Maxillofacial Surgery, and Dentistry, Brigham and Women's Hospital, and Professor of Oral Medicine, Harvard School of Dental Medicine, Boston, Massachusetts

Robert C. Wallach, M.D. Professor of Clinical Obstetrics and Gynecology, Department of Obstetrics and Gynecology, New York University School of Medicine, New York, New York

Reynold C. Wong, M.D. Clinical Associate Professor of Dermatology, Department of Dermatology, University of California, Davis, School of Medicine, Sacramento, California

Sook-Bin Woo, D.M.D., M.M.Sc. Attending Dentist, Division of Oral Medicine, Oral and Maxillofacial Surgery, and Dentistry, Brigham and Women's Hospital, and Instructor, Harvard School of Dental Medicine, Boston, Massachusetts

1

The Anatomy and Physiology of the Pregnant Woman

Marek Lewandowski
University of Bydgoszcz Medical Academy and City Hospital, Bydgoszcz, Poland, and The Ohio State University, Columbus, Ohio

Douglas J. Perkins
The Ohio State University, Columbus, Ohio

I. INTRODUCTION

The physiological processes essential for proper gestational development begin at conception and continue beyond parturition. Pregnancy is accompanied by adaptations within the maternal anatomy and physiology that are induced by changes within the hormonal milieu. During pregnancy, the development of a new endocrine gland, the placenta, assists in the secretion of a vast array of hormones that sustain fetal development. In addition, the maternal endocrine system also undergoes dramatic alterations during pregnancy. The interaction of various hormones from fetal and maternal sources imparts detectable changes within the maternal system that can be used for the diagnosis of pregnancy. Through proper diagnosis and prenatal care, the likelihood of a successful pregnancy is dramatically increased.

II. CONCEPTION AND EARLY EMBRYONIC DEVELOPMENT

A. Fertilization

The female must be in the ovulation phase of the menstrual cycle for fertilization to occur. Ovulation typically takes place around the fourteenth day of the menstrual cycle and involves the capture of the ovum by the fimbriae of the fallopian tube. Once captured, the fertilized ovum is then transported to the ampullar part of the fallopian tube by coordinated contractions of smooth muscle cells in the mesosalpinx and ciliary movements of epithelial cells. Activity within the mesosalpinx is modulated by the interaction of steroidal hormones produced by the corpus luteum during the luteal phase of the menstrual cycle. For example, estrogens enhance motility of the oviduct, whereas progesterone functions to inhibit oviduct motility. The interaction between estrogen and progesterone plays a major role in determining the site of fertilization within the fallopian tube (the typical fertilization location).

In addition to ovulation, fertilization requires the proper maturation and migration of sperm cells. The migration of sperm cells to the fertilization site usually takes place within a few hours following ejaculation. During ejaculation, fluid pressure provides sperm cells with the impetus to ascend into the uterus. While traveling from the vagina to the ampullar part of the fallopian tube, sperm cells undergo capacitation, a process which prepares the spermatozoa for fertilization. After reaching the uterus, contractions of the myometrium propel the sperm into the oviducts. The motile capacity of the sperm cells is an important factor in determining their ability to travel through the fallopian tube.

Fertilization typically occurs 14–15 days after last menstrual period and 12–24 hr after ovulation. If viable spermatozoa ascend successfully into the oviduct and come into contact with an ovulated oocyte, the spermatozoa attempt to insert their way into the cumulus mass of the oocyte (Fig. 1). This process requires the successful binding of spermatozoa to a human-specific glycoprotein sperm cell receptor located in the zona pellucida. Subsequent to receptor binding, the acrosome releases degradative enzymes such as hyaluronidase and acrosin that allow the sperm cell to separate and slough off the corona radiata and thus penetrate the zona pellucida. Once the spermatozoon penetrates the zona pellucida, the cell membranes of the spermatozoon and the oocyte fuse (Fig. 1). The fusion event promotes the release of cortical granules from beneath the cell membrane of the oocyte which prevents the penetration of the zona pellucida by additional spermatozoa. Subsequent to fertilization, the fertilized ovum is transported into the uterus.

During transportation of the ovum through the uterine tube, the zygote is cleaved into a blastomere. By 3–4 days, the embryo reaches the uterine cavity as a 16- to 32-cell–stage morula that becomes the developing embryoblast (see Fig. 1). After 4 days of development, the morula forms intracellular fluid-filled spaces between the blastomere which develop into the blastocyst cavity. The embryoblast cells aggregate to one side of the cavity (the embryonic pole) while the outer trophoblastic cell mass forms a single-layered epithelium. The resulting blastocyst then remains free inside the uterine cavity during next 2–3 days.

B. Implantation

Implantation typically occurs 7 days after ovulation (21 days after last menstrual period). The early phases of embryonic development are marked by hormonal

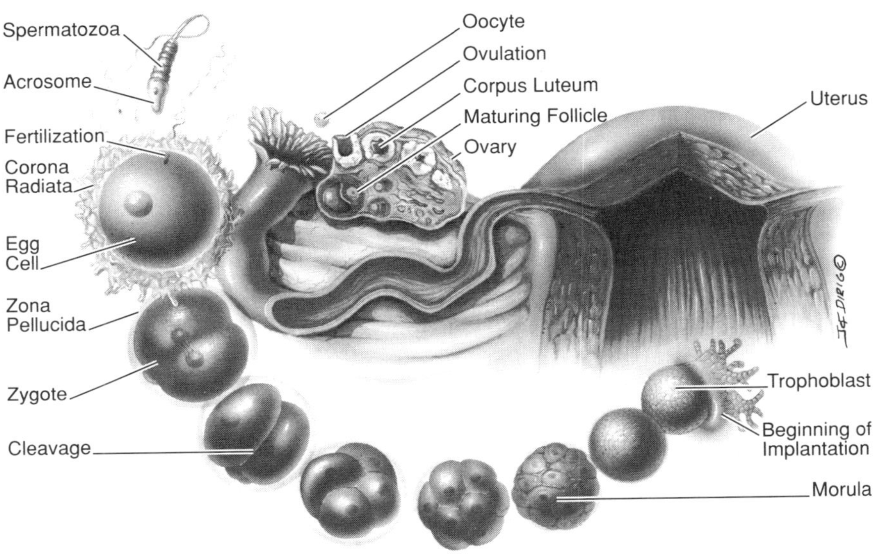

Figure 1 Fertilization and early embryonic development. Fertilization occurs when the spermatozoa penetrates and fuses with the egg cell. Following fusion of the two cells, the newly formed zygote goes through several divisions as it transverses the oviduct and enters the uterus.

secretions from the ovum that create alterations within the local and systemic embryonic environment. At present, the hormonal and enzymatic alterations accompanying embryonic development are only partially understood. Prior to implantation, the embryo has been shown to produce human chorionic gonadotropin (hCG), estradiol (E_2), and progesterone (1). Once implantation occurs, hCG is secreted at high levels from trophoblast cells. The release of hCG prevents the corpus luteum from degenerating and, therefore, prolongs the secretion of progesterone.

In addition to the release of hCG, trophoblast cells also produce proteolytic enzymes which digest the endometrial wall. Trophoblast cells penetrate the deep layers of the endometrium and allow for attachment of the embryo. The implanted conceptus is typically located on the anterior or posterior part of the uteral fundus. However, implantation may occur at abnormal sites such as the peritoneal cavity, oviduct, ovarian surface, or an alternate location within the uterus. Such ectopic pregnancies may provide a life-threatening situation for the mother.

C. Development of the Placenta

The tissue of the placenta is derived from the decidua basalis of the mother and fetal chorion. The chorionic membrane is composed of mesoderm and trophoblast cells which completely surround the conceptus. The embedded portion of the chorionic membrane is in intimate contact with the decidua basalis: the region of the decidua located under the site of implantation that participates in the formation of the mature placenta. During implantation, the trophoblast differentiates into two layers: an internal and external layer. The internal layer, the cytotrophoblast, gives rise to the external layer, the syncytiotrophoblast.

The cytotrophoblast expands to form radial columns that project into the decidua basalis. The central portion of the columns are supported by underlying connective tissue which eventually reaches the maternal tissue and develops into anchoring villi. Proliferation of the cytotrophoblast forms secondary and tertiary villi which are then invaded by angioblast cells. Tertiary villi are covered by a double-layered epithelium with an inner layer formed by the cytotrophoblast and an outer layer composed of the syncytiotrophoblast. Within the syncytiotrophoblast are lacunar spaces which surround the placental villi and anastomose with the maternal capillaries. At about 15 days postfertilization, maternal blood enters the lacunar spaces and completes the placental circulation. The maternal blood is separated from the fetal circulation by a "barrier" formed by the trophoblast, intervillous connective tissue, and the fetal capillary wall.

During the second month of development, the villi aggregate to form the so-called leafy tree (chorion frondosum), which is the fetal component of the placenta associated with the decidua basalis. Some of the relevant structures associated with blood flow in the maternal-fetal unit are shown in Figure 2. The placental villi continue to proliferate throughout the remainder of gestation until connective tissue is eventually replaced by capillaries which allow communication between the fetal and maternal blood. The general morphological correlates between the developing fetus and the mother are shown in Figure 3 at the sixth week of gestation.

III. THE ENDOCRINOLOGY OF PREGNANCY

A. Placental Hormones

1. Placental Peptide Hormones

a. Human Chorionic Gonadotropin. Human chorionic gonadotropin (hCG), a 39-kD glycosylated protein dimer composed of one alpha and one beta subunit, is a placental hormone secreted by the syncytiotrophoblast. The alpha subunit of hCG shares a high degree of homology with many other glycoproteins, whereas the beta subunit has a relatively unique structure. As such, expression of the beta subunit is often used for the diagnosis of pregnancy.

During gestation, increased levels of hCG first become detectable in the maternal plasma and urine approximately 9 days after conception (2). As with other placental hormones, levels of hCG change throughout the course of pregnancy (Fig.

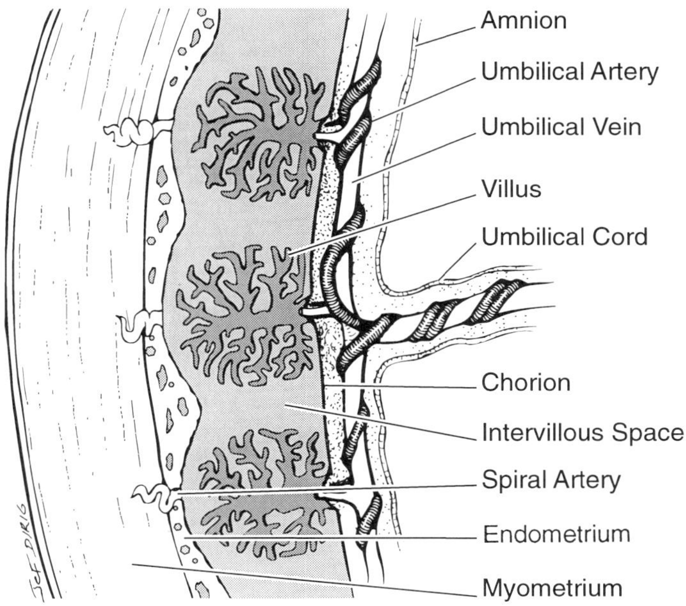

Figure 2 Cross-sectional representation of the relevant structures involved in placental circulation.

4). Serum levels of hCG increase rapidly during the first several weeks of pregnancy and then peak at 108,000 IU/L during the tenth week of gestation. After reaching maximal values, hCG levels decline rapidly to approximately 25% of the peak value between weeks 16–22 where they remain constant throughout the last trimester until parturition (3).

From a functional standpoint, hCG has been reported to prolong the life of the corpus luteum and increase the ovarian secretion of steroids during the early stages of pregnancy (4). However, after the fifth week of gestation, some investigators have reported that rapidly increasing levels of hCG have very little effect on prolongation of the corpus luteum (5). Although the mechanism for prolongation remains unclear, interactions of hCG with human chorionic somatomammotropin (hCS) appear to be important. After 8 weeks of gestation, function of the corpus luteum declines as the level of hCG rises to a maximal value. At present, the possible relevance of this inverse relationship remains elusive.

Although many facts about hCG have been reported, the actual role of the molecule in pregnancy is only partially understood. One important function often associated with hCG is activation of the thyroid gland through stimulation of intrinsic thyrotropic activity (6,7). Second, hCG appears to be important in stimu-

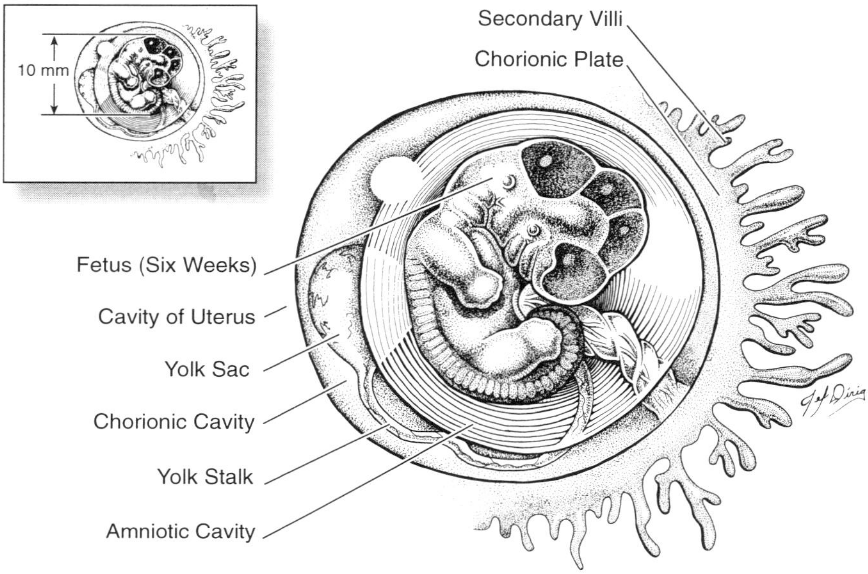

Figure 3 Structural relationship between the fetus and uteral wall at the sixth week of gestation.

lating the testes to produce testosterone. Third, hCG appears to regulate immunological functions by inhibiting the effect of maternal lymphocyte activity against trophoblastic cells (7,8).

b. Human Chorionic Somatomammotropin. Human chorionic somatomammotropin (hCS), also known as human placental lactogen (hLP), is a hormone secreted by the syncytiotrophoblast that reaches detectable levels in the maternal plasma between weeks 5 and 6 of gestation. The level of hCS rises throughout the course of pregnancy with values typically in the range of 6–7 μg/ml at term (see Fig. 4). hCS is a single-chain polypeptide of 191 amino acids held together by two disulfide bonds. Therefore, hCS is structurally similar to human growth hormone (hGH) produced by the pituitary gland. Moreover, hCS has many growth hormone–like effects on maternal metabolism during pregnancy (7).

Although the role of hCS in pregnancy is only partially understood, it is clear that hCS stimulates lipolysis, nitrogen-retaining activity, and calcium retention. In addition, hCS increases lactogenic activity in experimental animals. The definitive role of hCS in human lactogenic activity, however, has not been established. In the maternal system, hCS induces insulin resistance and carbohydrate intolerance (7). As such, hCS provides the fetus with increased levels of glucose throughout pregnancy by decreasing the maternal glucose uptake and insulin activity.

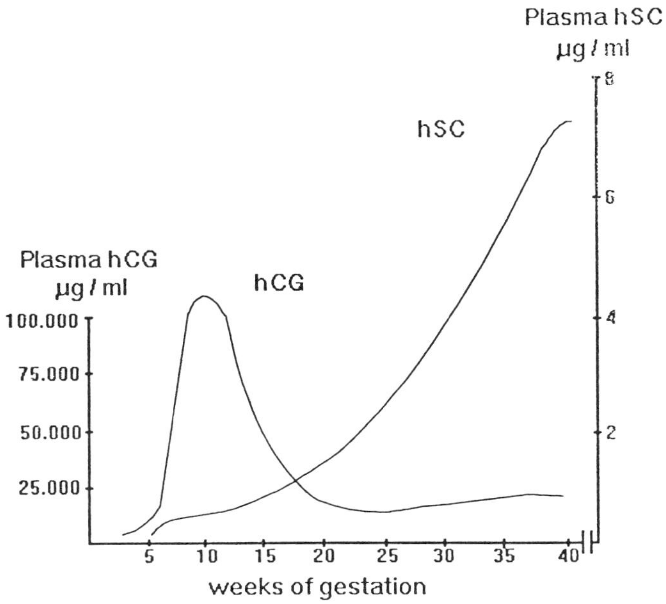

Figure 4 Plasma concentration levels of human chorionic gonadotropin (hCG) and human chorionic somatomammotropin (hCS) during pregnancy. (From Ref. 7.)

c. Relaxin. Relaxin is a peptide hormone produced by the persistent corpus luteum. The hormone is composed of two peptide chains of 24 and 29 amino acids linked by disulfide bridges. Plasma levels of relaxin rise in the first trimester when the corpus luteum is dominant and then decline during the second trimester of pregnancy (9). The major effect of relaxin appears to be softening of the cervix, inhibition of uterine contractions, and relaxation of the pubic symphysis. Although relaxin certainly appears to be important during pregnancy, studies in women with donated oocytes (i.e., without corpora lutea) suggest that relaxin is not an absolutely essential element for the maintenance of pregnancy.

d. Human Chorionic Thyrotropin. Human chorionic thyrotropin (hCT) is a thyrotropic substance secreted in small amounts by the placenta. The size and function of hCT are similar to pituitary TSH. However, hCT appears to be different from most other glycoproteins in that it does not share the common alpha subunit. Through a complex and poorly characterized mechanism, hCT interacts with hCG to increase thyroid hormone levels during pregnancy.

e. Human Chorionic Adrenocorticotropin. Throughout pregnancy the secretion of adrenocorticotropin (ACTH) and corticotropin-releasing hormone

(CRH) by the placenta causes a consistent rise in maternal cortisol levels (10,11). Since elevated maternal cortisol levels are resistant to suppression by dexamethasone, at least some of the maternal ACTH and CRH is not derived solely from maternal pituitary sources. The decreased suppression of cortisol by maternal ACTH during pregnancy is likely the result of an increased set-point of the pituitary-hypothalamic feedback mechanism. Although increased hormonal secretion is common, abnormally large increases in CRH values have been associated with such pathological conditions as premature labor, hypertension, fetal asphyxia, and intrauterine growth retardation (12).

2. *Steroid Hormones*

a. Estrogens: Estrone, Estradiol, Estriol. During the first 4–6 weeks of pregnancy, estrogens are produced by the corpus luteum. However, throughout the remainder of gestation, the placenta utilizes precursor molecules supplied from maternal and fetal origins for the production of estrogens. Estrone (E_1) and estradiol (E_2) are derived from maternal and fetal dehydroepiandrosterone sulfate (DHEAS) precursors, whereas estriol (E_3) is aromatized from 16OH-DHEA. The plasma concentration levels of E_1 remain relatively constant in early pregnancy before increasing rapidly in the tenth week of gestation, where levels remain elevated until term. Levels of E_1 are approximately 0.15 ng/ml at week 3, 2.25 ng/ml at week 13, and 2–30 ng/ml at term (13). The serum concentration of E_2 rises rapidly between weeks 16–20, plateaus between 20–30 weeks, and then rises to an average of 30 ng/ml at the end of the third trimester (5,14). E_3 plasma concentration values range from 0.01–0.05 ng/ml until approximately week 11, where the levels then slightly increase (5,13). The most pronounced elevation in E_3 plasma concentration is between weeks 35 and 40, with maximal levels peaking at about 15 ng/ml. After reaching peak values, E_3 plasma concentration remains elevated until term.

Estrogens have a multitude of functions in gestation and labor. A deficiency in the production of E_2 and E_3 may result in profound negative effects on the fetoplacental unit. Furthermore, estrogens are responsible for inducing changes within the maternal reproductive system, including enlargement of the uterus and breasts. E_1 plays an important role in increasing the flow of uterine blood, stimulating the renin-angiotensin-aldosterone system, and inducing the production of binding proteins in the liver.

Additionally, the process of parturition also requires the production of estrogens. During the last several weeks of pregnancy when plasma concentration levels of estrogens are elevated, these hormones induce the formation of binding sites for oxytocin in the myometrial layer of the uterus. In part, the increase in binding sites sets the stage for contraction of the uterus and the beginning of labor. Finally, estrogens relax the pelvic ligaments and prepare the maternal system for expulsion of the fetus.

b. Progesterone. The formation of progesterone takes place in the placenta with maternal cholesterol as the primary precursor. Prior to implantation, secretion of progesterone from the conceptus induces the relaxation of maternal tubal musculature. Moreover, progesterone also stimulates decidualization of the endometrium and inhibition of myometrial contractions. During the early stages of gestation, the main source of progesterone is via the maternal circulation by way of the persistent corpus luteum. The secretion of progesterone during the luteal phase of the menstrual cycle is about 25 mg/day, whereas the maternal plasma concentration is approximately 13.8 ng/ml. Although the production of progesterone by the ovaries persists until delivery, once the early stages of gestation have passed, the placenta is the main source of progesterone production (15). After the eighth week of gestation, bilateral luteectomy does not induce abortion due to the substantial supply of progesterone produced by the placenta (16). The production of progesterone rises throughout gestation to reach approximately 250 mg/day by term, with plasma concentration values in the range of 100–300 ng/ml (13). The rise in progesterone between weeks 36 and 40 occurs concomitant with the rapid increase in estradiol and estriol. The biochemical importance of the relationship, however, remains unclear.

Progesterone mediates many of the functionally important alterations that are necessary for the maintenance of pregnancy. In general, progesterone relaxes smooth muscle tissue within the maternal body. The inhibitory action of progesterone on contractile activity in the myometrium may provide a mechanism for the prevention of abortion. Together with estrogen, progesterone is responsible for regulating uterine growth. Progesterone is capable of inhibiting the stimulatory effect that estrogens have on uterine blood flow. In addition, high concentrations of progesterone have been shown to block the secretion of hCG while having little, if any, effect on the production hCS (17). Finally, progesterone appears to play a role in regulating the maternal metabolic activities by increasing sodium excretion in the renal tubule and elevating blood flow to the kidney.

B. Maternal Endocrine System

1. Pituitary Gland

The pituitary gland enlarges significantly during normal pregnancy. Magnetic resonance imaging of normal gravidas and nonpregnant controls reveals that the size of the pituitary gland increases as much as 136% at term (18). In addition, pregnancy is also marked by an increase in the release of pituitary growth hormone (PGH) which appears to be regulated, at least in part, by hCS. The release of PGH from the pituitary gland is antagonized by hCS.

Serum pituitary prolactin levels begin increasing in the first trimester and continue to elevate until term. The activity of prolactin appears to be the most important factor in determining lactation. The stimulation of lactogenesis by prolactin requires a decline in the levels of estrogen and progesterone. After delivery, prolactin concentration decreases in lactating and nonlactating women. However, somatosensory pathways induced by suckling are capable of inducing the release of prolactin and, therefore, maintaining the elevated plasma prolactin levels necessary for lactation.

2. *Thyroid Gland*

The thyroid gland undergoes a slight enlargement (approximately 13%) during pregnancy that is generally not detectable on palpation (19). Enlargement of the thyroid during pregnancy is due to hyperplasia of follicular tissue and an increase in glandular blood flow. In addition, glandular size is also increased by a rise in thyroxine (T_4)–binding globulin (TBG) concentration coupled with a decrease in the concentration of circulating extrathyroidal iodine in the maternal blood. During pregnancy, an increase in the clearance of iodine occurs in the maternal thyroid and kidney. The elevation of iodine in the maternal plasma prompts the passage of iodine through the placenta into the fetus. The subsequent rise of iodine in the fetal circulation triggers the developing fetus to synthesize fetal thyroid hormone.

The basal metabolic and resting pulse rate are elevated in the maternal thyroid gland during pregnancy. These changes are likely induced by the activity of hCG and placental thyrotropin. Additionally, the influence of high levels of estrogens indirectly causes TBG to rise from about 7.1 mg/dl in the first trimester to 8.9 mg/dl by term. The increase in TBG levels results from an elevation in the concentration of total triiodothyronine (TT_3) and total thyroxine (TT_4) (20). The plasma concentration of the active hormones free T_3 (FT_3) and free T_4 (FT_4) are unchanged throughout pregnancy.

The hypothalamic-pituitary-thyroid relationship does not appear to undergo dramatic alterations throughout the course of pregnancy. However, serum thyroid-stimulating hormone (TSH) levels appear to decrease in the early phases of pregnancy and then return to nonpregnant values by the end of the first trimester (21). Values of thyroid-releasing hormone (TRH) seem to remain relatively constant during gestation.

3. *Parathyroid Hormone and Calcium Metabolism*

Parathyroid hormone (PTH) concentration declines slightly in the maternal plasma during the first trimester and then increases in the second trimester to values approximately 50% higher than those observed in the nonpregnant state. Elevation of PTH is contingent on an increase in plasma volume, a rise in glomerular filtration, and transportation of ionized calcium through the placenta into the fetus (22).

The concentration of total calcium in the maternal system decreases from approximately 10.3 mg/100 ml in the first trimester to around 9.8 mg/ml in the last month of gestation (23). Figure 5 demonstrates the decline in total maternal calcium (mg/100 ml) which parallels the decreasing level of maternal albumin (g/100 ml). The level of ionized maternal calcium declines during pregnancy from 2.33 mEq/L at the onset of gestation to 2.24 mEq/L at term (24). The decrease in ionized calcium induces a feedback mechanism that regulates the secretion PTH. Therefore, physiological hyperparathyroidism is observed at term.

The only organs that undergo increased calcium reabsorption during pregnancy are the intestines and kidney. The high levels of PTH that are produced during pregnancy have little impact on the maternal bones, because elevated levels of estrogen prevent calcium reabsorption. In addition, reabsorption of calcium in the maternal bones is further restricted by elevated levels of calcitonin in the maternal plasma. Throughout gestation, the level of calcitonin in the maternal circulation remains lower than that of the fetal circulation (25).

4. *Adrenal Glands*

The overall size of the adrenal glands does not change significantly during pregnancy. However, an increase in the width of the zona fasciculata is common during gestation (26). In the pregnant woman, there is an increase in the release of cortisol, deoxycorticosterone, and aldosterone by the adrenal glands. The level of

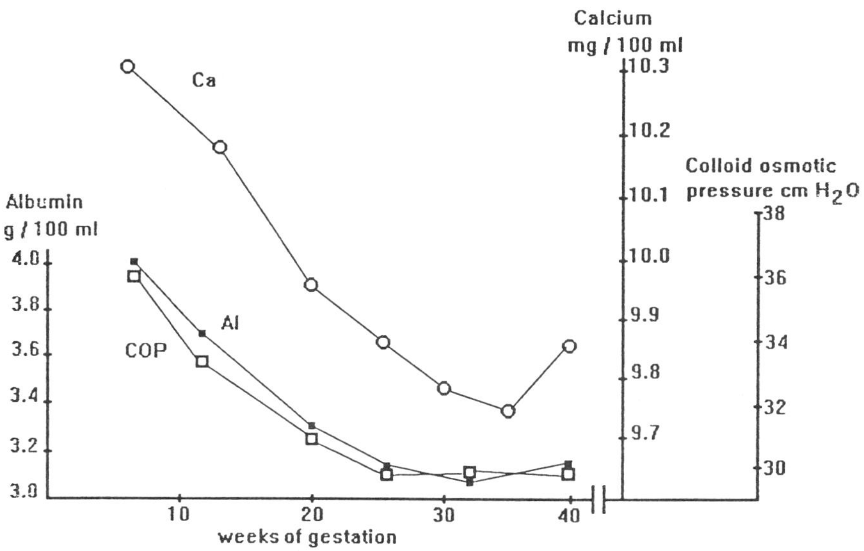

Figure 5 Relationship between colloid osmotic pressure, and plasma concentration levels of total calcium and albumin. COP, colloid osmotic pressure; Ca, total calcium; Al, Albumin. (From Refs. 23 and 24.)

hormone-binding globulin also increases during pregnancy owing to the stimulatory effect of elevated estrogen levels.

An increase in the secretion of ACTH usually occurs around 12 weeks of pregnancy, at which it continues to rise until the end of gestation, with levels approximately threefold higher than in the nonpregnant state. The secretion of ACTH appears to be regulated, at least in part, by progesterone. The addition of progesterone to pituitary cells in vitro inhibits the secretion of ACTH.

a. Cortisol. The plasma concentration level of free cortisol decreases slightly during pregnancy, because of an elevation in the amount of cortisol in the bound form. However, the production of cortisol does not change significantly during pregnancy. The elevation of cortisol plasma levels appears to be due to a reduced clearance of the hormone and prolongation of the molecule's half-life. The mean amplitude of episodic secretion between the single minimum and maximum plasma cortisol levels is markedly higher in pregnant women, whereas the normal rhythm of cortisol secretion remains unchanged. Throughout gestation, the levels of transcortin increase as a result of the altered estrogen levels. If, however, the value of estradiol remains below 130 ng/dl and the level of estrone does not exceed 50 ng/dl, the amount of bound cortisol does not rise substantially during pregnancy (27).

b. Aldosterone. The secretion of aldosterone increases around 8 weeks of gestation, reaches a plateau during the second trimester, and rises substantially in the last trimester to reach plasma concentrations levels of 59.4 ng/100 ml (10-fold higher than nonpregnant values) (14). The elevation of aldosterone values coincides with the observed increase in the renin-angiotensin system that imparts compensatory mechanisms for the effect of progesterone on natrium metabolism. For additional information on the relationship between aldosterone and plasma progesterone levels, refer to Wilson et al. (14).

c. Androstenedione. During pregnancy, the plasma levels of androstenedione are largely determined by the relative increase in testosterone and sex hormone–binding globulin. The placenta utilizes maternal androstenedione for the production of estradiol. Since the clearance rate of androstenedione is greater in the gestational state, circulating plasma levels of the compound are elevated relative to nonpregnant controls.

IV. MATERNAL ADAPTATIONS DURING PREGNANCY

A. Genital Tract

1. Uterus

The uterus of the nonpregnant female is a pear-shaped, thick-walled muscular organ that measures 7–9 cm in length, 5–6 cm in breath, and 2.5 cm in thickness.

The dome of the uterus superior to the ostia of the fallopian tubes is known as the fundus. The largest two-thirds of the uterus (superior portion) is termed the body, or corpus. During gestation, the uterus undergoes physiological and anatomical changes that are, in part, mediated by the levels of estrogen and progesterone. In addition, uterine tissue is also influenced by placental hormones. During the first several weeks of pregnancy, the fundus and corpus become more globular in shape. The size of the uterus doubles by about the tenth week of pregnancy and, from the first trimester onward, can be palpated above the symphysis pubis. Protrusion of the abdomen can be observed as the uterus pushes against the anterior abdominal wall. The magnitude of abdominal enlargement is partially determined by the height and weight of the pregnant woman. In addition, variations in the amount of amniotic fluid and positioning of the fetus also contribute to differences in the degree of abdominal enlargement.

During the second trimester, the uterus transforms into a more spherically shaped organ. The change in anatomical shape results from a more rapid expansion of the uterus in length than in width. As fetal development proceeds, the uterus undergoes dextrorotation, because of pressure exerted from the rectosigmoid colon located on the left side of the maternal body. The fundus of the uterus ascends superiorly during each successive week of fetal maturation (Fig. 6). As such, the fundus can be palpated through the anterior abdominal wall. Palpation of the fundus is a useful technique for determining the gestational age of the fetus.

From the thirty-second week until term, uterine growth proceeds slowly with the fundus peaking in height approximately 4 weeks prior to term. After reaching a maximum upward displacement, the uterus descends a few centimeters prior to parturition. The weight of the uterus increases dramatically during pregnancy from 70 to 100 g prior to conception to approximately 1100 g at term. The tremendous increase in size results from hypertrophy and hyperplasia of myometrial cells. Hyperplasia predominates in the early stages of pregnancy, whereas hypertrophy is most common during the later stages of gestation. Individual myometrial cells grow as much as 100 times in length to reach a total length of 500 μm at term. Furthermore, collagenous connective tissue and intercellular ground substance are also increased. The thickness of the myometrium increases throughout the first two trimesters and then decreases in the last trimester as a result of pressure exerted by the growing fetus.

2. *Cervix*

The inferior third of the uterus continuous with the superior corpus is known as the cervix. The cervix projects into and communicates with the vagina via the uterine ostium. The uterine cervix, composed mainly of collagenous tissue, contains substantially less smooth muscle than the corpus. Vascularity, hyperplasia, and hypertrophy of the cervical glands are dramatically increased at the onset of

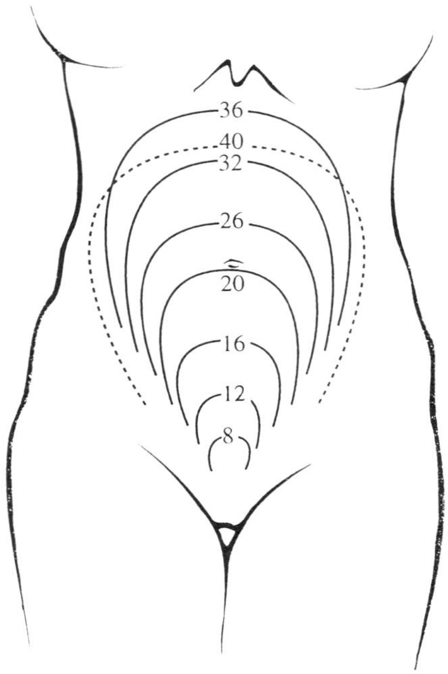

Figure 6 Height of the uteral fundus during the successive weeks of pregnancy.

pregnancy. Together these processes induce softening and cyanosis of the cervix. Moreover, eversion of the endocervical epithelium is also common during gestation. Glands of the cervical mucosa, under the influence of progesterone, proliferate near term to produce a mucous plug. During the early stages of labor, dilation of the cervix appears to be largely determined by prostaglandin E_2 (PGE_2). Although the cervix does contain prostaglandin receptors, the underlying biochemical mechanism responsible for cervical dilation is poorly understood.

3. Vagina

The vagina is the musculomembranous tube which forms the inferior portion of the female genital tract. The vagina is typically 7–9 cm in length and extends from the vestibule of the perineum to the cervix uteri. The pH of the vagina is acidic (4–5.0) owing to lactic acid produced in the breakdown of glycogen by Dorderlein bacilli. Vaginal acidity assists in protecting the genital tract by retarding the growth of various pathogens. The vascularity of the vagina increases during pregnancy and produces a violetlike color in the vaginal mucosa. Throughout gestation, the vaginal walls thicken and vaginal secretions are elevated.

B. Breasts

Some of the earliest physical manifestations characteristic of pregnancy can be observed in the breasts. Typically, tenderness, tingling, and heaviness of the breasts can be recognized in the pregnant female 4–6 weeks after the last menstrual period. From the eighth week of gestation onward, the breasts grow rapidly and their superficial venous network becomes visible. During pregnancy, the areolae increase in size and change from a pink color in white nulliparous women to a deep brown to black color depending on skin pigmentation. The circumference of the areolae increases from about 34–36 mm in the nonpregnant state to about 50–52 mm just after delivery. The diameter of the nipples ranges from 9.5–11.5 mm in primigravidas to 10.0–12.5 mm in multigravidas. The total increase in breast tissue during pregnancy is approximately 400 ml.

Changes that take place in the breasts during pregnancy are stimulated by a vast array of hormones, including estradiol, progesterone, placental lactogen, prolactin growth hormone, and thyroid hormone. The exact in vivo role of most of these hormonal substances is only partially understood in the gestational state. However, one function known to have multiple hormonal influences that is, at least, partially understood is lactogenesis. Growth of the lactiferous ducts for the preparation of milk production appears to be mediated by estradiol, whereas progesterone appears to be responsible for the increase in alveolar growth and the inhibition of proliferating prolactin receptors (28). The growth of the breasts for the preparation of milk production is presented in Figure 7. In order for lactogenesis to begin, the withdrawal of estrogen and progesterone is necessary. After delivery, levels of progesterone decrease to allow the proliferation of prolactin receptors and the onset of lactation (29). Prior to lactation in the last trimester, the mammary glands secrete a white to yellowish pre–milk fluid known as colostrum.

C. Cardiovascular System

1. *Anatomical Adaptations of the Heart*

The relative position and overall size of the heart changes throughout the course of pregnancy. During gestation, the heart moves superiorly and to the left as a result of the progressive elevation of the diaphragm. The amount of upward displacement of the diaphragm is determined by the amount of uterine expansion, maternal weight, and maternal height. In the pregnant woman, the heart undergoes a slight hypertrophy that can be visualized in radiographs. Cardiac hypertrophy results from an increase in blood volume and cardiac output. Additionally, the heart may also display atrial dilatation during pregnancy that is not necessarily suggestive of mitral valvular disease.

In the later stages of pregnancy, displacement of the heart coupled with an increase in blood volume causes auscultatory changes such as systolic ejection

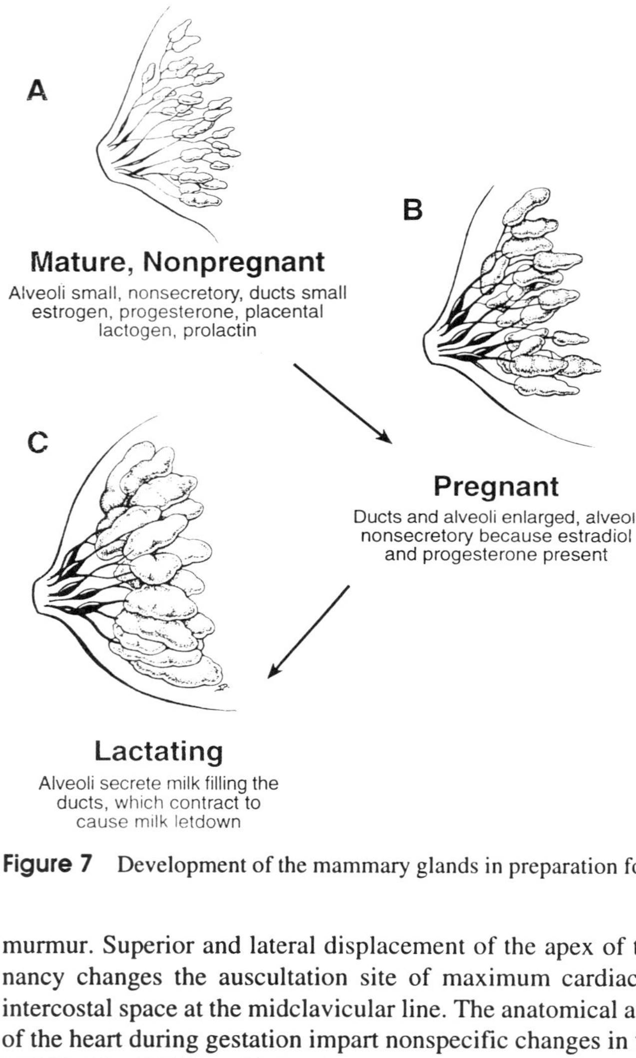

Figure 7 Development of the mammary glands in preparation for lactogenesis.

murmur. Superior and lateral displacement of the apex of the heart during pregnancy changes the auscultation site of maximum cardiac action to the fourth intercostal space at the midclavicular line. The anatomical and functional changes of the heart during gestation impart nonspecific changes in the electrocardiogram (ECG). The ECG profile in the pregnant woman may show left axis deviation, nonspecific depression of the S-T segment, and lower voltage in QRS complexes (30).

2. *Hemodynamic Adaptations*

a. Blood Volume. The total maternal blood volume rises about 30% during normal singleton pregnancy. The magnitude of the increase in maternal blood volume is determined by changes in plasma volume and red cell volume. Plasma volume rapidly elevates until 30–34 weeks of pregnancy, where levels remain constant until term. After delivery, plasma volume quickly decreases to the nonpregnant or slightly lower value. The maximal increase in plasma volume over nonpregnant values is about 30% (1000 ml) if iron supplementation accompanies the pregnancy (31,32). The red cell volume rises throughout pregnancy, with peak values occurring around week 30.

b. Cardiac Output. The most significant hemodynamic change that takes place during pregnancy is the 40% increase (1.5 L/min) in maternal cardiac output (32). A rise in cardiac output results from an elevation of heart rate and stroke volume. In addition, the placental circulation (or peripheral vascular resistance) creates an alteration in the maternal cardiac output. The cardiac output rises persistently until 16–22 weeks of gestation, at which levels remain steady until delivery. The stroke volume increases around 30% (from 64 to 71 ml) throughout the course of pregnancy. The maximal stroke volume values occur between weeks 20 and 24, with values either maintaining a plateau or slightly declining prior to delivery (33).

During gestation, the heart rate increases about 15 beats per minute prior to week 28, and from that time onward, the heart rate remains relatively constant. At present, it is not clear why an increase in cardiac output takes place during the early stages of pregnancy prior to the dramatic rise in uterine blood flow. In general, the distribution of blood to the various organs is unchanged throughout gestation. However, a few exceptions should be noted: (a) the uterus receives about 3% of the cardiac output in the first trimester and approximately 17% of the cardiac output in the later stages of pregnancy, (b) the distribution of cardiac output to the kidneys rises approximately 40%, and (c) blood flow to the breasts increases slightly (34). The dramatic elevation in uterine and renal blood flow is compensated for by alterations in the cardiac output.

c. Blood Pressure. The peripheral vascular resistance of the pregnant female declines until week 24 of gestation, because of the relaxing influence imparted by elevated progesterone levels. Accompanying the decline in peripheral vascular resistance is a decrease in blood pressure by approximately 10 mmHg. In normal pregnancies, blood pressure returns to nonpregnant values during the last trimester. Blood pressure in the pregnant woman is maximal when she is either seated or when she is lying in the supine position. The minimum blood pressure value can be achieved when the pregnant female is in the lateral recumbent position. An increase in blood pressure is due to compression of the pelvic and abdominal vessels by the enlarged uterus. Enlargement of the uterus causes the partial occlusion of venous blood return from the lower extremities. A progressive rise in venous blood pressure often occurs in the lower limbs during pregnancy with values doubling around week 10 (35). Occlusion of the vena cava and pelvic veins by the enlarged uterus is especially prominent in the later stages of pregnancy. These partial blockages frequently result in hemorrhoids, edema, and varicose veins in the lower extremities.

3. *Hematological Changes*

a. Red Blood Cells and Iron Metabolism. Since the requirement for oxygen is dramatically increased during pregnancy, an increase in red blood cells (RBC) is necessary for the transport of oxygen to the maternal viscera and fetus. Red blood cell volume rises progressively during gestation, with maximal values peaking near term. Accompanying the rapid rise in RBC production is the demand for increased iron intake in the maternal diet. During pregnancy, the red blood cell mass increases as much as 20–30% (250–400 ml) with iron supplementation and 17% when additional iron is not added to the maternal diet. The total intake requirement for iron throughout the course of pregnancy is around 1000 mg. Of that 1000 mg, the pregnant woman utilizes about 500 mg, transfer to the fetus accounts for 300 mg, and approximately 200 mg is lost through excretion. The average daily iron requirement during pregnancy is between 6 and 7 mg (36).

During the first two trimesters, a decline in hematocrit results in anemia. This is largely because red cell mass increases at a slower rate than plasma volume. The normal pregnant woman can absorb about 20% of the iron that she ingests, whereas gravidas with iron deficiency anemia are capable of absorbing much more. Importantly, fetal iron stores are not reduced during maternal iron deficiency anemia.

b. Leukocytes and Platelets. The white blood cell count increases from 3,000 to 15,000/mm^3 in nonpregnant women to 6,000 to 16,000/mm^3 in pregnant women. The white blood cell count usually peaks during labor at levels as high as 30,000/mm^3 and then rapidly returns to normal levels after delivery (37). The increase in white blood cells is largely determined by elevated circulating neutrophil polymorphonuclear cells (granulocytes).

Although past reports of platelet count have been conflicting, the availability of automated cell counters has now made reports more reliable. It appears that a slight decline in platelet count may take place during the second trimester, because of the increase in plasma volume.

c. Coagulation Factors. Several coagulation factors are increased during gestation, whereas others either remain unchanged or even decrease. Table 1 shows the physiological alterations in the coagulation factors during the third trimester. Plasma fibrinogen (factor I) rises approximately 50% from a range of 200–300 mg/dl in nonpregnant woman to a range of 300–600 mg/dl at term. In addition, factors VII (proconvertin), VIII (antihemophilic globulin), IX (Christmas factor), XII (Hageman factor), and X (Stuart factor) are also significantly elevated. In contrast, the levels of factors XI (plasma thromboplastin) and XIII

Table 1 Physiological Changes in Coagulation Factors During the Third Trimester

Coagulation factors	Factor no.	Change from nonpregnant level (%)
Fibrinogen	I	Increased (50)
Prothrombin	II	Unchanged
Proaccelerin	V	Unchanged
Proconvertin	VII	Increased (106)
Antihemophilic factor (AHF)	VIII	Increased (92)
Christmas factor	IX	Increased (140)
Stuart factor	X	Increased (65)
Plasma thromboplastin	XI	Decreased (60)
Hageman factor	XII	Increased
Fibrin-stabilizing factor	XIII	Increased (50)

Source: Data from Refs. 38 and 39.

(fibrin-stabilizing factor) are slightly decreased during pregnancy. Although the values of factors V (proaccelerin) and II (prothrombin) are relatively constant during gestation, some investigators have reported a slight increase in the concentration of Iiprothrombin (38,39). Finally, fibrinolytic activity increases during early gestation and then declines in the last trimester with accompanying thrombosis.

D. Respiratory System

1. Anatomical Adaptations of the Thoracic Cage

The anatomical changes that take place within the thoracic cage during gestation are partially induced by mechanical pressure of the growing uterus. The transverse diameter of the thoracic cage increases about 2 cm and the thoracic circumference increases up to 6 cm. Interestingly, these changes begin during the first trimester before the uterus can elevate the diaphragm and change the dimensions of the thorax. The mechanism responsible for the early changes in the dimensions of the thorax is only partially understood. One key factor that appears to be involved in thoracic enlargement is progesterone. The elevated levels of progesterone which accompany gestation are capable of softening the thoracic ligaments and cartilaginous attachments of the ribs. In addition, muscles of the anterolateral abdominal wall prepare for thoracic enlargement by becoming more relaxed. As a final step in expansion of the thorax, maternal respiration becomes more diaphragmatic and thus allows the dissipation of abdominal breathing as the pregnancy progresses.

2. *Physiological Adaptations of Pulmonary Function*

The widespread physiological changes which occur in the respiratory system during pregnancy are necessary to compensate for an increase in oxygen consumption by the fetus and mother (Fig. 8). In the pregnant female, basal oxygen consumption rises 30–40 ml/min (15–20% over the nonpregnant state). The elevation in O_2 consumption is influenced by alterations in maternal renal reabsorption, cardiac output, and respiration (40).

The products of conception, namely, the fetus and placenta, consume about 14–18 ml/min of oxygen. The amount of oxygen consumed varies according to metabolic demand and fetal weight. By measuring pulmonary volume and capacity, pulmonary functions can be characterized. Alterations in lung volume and capacity during normal pregnancy are presented in Table 2. During gestation, the pregnant female breathes deeper and therefore increases tidal volume (TV) by approximately 30–40% and inspiratory capacity (IF) by about 5%. In contrast, functional residual capacity (FCC), residual volume (RV), and expiratory reserve volume (ERV) are reduced around 20%. The respiratory rate (RR) and vital capacity (VC) remain constant throughout gestation. In addition, forced expiratory volume (FEV) also appears relatively unchanged, with the normal range of 80–85% of the vital capacity being maintained until term (40). The minute ventilation rises about

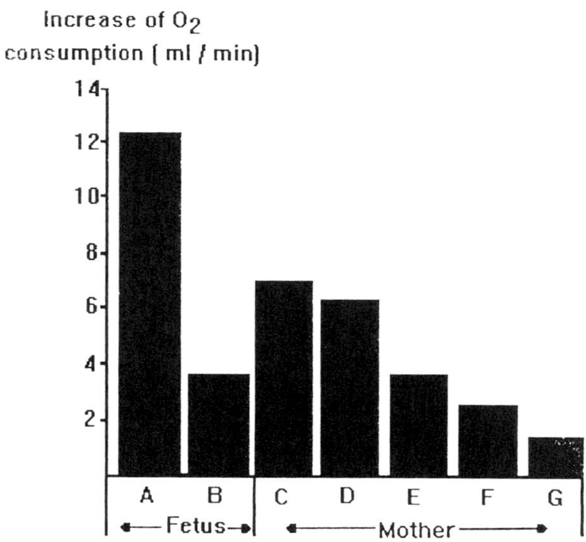

Figure 8 Distribution of oxygen consumption at the end of the last trimester. Fetal compartment: A, fetus; B, placenta. Maternal compartment: C, kidney; D, cardiac output; E, myometrium; F, respiration; and G, breasts. (From Ref. 40.)

Table 2 Changes in Lung Volume and Capacity During Normal Pregnancy

Lung volumes and capacities	Abbreviations	Changes during pregnancy (%)
Vital capacity	VC	Unchanged
Tidal volume	VT	Increased (30–40)
Functional residual capacity	FRC	Decreased (20)
Residual volume	RV	Decreased (20)
Expiratory reserve volume	ERV	Decreased (20)
Inspiratory reserve volume	IRV	Unchanged
Inspiratory capacity	IC	Increased (5)
Respiratory rate	RR	Unchanged
Forced expiratory volume	FEV1	Unchanged

Source: Data from Ref. 40.

30–40% during gestation from 7.5 L/min in the nonpregnant state to 10.5 L/min in the second trimester, where levels are maintained until delivery. The minute ventilation is contingent on the RR and TV values.

Because of the 20% rise in O_2 consumption and the 40% increase in minute ventilation, respiratory alkalosis is frequently observed during gestation. The arterial blood gas changes during normal pregnancy are presented in Table 3. An increase in respiratory effort during pregnancy results in a decrease of maternal Pco_2 from normal levels of 35–40 mmHg to levels of 30 mmHg (40). The decrease in maternal Pco_2 is compensated for by an increase in renal bicarbonate excretion. The increase in renal bicarbonate excretion subsequently assists in maintaining the maternal pH at the normal value of 7.40.

Table 3 Arterial Blood Gas Changes During Normal Pregnancy

Arterial blood gas	Nonpregnant women	Pregnant women
Po_2	85–90 mmHg	85–90 mmHg
Pco_2	35–40 mmHg	30 mmHg
pH	7.40	7.40
Hco_3	24 mEq/L	21 mEq/L

Source: Data from Ref. 40.

3. *Pulmonary Hemodynamics*

Pulmonary blood flow rises from 4.88 L/min in the nonpregnant state to 7.19 L/min during gestation (41). However, since vascular resistance declines from the first trimester onward on account of elevated levels of estrogens, progesterone, and prostacyclin, the pulmonary arterial pressure does not change significantly during pregnancy.

E. Urinary System

1. *Anatomical Changes*

Both the size and weight of the kidneys are enhanced during pregnancy. The length of each kidney increases about 1.0–1.5 cm. The renal pelvices, calices, and ureters begin dilating at the end of the first trimester. These changes in renal anatomy are especially pronounced on the right side owing to compression of the ureter against the bony pelvis by the enlarged uterus and ovarian venous plexus. Compression of abdominal contents by the uterus is greater on the right side owing to rotation of the organ to the right.

The relaxing effect of progesterone on smooth muscle tissue contributes to dilation of the collecting system. As such, changes within the urinary bladder are common during pregnancy. The urinary bladder becomes flattened in the sagittal plane owing to compression exerted by the expanding uterus. In addition, the trigone of the bladder is widened and elevated superiorly resulting in a decrease in volume capacity. The anatomical changes that occur in the urinary system during pregnancy may cause urinary frequency and nocturia. Further exacerbation of urinary problems may result from elevated levels of progesterone that relax the urethral sphincter and tone of the bladder.

2. *Physiological Changes in Renal Function*

In the gestational state, renal plasma flow (RPF) increases about 75% and glomerular filtration rate (GFR) rises around 50% (42,43). The RPF and GFR increase rapidly during the first trimester, slightly during the second trimester, and then decline throughout the third trimester until parturition (Fig. 9). In addition, endogenous creatinine clearance (CC) begins rising in the sixth week of gestation and plateaus at maximal values throughout most of pregnancy until several weeks prior to term, at which levels slightly decrease. The total increase in CC during gestation is approximately 45%. The regulatory mechanisms responsible for these physiological changes are largely unknown. However, the relative position of the pregnant female appears, at least in part, to influence physiological alterations. In the supine position, the uterus compresses the inferior vena cava inferiorly and reduces venous blood return to the heart. The resulting reduction in cardiac output imparts a decrease in RPF and GFR. In contrast, in the lateral recumbent position, the RPF

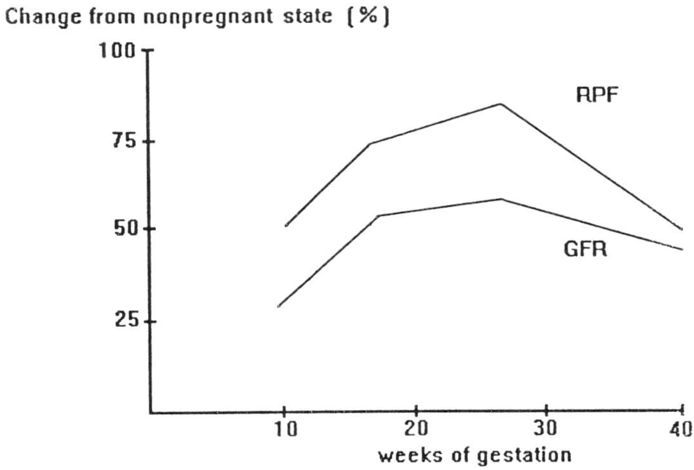

Figure 9 Physiological changes in renal hemodynamics throughout pregnancy. GFR, glomerular filtration rate; RPF, renal plasma flow. (From Ref. 43.)

and GFR are increased, with differences between the pregnant and nonpregnant state being dramatically reduced.

Functional changes in the renal system during pregnancy produce alterations in sodium metabolism. The dramatic increase in body water of the pregnant woman results in the retention of about 800–900 mEq of sodium. The tubular reabsorption of sodium is increased by elevated levels of aldosterone, deoxycorticosterone, and estrogens. However, despite dramatic alterations in sodium reabsorption, pregnant women are able to maintain a normal serum sodium concentration over a wide range of sodium diets. Therefore, the kidney of the pregnant woman is capable of maintaining sodium balance and tonicity.

In addition to the effect on sodium reabsorption, alerted renal tubular function also induces the excretion of glucose. From early gestation onward, the loss of glucose is not compensated for by tubular reabsorption. Therefore, physiological glucosuria increases throughout pregnancy until term.

F. Gastrointestinal Tract

1. Stomach. Gastric emptying time is prolonged during pregnancy owing to relaxation of the muscular layer of the stomach by progesterone. Functional secretions of the stomach are altered from the early weeks of conception until term. The production and secretion of gastrin from the gastric mucosa are substantially elevated during pregnancy. Therefore, fluctuations in the level of gastric acidity are common. Gastric reflux (heartburn) frequently occurs in the pregnant woman owing to a reduction in the tone of the gastroesophageal sphincter. In addition, displacement and compression of the stomach by the growing uterus, particularly during later stages of pregnancy, also contributes to gastric reflux.

2. Large and Small Intestines. The small intestine of the pregnant female is displaced superiorly and laterally by the expanding uterus. In addition, compression of the large intestine is also common as the uterus increases in size. Displacement of the appendix superiorly and laterally to the right flank is frequently observed during pregnancy. Mechanical obstruction of the large bowel and, hence, constipation is especially prominent in the later stages of pregnancy. The elevated anatomical pressure below the pelvic brim and rectal venous plexus may result in hemorrhoids. Although significant anatomical alterations occur in the large and small intestines, the absorption of nutrients is relatively unchanged. However, absorption of iron from the small intestine becomes more efficient during gestation, and the absorption of water and sodium by the large intestine is increased as well.

3. Liver and Gallbladder. The position and morphology of the liver remain stable throughout pregnancy. During gestation, the flow of hepatic blood is either unchanged or slightly increased. The production of binding proteins (ceruloplasmin and transcortin), globulins, and serum alkaline phosphatase are all elevated during pregnancy. In contrast, the production of albumin is markedly decreased throughout gestation.

The functional characteristics of the gallbladder change dramatically in gravidas owing to relaxation of the smooth musculature by progesterone. Since the emptying time of the gallbladder is prolonged during pregnancy, the formation of gallstones is common.

G. Metabolic Changes

1. Weight Gain

The average weight gain during pregnancy should be in the range of 10–12 kg by term. During the first trimester, the average weight gain should amount to about 1 kg. Around 12 weeks of gestation, the amount of weight gained should increase more rapidly. The total amount of weight gained during each of the last two trimesters should be approximately 5 kg. Throughout the last trimester, the maternal body weight increases about 0.35–0.4 kg per week (44). The total amount of weight gained during pregnancy is largely determined by the increase in size of the individual organs and tissues. Some individual components contributing to the total weight gain at term are presented in Figure 10. The greatest contribution to the total weight gain during pregnancy is from the growing products of conception. On average, the fetus weighs about 3–4 kg by term, the amniotic fluid weighs about 0.8 kg, and the placenta weighs approximately 0.65 kg. The weight gain in the maternal body is due to a 3.5-kg increase in fat tissue, a 1.3-kg elevation in total

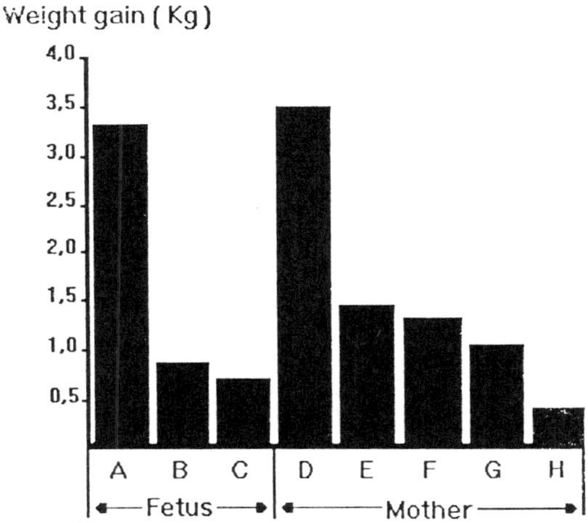

Figure 10 Distribution of fetal and maternal weight gain by term. Fetal compartment: A, fetus; B, amniotic fluid; C, placenta. Maternal compartment: D, fatty tissue; E, extracellular fluid (without leg edema); F, total plasma volume; G, uterus; H, breasts. (From Refs. 44 and 45.)

blood volume, a 1.1-kg increase in uterine size, and a 0.45-kg rise in breast tissue (45). The contribution of extracellular fluid to the total increase in weight gain during pregnancy is approximately 1.5 kg. The increase in body weight during pregnancy appears to be more pronounced in younger women that in older women.

2. *Protein Metabolism*

The total amount of protein in the maternal serum decreases during early pregnancy, reaches a plateau between weeks 10–20, and returns to nonpregnant values in the last trimester. Plasma protein concentration declines in the early stages of gestation from values of 6 to 7 g/100 ml in the nonpregnant state to gestational values of 5–6 g/100 ml (46). Once the decrease in plasma protein concentration stabilizes, values remain constant until term owing to an increase in plasma volume.

a. Albumin, Globulin, and Fibrinogen. The concentration of albumin decreases from 3.5 g/ml in the nonpregnant state to approximately 1 g/ml in week 32 of pregnancy, at which the levels of albumin then slightly increase prior to term (46). The overall decline in serum albumin levels results from a drop in total serum protein by approximately 20% (23). In addition, lowered plasma albumin levels induce a decline in the colloid osmotic pressure (COP) (see Fig. 5).

Additional proteins such as globulin and fibrinogen decline during pregnancy and therefore further contribute to a decrease in COP. The reduction in albumin, globulin, and fibrinogen elicits the redistribution of water from the vasculature into the maternal cells. Edema formation is therefore common during the last trimester of pregnancy.

3. Lipid, Salt, and Water Metabolism

The concentration of plasma lipids, triglycerides, phospholipids, and cholesterol rise sharply during gestation. An increase in serum lipids results from the elevation in placental steroid hormones. After delivery, the concentration of serum lipids returns to nonpregnant values.

The retention of sodium and water is common in pregnant females. During normal pregnancies, sodium metabolism is controlled by numerous hormones, including progesterone, aldosterone, deoxycorticosterone, and estrogens. An elevation in the level of progesterone induces natriuresis. The rise of progesterone coupled with an elevation in GFR promotes the loss of sodium. To compensate for sodium loss, renal tubules markedly increase sodium reabsorption. An elevation in the levels of aldosterone, deoxycorticosterone, and estrogens assist in enhancing the reabsorption of sodium.

The renin-angiotensin system undergoes dramatic changes during pregnancy. Renin levels rise 5–10 times in gravidas, whereas angiotensin and angiotensinogen (renin-substrate) values increase four- to fivefold. The result of these elevated parameters is a rise in the production of aldosterone and the subsequent maintenance of sodium homeostasis.

In addition to changes in sodium metabolism, the pregnant woman also experiences changes in water retention. During pregnancy, the total water volume increases about 6.1 L. The increase in water content is primarily localized within extracellular tissue space. Together the fetus, placenta, and amniotic fluid contain about 3.7 L of H_2O. The blood plasma contains about 1.1 L of water (extracellular H_2O) and red blood cells contain about 0.2 L of water (intracellular H_2O) (45). Finally, the mammary glands have approximately 0.15 L of extracellular H_2O and 0.15 L of intracellular H_2O.

4. Drug Metabolism

Before deciding to use pharmacological intervention in the pregnant woman, the physician must determine the effect that the compound(s) will have on the maternal and fetal bodies. Caution should always be exercised when prescribing medication to the pregnant woman owing to the teratogenic side effects of many medications on the fetal unit. A large percentage of infant deaths, spontaneous abortions, and congenital abnormalities are the result of improper usage of pharmacological and chemical compounds. Throughout the last several years, our understanding of transport from maternal to fetal sources has rapidly expanded. Since many compounds cross the placenta by simple diffusion, it is important to realize that a concentration gradient exists between the maternal and fetal organism. In addition, the ionization and molecular weight of the molecules appear to be important in determining the degree of placental transport. In general, nonionized compounds cross the placental border more readily than ionized forms, and compounds with low molecular weights are better able to penetrate the placenta than compounds with high molecular weights.

In addition to passive diffusion, active transport and facilitated diffusion are also utilized by the placenta. Active transport allows the movement of compounds against a concentration gradient form maternal to fetal stores. The transport of glucose across the placenta takes place by way of facilitated diffusion. This process allows the movement of compounds in a more precise and rapid manner than does simple diffusion.

H. Musculoskeletal System

From early pregnancy onward, elevated levels of progesterone and relaxin produce secondary changes that induce relaxation of the pelvic joints and ligaments. The induction of elasticity and the softening of ligaments is especially pronounced in the later stages of pregnancy at the sacroiliac joints and the symphysis pubis. Therefore, the pregnant woman has an increased pelvic capacity shortly before delivery.

In addition to the relaxation of ligaments, relaxation of the abdominal wall musculature is important during gestation. An increase in pressure within the abdominal cavity by the expanding uterine contents is compensated for by relaxation of anterior abdominal wall musculature. Even though compression and relaxation of the abdominal muscles is present during the later stages of pregnancy, the rectus abdominis muscle is still capable of being separated.

Musculoskeletal changes in the vertebral column are also common during pregnancy. To compensate for the growing uterus moving away from the center of gravity, the pregnant female must make postural adjustments. These postural changes increase lumbar lordosis and contribute to difficulty in walking. Moreover, postural rearrangements commonly cause lower back pain (especially in the later stages of pregnancy).

V. THE DIAGNOSIS OF PREGNANCY

Prior to delivering treatment to women of reproductive age, the possibility of pregnancy must always be considered. Irrespective of the clinical interest and/or specialty of the practicing physician, a proper diagnosis of pregnancy is crucial. In most instances, the diagnosis of pregnancy is relatively straightforward. The diagnosis of pregnancy, however, may often be difficult, particularly in women with irregular menstrual periods. In addition, many of the characteristics typically associated with pregnancy also occur in various pathological conditions. The diagnosis of pregnancy must therefore be based on the manifestation of symptoms and signs that are determined by physiological and anatomical changes in the maternal body. The clinical criteria for the diagnosis of pregnancy can be classified into three groups: presumptive, probable, and positive evidence of pregnancy.

A. Presumptive Evidence of Pregnancy

The presumptive evidence of pregnancy is largely based on subjective symptomatology presented by the patient during a medical history intake interview. Generally, the presumptive evidence of pregnancy is detected by women prior to visiting their physician. The presumptive signs of pregnancy are not exclusive to gestation and must therefore be coupled with positive symptoms and signs of pregnancy for a conclusive diagnosis. A list of the common presumptive symptoms and signs of pregnancy include (a) amenorrhea, (b) nausea with and without vomiting, (c) fatigue, (d) micturition and nocturia, (e) changes in the breasts, (f) fetal movement, and (g) elevation of body temperature.

1. Amenorrhea

The most common and often earliest sign of pregnancy is the cessation of menses (amenorrhea). Amenorrhea is a fairly reliable indication of conception in women with regular menstrual cycles. However, the diagnostic value of amenorrhea is not a reliable indicator of pregnancy until 10 or more days after the expected onset of menses owing to variations in the menstrual cycle. It should be noted that vaginal bleeding occurs in approximately 8% of all pregnancies at expected date of menses. The diagnosis of pregnancy based on amenorrhea is further complicated because cessation of menses is a common phenomenon in various disease states. As such, amenorrhea should not be used in isolation as the only prognosticator of pregnancy.

2. Nausea with or Without Vomiting

Nausea, which may or may not include vomiting, is a common presumptive sign of gestation. The production of nausea appears to be largely induced by an elevation in placental hormones such as hCG. In addition, nausea may also result from psychogenic components. Nausea commonly appears between weeks 6 and 12 in approximately 50% of all pregnancies. Typically, nausea occurs in the morning (commonly referred to as morning sickness), and occasionally these symptoms are also present during the night. In most cases, nausea and vomiting disappear abruptly after the twelfth week of gestation.

3. *Fatigue*

Fatigue is a common characteristic sign of early pregnancy. However, since the manifestation of fatigue has numerous origins independent of gestation, this sign is of poor diagnostic quality. Fatigue is likely caused by high levels of progesterone that induce relaxation of smooth muscle tissue within the maternal body.

4. *Micturition and Nocturia*

Additional presumptive signs of gestation include micturition and nocturia. Pressure exerted on the bladder from the growing uterus inevitably causes difficulty in controlling urination. As the fetus grows in size, micturition and nocturia become more prevalent. Micturition and nocturia are further exacerbated by a rise in progesterone levels that relax the urethral sphincter and tonality of the bladder.

5. *Changes Within the Breasts*

Throughout the course of pregnancy, anatomical and physiological changes occur in the breasts. During the early stages of gestation, tingling and tenderness of the breasts is particularly well perceived by primigravidas. Changes in the breasts are largely determined by alterations in such hormones as estrogens, progesterone, placental lactogen, prolactin, growth hormone, and thyroid hormone (see Fig. 7). However, independent of pregnancy, pathological changes may occur in the breasts of women with prolactin-secreting pituitary tumors.

6. *Fetal Movement*

Fetal movements are first recognized at 18–20 weeks in primigravidas and 14–16 weeks in multigravidas. Fetal activity (movement) is often misinterpreted as active peristalsis in primigravidas. The detection of fetal movement used in isolation provides very little value in diagnosing pregnancy.

7. *Elevation of the Basal Body Temperature*

The elevation of basal body temperature over a 3-week period may be used as a presumptive sign to indicate pregnancy. The elevation of body temperature, however, is a nonspecific method of detecting pregnancy and is by no means diagnostic.

B. Probable Evidence of Pregnancy

The probable evidence of pregnancy includes symptoms and signs which can be identified during a physical examination. The probable evidence of pregnancy is the result of changes within the maternal anatomy and physiology. As such, the probable evidence of pregnancy can provide a relatively accurate diagnosis of pregnancy. A definitive diagnosis of pregnancy, however, should never be concluded without evaluating the positive symptoms of pregnancy. The probable symptoms and signs of pregnancy include (a) changes in skin pigmentation, (b) changes in the uterus, (c) uterine contractions, (d) changes in the cervix, and (e) enlargement of the abdomen.

1. Skin Pigmentation

A change in the skin pigmentation of the nipples occurs several weeks after conception. During pregnancy, the areolae increase in size and change from a pink color in white nulliparous women to a deep brown to black color depending on skin pigmentation. In addition, pregnancy is also marked by a darkening of the skin in the lower abdomen (linea alba). Changes in the pigmentation of the skin during pregnancy, although common, are not always present. An increase in skin pigmentation may occur due to the ingestion of estrogen-progestin contraceptives.

2. Changes in the Uterus

After the fifth week of gestation, irregular softening of the fundus occurs at the site of implantation (Von Fernwald sign). If the site of implantation is located at the cornu of the uterus, softening of the fundus occurs in that area (Piskacek sign). At approximately the sixth week of gestation, a softening of the uterocervical junction in the anterior midline may be detected (Ladin sign). Between weeks 6 and 8 of pregnancy, a zone of softness in the isthmus may be detected during bimanual examination owing to the compressibility of the uterus (Hegar sign). During that same time period, the uterus is easy flexed at the uterocervical junction (McDonald sign).

3. Uterine Contractions

Irregular uterine contractions (Braxton Hicks contractions) are manifested by pregnant women as a tightening sensation in the abdomen. From approximately week 28 of gestation onward, uterine contractions increase as the pregnant woman approaches term. During the more advanced stages of gestation, uterine contractions can be palpated on physical examination.

4. Changes in the Cervix

Visual examination of the cervix may reveal cyanosis of the vagina and cervix (Chadwick sign) around 6 weeks of gestation. During the same time period, softening of the cervix may also be present.

5. *Enlargement of the Abdomen*

During the early stages of gestation, enlargement of the abdomen is not a useful sign for the diagnosis of pregnancy. However, after the first trimester, the fundus of the uterus can be palpated above the symphysis pubis on the anterior abdominal wall. As the pregnancy proceeds, the fundus rises during each successive week of gestation (see Fig. 6). Elevation of the fundus can be used as a reliable indication of the gestational age of the fetus. Approximately 4 weeks prior to delivery, the fundus descends several centimeters.

C. Positive Evidence of Pregnancy

The only way to reach a definitive conclusion concerning the presence or absence of pregnancy is by evaluating the positive symptoms and signs of gestation. The positive symptoms and signs of pregnancy are based on criteria that are clearly identifiable through physical examination or biochemical assays. Many of the positive symptoms and signs of pregnancy are elicited by the identification of fetal characteristics such as the fetal heart rate. Other positive symptoms and signs of pregnancy rely on the biochemical detection of relatively specific hormonal cues elicited only in the pregnant state. The positive symptoms and signs of pregnancy are (a) identification of the fetal heart rate, (b) ultrasonographic recognition, (c) recognition by radiography, and (d) pregnancy tests.

1. *Identification of Fetal Heart Action*

The earliest that the action of the fetal heart can be detected by echocardiography is 48 days after the last menstrual period (47). Doppler ultrasound is capable of detecting the fetal heartbeat at about 8–10 weeks of gestation, and auscultation with the fetoscope can successfully detect the fetal heartbeat at 17–19 weeks. Recognition of the fetal heart rate during physical examination can be easily discriminated from the maternal heart rate owing to their disproportionate ranges. The fetal heartbeat ranges from 120 to 140 beats/min, whereas the normal maternal heart rate ranges from 60 to 90 beats/min.

2. *Ultrasonographic Recognition*

Vaginal ultrasonography is a reliable method of fetal recognition during the early and late stages of gestation. The small characteristic gestational sac becomes detectable during the fourth week of gestation (47). In addition, ultrasonography can visualize the yolk sac when it first appears at about the fifth week of gestation (see Fig. 3). Shortly thereafter, ultrasonography can detect the fetal heart action in the sixth week of pregnancy (48).

In addition to vaginal ultrasonography, Doppler ultrasound can also be used to identify these structures. However, recognition of embryonic structures with Doppler ultrasound occurs at later time points. For example, the small characteristic gestational ring can be identified using the Doppler principle after the sixth week of gestation, whereas vaginal ultrasonography recognizes the same structure approximately 4 weeks after the last menstrual period.

3. *Recognition by Radiography*

The use of x-ray radiography should only be considered in pregnant women under extreme circumstances. The ionizing radiation produced by x-rays may be extremely detrimental to the maturation and development of the fetus. However, radiological examination is occasonally done when a pregnancy goes undetected. In these circumstances, fetal recognition is possible only after the sixteenth week of gestational development when the fetal bones have begun to ossify.

4. *Pregnancy Tests*

The most common and sensitive tests for detecting a pregnancy within the early stages measure changes in the hormonal level of hCG. hCG can be detected in the maternal serum and urine as early as 9 days after ovulation (1 day after implantation). hCG is composed of two subunits, one alpha and one beta. Based on the unique molecular structure of the beta subunit, this monomer is commonly used as a diagnostic indicator of pregnancy. Since the beta subunit undergoes a specific interaction with the target molecule, detection of this subunit provides accurate and reliable results.

To date, many different commercial home pregnancy tests are available. These commercial pregnancy tests rely on the recognition of hormones in the maternal urine that reach detectable levels approximately 4–5 weeks after the last menstrual period. Unfortunately, many of those who choose to use home pregnancy tests do not follow the directions for proper usage and therefore false-negative results are relatively high.

VI. SUMMARY

The anatomical and physiological changes that take place within the pregnant woman begin at conception and continue well beyond term. Subsequent to fertilization and embryonic implantation, a new endocrine gland, the placenta, is formed. Throughout the course of pregnancy, the myriad of hormones which support the developing fetus are derived from placental and maternal sources. Although some hormones such as hCG originate solely from the placenta, others, including estrogens and progesterone, have a shared placental and maternal descent.

Although many of the biochemical mechanisms responsible for proper gestational development are poorly defined, it is clear that changes within the hormonal milieu impart anatomical and physiological alterations in the maternal body. In the gravida, profound biological alterations occur in the genital tract and breasts. In addition, significant adaptations also occur in the cardiovascular, respiratory, urinary, digestive, and musculoskeletal systems. The physiological changes that accompany pregnancy also contribute to variations within the maternal metabolism. In conclusion, the successful maintenance of pregnancy requires a well-coordinated interaction between maternal and fetal systems.

The changes in endocrinology, anatomy, and physiology that arise during gestation can be used for the diagnosis of pregnancy. The symptoms and signs of pregnancy can be grouped into three categories: presumptive, probable, and positive evidence of pregnancy. The symptoms and signs of pregnancy may be recognized through physical examination and biochemical assays. The proper diagnosis and identification of pregnancy is essential for increasing the likelihood of a healthy mother and infant.

REFERENCES

1. D. A. Shutt and A. Lopata. The secretion of hormones during the culture of human preimplantation embryos with corona cells, *Fertil. Steril. 35*:413 (1981).
2. T. Kosasa, L. Levesque, D. P, Goldstein, and M. L. Taymor. Early detection of implantation using a radioimmunoassay specific for human chorionic gonadotropin, *J. Clin. Endocrinol. Metab. 36*:622 (1973).
3. D. L. Hay. Placental histology and the production of human chorionic gonadotrophin and its subunits in pregnancy, *Br. J. Obstet Gynecol. 95*:1268 (1988).
4. R. J. Stock, J. B. Josimovich, B. Kosor, et al. The effect of chorionic gonadotropin and chorionic somatomammotropin on steroidogenesis in the corpus luteum, *J. Obstet. Gynecol. Br. Common. 78*:549 (1971).
5. D. Tulchinsky and C. J. Hobel. Plasma human chorionic gonadotropin, estrone, estradiol, estriol, progesterone, and 17 α-hydroxyprogesterone in human pregnancy, *Am. J. Obstet. Gynecol. 117*:884 (1973).
6. J. G. Kenimer, J. M. Hershman and H. P. Higgins. The thyrotropin in hydatidiform moles is human chorionic gonadotropin, *J. Clin. Endocrinol. Metab. 40*:482 (1975).
7. R. B. Jaffe. Protein hormones of the placenta, decidua, and fetal membranes, *Reproductive Endocrinology, Physiology, Pathophysiology and Clinical Management* (S. S. C. Yen and R. B. Jaffe, eds.), Saunders, Philadelphia, 1986, pp. 760–763.
8. E. W. Adcock III, F. Teasdale, CH. S. August, et al. Human chorionic gonadotropin: Its possible role in maternal lymphocyte suppression, *Science 181*:845 (1973).
9. J. Quagliarello, B. G. Steinetz, and G. Weiss. Relaxin secretion in early pregnancy, *Obstet. Gynecol. 53*:62 (1979).
10. L. H. Rees, C. W. Buarke, S. W. Evans, and A. T. Letchorth. Possible placental origin of ACTH in normal human pregnancy, *Nature 254*:620 (1975).
11. R. S. Goland, S. L. Wardlaw, M. Blum, et al. Biologically active corticotropin-releasing hormone in maternal and fetal plasma during pregnancy, *Am. J. Obstet. Gynecol. 159*:884 (1988).

12. C. D. A. Wolfe, S. P. Patel, E. A. Linton, et al. Plasma corticotropin releasing factor (CRH) in abnormal pregnancy, *Br. J. Obstet. Gynecol. 95*:1003 (1988).
13. J. E. Buster and S. A. Carson. Placental endocrinology and diagnosis of pregnancy, *Obstetrics, Normal and Problem Pregnancies* (S. G. Gabby, J. R. Niebyl, and J. L. Simpson, eds.), Churchill Livingstone, New York, 1991, pp. 79, 80.
14. M. Wilson, A. A. Morganti, I. Zervoudakis, et al. Blood pressure, the renin-aldosterone system and sex steroids throughout normal pregnancy, *Am. J. Med. 68*:97 (1980).
15. A. Klopper. Steroids in pregnancy, *Clinical Reproductive Endocrinology* (P. Sherman, ed.), Churchill Livingstone, New York, 1985, p. 213.
16. A. I. Csapo and M. Pulkkinen. Indispensability of the human corpus luteum in the maintenance of early pregnancy luteectomy evidence, *Obstet. Gynecol. Surv 33*:69 (1978).
17. E. A. Wilson, M. J. Jawad, and L. R. Dickson. Suppression of human chorionic gonadotropin by progestational steroids, *Am. J. Obstet. Gynecol. 138*: 708 (1980).
18. J. G. Gonzales, G. Elizondo, Saldivar P. D. et al. Pituitary gland growth during normal pregnancy: an in vivo study using magnetic resonance imaging, *Am. J. Med. 85*:217 (1988).
19. M. Nelson, G. G. Wickus, R. H. Caplan, and E. A. Beguin. Thyroid gland size in pregnancy: an ultrasound and clinical study, *J. Reprod. Med. 32*:888 (1987).
20. C. Mulaisho and R. D. Utiger. Serum thyroxine-binding globulin determination by competitive ligand-binding assay in thyroid disease and pregnancy, *Acta Endocrinol. 85*:314 (1977).
21. A Harada, J. M. Hershman, A. W. Reed, et al. Comparison of thyroid stimulators and thyroid hormone concentrations in the sera of pregnant women, *J. Clin. Endocrinol. Metab. 48*:793 (1979).
22. R. M. Pitkin, W. A. Reynolds, G. A. Williams, and G. K. Hargis, Calcium metabolism in normal pregnancy: A longitudinal study, *Am. J. Obstet. Gynecol. 133*:781 (1979).
23. E. G. Robertson and G. A. Cheyne. Plasma biochemistry in relation to oedema of pregnancy, *J. Obstet. Gynecol. Br. Common. 79*:769 (1972).
24. R. M. Pitkin and M. P. Gebhardt. Serum calcium concentrations in human pregnancy, *Am. J. Obstet. Gynecol. 127*:775 (1977).
25. R. M. Pitkin. Calcium metabolism in pregnancy: A review, *Am. J. Obstet. Gynecol. 121*:724 (1975).
26. J. H. Whiteley and H. B. Stoner. The effect of pregnancy on the human adrenal cortex, *J. Endocrinol. 14*:325 (1957).
27. R. E. Peterson, Corticosteroids and corticotropins, *Endocrinology of Pregnancy* (F. Fuchs and A. Klopper, eds.), Harper & Row, Philadelphia, 1983, p. 120.
28. Y. J. Topper and C. S. Freeman. Multiple hormone interactions in the developmental of the mammary gland, *Physiol. Rev. 60*:1049 (1980).
29. J. Djiane and P. Durand. Prolactin-progesterone antagonism in self regulation of prolactin receptors in the mammary gland, *Nature 266*:641 (1977).
30. M. L. Barclay. Physiology of pregnancy, *Gynecology and Obstetrics*, Vol. 2 (P. V. Dilts and J. J. Sciarra, eds.), Lippincott, Philadelphia, 1994, p. 7.
31. R. C. Benson and M. L. Pernoll (eds.). Maternal physiologic adjustment to pregnancy, *Handbook of Obstetrics and Gynecology*, Lange, Los Altos, CA, 1994, p. 98.
32. R. Pesnic and R. A. Barce. Physiology of pregnancy, *Best and Taylors, Physiological*

Basis of Medical Practice (J. B. West, ed.), Williams & Wilkins, Baltimore, 1990, pp. 892–893.

33. M. de Swiet. Cardiovascular system, *Clinical Physiology in Obstetrics* (F. E. Hytten and G. Chamberlain, eds.), Blackwell Scientific, Boston, 1991, p. 10.
34. T. R. Moore. Maternal adaptation to pregnancy, *Gynecology and Obstetrics* (T. R. Moore and R. C. Reiter, eds.), Churchill Livingstone, New York, 1993, p. 228.
35. D. P. Cruikshank and P. M. Hays. Maternal physiology in pregnancy, *Obstetrics, Normal and Problem Pregnancies* (S. G. Gabby, J. R. Niebyl, and J. L. Simpson, eds.), Churchill Livingstone, New York, 1991, pp. 136, 138–139.
36. N. F. Grant and G. Cunninghams (eds.), Maternal adaptations to pregnancy, *Basic Gynecology and Obstetrics*, Appleton and Lange, Norwalk, CT, 1993, pp. 283–284.
37. J. A. Pritchard, R. M. Baldwin, Dickey, et al. Blood volume changes in pregnancy and the puerperium, *Am J Obstet Gynecol. 84*:1271 (1962).
38. E. Letsky. The hematological system, *Clinical Physiology in Obstetrics* (F. Hytten and G. Chamberlain, eds.), Blackwell Scientific, Boston, 1980, pp. 69–70.
39. C. K. Kasper, M. S. Hoag, P. M. Aggeler, and S. Stone. Blood clotting factors in pregnancy: Factor VIII concentrations in normal and AFH-deficient women, *Obstet. Gynecol. 24*:242 (1964).
40. M. de Swiet. The respiratory system, *Clinical Physiology in Obstetrics* (F. E. Hytten and G. Chamberlain, eds.), Blackwell Scientific, Boston, 1991, pp. 86–87, 92–94.
41. S. C. Robson, S. Hunter, R. H. Boys, and W. Dunlop. Serial changes in pulmonary haemodynamics during human pregnancy: A non-invasive study using Doppler echocardiography. *Clin. Sci. 80*:113 (1991).
42. W. Dunlop. Serial changes in renal haemodynamics during normal human pregnancy. *Br. J. Obstet. Gynecol. 88*:1 (1981).
43. C. Baylis and J. Davidson. The urinary system, *Physiology of Human Pregnancy* (F. Hytten and G. Chamberlain, eds.), Blackwell, Boston, 1991, p. 249.
44. R. M. Pitkin. Obstetrics and gynecology, *Nutritional Support of Medical Practice* (H. A. Schneider, C. E. Anderson, and D. B. Coursin, eds.), Harper & Row, Philadelphia, 1983, p. 492.
45. F. E. Hytten. Weight gain in pregnancy, *Clinical Physiology in Obstetrics* (F. Hytten and G. Chamberlain, eds.), Blackwell Scientific, Boston, 1991, pp. 177–188, 193.
46. F. E. Hytten. Nutrition, *Clinical Physiology in Obstetrics* (F. E. Hytten and G. Chamberlain, eds.), Blackwell Scientific, Boston, 1991, pp. 161–162.
47. G. Bernaschek, R. Rudelstorfer, and P. Csaicsich. Vaginal sonography versus serum human chorionic gonadotropin in early detection of pregancy, *Am. J. Obstet. Gynecol. 158*:608 (1988).
48. E. Timor-Tritsch, Z. Blumenfeld, and Sh. Rotten. Sonoembryology, *Transvaginal Sonography* (I. E. Timor-Tritsch and S. H. Rotten, eds.), Elsevier, New York, 1991, p. 296.

2

Physiological Skin Changes in Pregnancy

Reynold C. Wong
University of California, Davis, School of Medicine, Sacramento, California

I. INTRODUCTION

The human skin undergoes dramatic changes during pregnancy owing to numerous metabolic, endocrinological, and immunological adjustments. Certain types of skin changes are so common that they could be considered normal or physiological. Indeed, these "physiological" changes are normal or pathological and occur in the normal population but are increased in frequency among pregnant women. These physiological changes include pigmentation, increased vascularity, striae, pruritus, and changes in the hair and nails (1–7). Some recently described skin changes have been described in such small numbers of women that clinical significance is uncertain (8–16). Physiological skin changes have trivial, if any, systemic or fetal significance, and reassurance is in order for the anxious mother; safe and effective treatments, albeit sometimes temporary, are often available. Since dermatologists, obstetricians, and gynecologists are often called to evaluate patients regarding the significance and prognosis of these skin changes, familiarity with their presentation, cause, and treatment is recommended.

II. PIGMENTARY CHANGES

Hyperpigmentation occurs in up to 90% of pregnant women. It is mild and either localized or generalized, and it is most marked in dark-haired, dark-complexioned women. Accentuation occurs in normally hyperpigmented regions such as the areolae, nipples (Fig. 1), axillae, genitalia, perineum, anus, and inner thighs. The increased pigmentation of the skin surrounding the areolae produces the so-called secondary areolae, and in the linea alba (the tendinous median line in the anterior abdominal wall) produces the linea nigra (Fig. 2), which can extend from the symphysis pubis to the xiphoid process. Hyperpigmentation occurs during the first trimester, increases until delivery, and mostly resolves postpartum, although the skin does not return to its exact previous color (1–6, 17–21). Longitudinal melanonychia of the fingernails and group B natural pigmentary demarcation lines of the legs have been described in a few women (11–13). The group B pigmentary lines do not always resolve postpartum (11).

Freckles, lentigines, nevi, and recent scars occurring a few months before or during pregnancy can darken and even enlarge during pregnancy (1,2,4–6,21). About 10% of pregnant women report changes in their pigmented nevi during pregnancy, especially in the first trimester (22). An increase in the size or change in color of a nevocellular nevus is always of concern, but histological evaluation of nevi in pregnancy reveals little in the way of atypia. However, nevi cells in pregnant women or those on oral contraceptives have markedly increased numbers of estrogen- and progesterone-binding sites similar to those observed in melanoma

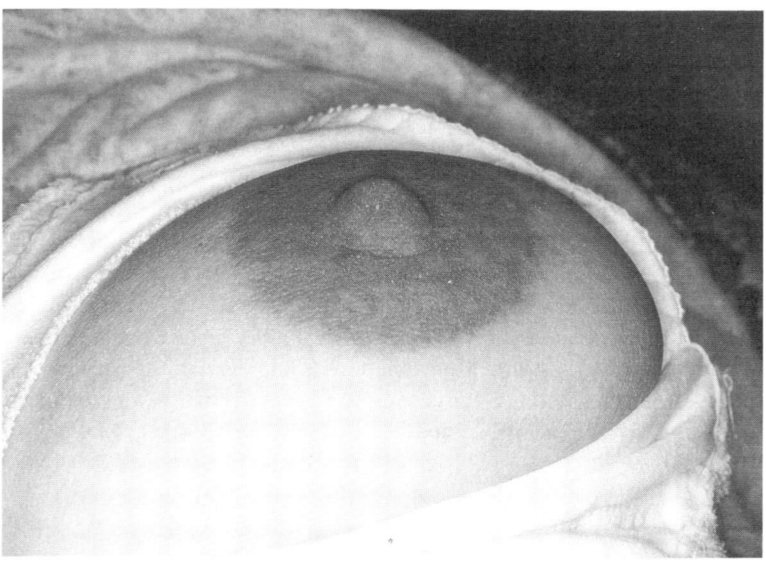

Figure 1 Hyperpigmented nipple and areola, Montgomery's tubercles.

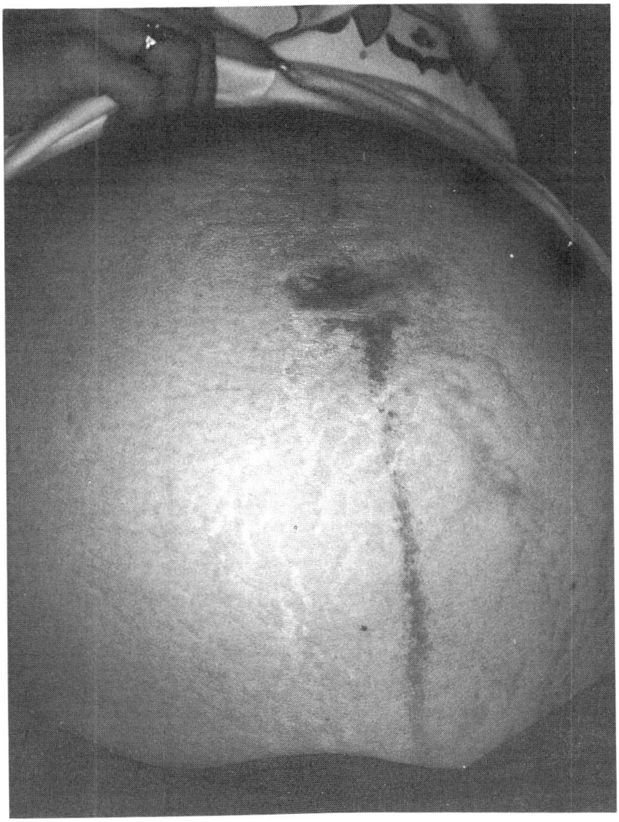

Figure 2 Linea nigra.

and atypical moles, and these sites may account for the hormone-induced changes (2,4,5,23,24). The question of whether pregnancy increases melanoma incidence still remains unanswered (5).

The cause of hyperpigmentation is still unclear, but it is probably due to increased levels of melanocyte-stimulating hormone (MSH), estrogen, and/or progesterone, which are strong melanocytic stimulants (6,25–30). The importance of MSH in causing hyperpigmentation is controversial, because hyperpigmentation begins during the first trimester of pregnancy, whereas levels of plasma alpha-MSH are high only during late pregnancy (29). In addition, there is no difference in levels of plasma beta-MSH in late pregnancy and after parturition (28).

Melasma (chloasma) consists of symmetrical, irregular but well-demarcated light to dark brown hyperpigmentation on the face that occurs in up to 75% of pregnant women and 30% of women on birth control pills (Fig. 3). It is more frequent in dark-haired, dark-complexioned women and tends to appear during the second trimester (1,2,5,6,17–19). There are three clinical patterns of melasma (31), with the most common being the centrofacial pattern in 63% of all cases. It involves the cheeks, forehead, upper lip, nose, and chin. The malar pattern is limited to the cheeks and nose, and it is seen in about 21% of cases. The least common type of melasma is mandibular type (16%), which involves the ramus of the mandible.

Two histological patterns of pigmentation are seen in melasma: an epidermal type where melanin is seen in the melanocytes and suprabasal layers and a dermal type with melanin in macrophages (19). There are four clinical types of melasma distinguished by Wood's light (31). The epidermal type occurs in 72% of cases and

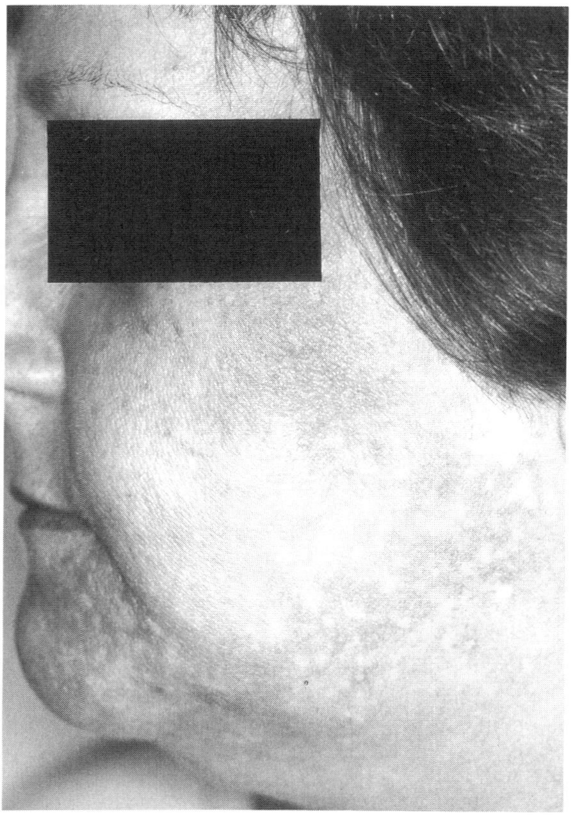

Figure 3 Melasma postpartum.

is light brown in natural light. When examined under Wood's light, it will show enhancement of the color. The melanin is located primarily within the epidermis. The dermal type occurs in 13% of patients and appears blue-gray in natural light. There is no enhancement with Wood's light. The mixed type (5%) is deep brown and shows spotty enhancement with Wood's light. The inapparent type (9%) occurs in very dark women and is "inapparent" with Wood's light. The melanin is located primarily in melanophages.

The cause of melasma is unknown. Hormonal factors include elevated levels of estrogens, progesterone, and MSH. Contributing factors include pregnancy, birth control pills, genetics, race, sunlight, and cosmetics (31–33).

My approach to melasma during pregnancy is to recommend avoidance of the sun, suntanning, cosmetics (especially perfumed preparations), and trauma and the liberal use of sunscreens (1,2,6). Improvement within a year postpartum is usual, but melasma may persist in 30% of cases (6,19,25). For persistent melasma postpartum, hydroquinone 5% and/or tretinoin with or without 2.5% hydrocortisone cream can be partially effective, even for the dermal type of melasma (1,2,6,34). A recent report describes satisfactory results in 65% of patients with melasma treated with 20% azelaic acid, a competitive inhibitor of tyrosinase (35).

III. VASCULAR AND HEMATOLOGICAL CHANGES

Vascular changes are very common during pregnancy, often beginning during the second trimester, and are related to distention, fragility, and proliferation of vessels. Two-thirds of white pregnant women and 11% of black pregnant women develop vascular spiders (spider angiomas, arterial spiders, nevi aranei, spider nevi) (1,2,4, 5,17–19,36). Spider angiomas are most commonly found in areas drained by the superior vena cava, such as the neck, throat, face, upper chest, arms, and hands (Fig. 4) (1,2,5,6,17–20,37). Spider angiomas are macular or slightly papular, small red arteriolar telangiectatic puncta with tortuous dilated branches and surrounding erythema (1,2,5,6,18). Even though there is a tendency for the number and size of spider angiomas to increase during pregnancy, I avoid treatment during pregnancy, since about 75% of spider angiomas fade within 3 months postpartum (1,2,5,6,18, 36,38). They rarely digress completely. Enlargement during subsequent pregnancies have been reported (19). Persistent lesions can be treated with electrodesiccation at low voltage with the use of a fine needle applied to the punctum (1,2,5,6).

Palmar erythema (Fig. 5) occurs in about two-thirds of pregnant white women and one-third of pregnant black women, beginning around the first trimester (1,2,17,20,36). Erythema of the palms and fingerpads, as well as diffuse mottling of the entire palm with cyanosis and pallor, clinically indistinguishable from that seen in hyperthyroidism and cirrhosis, are seen (1,2,4,6,17–19,37). There is no treatment for palmar erythema and, besides, it generally regresses postpartum (1,2,5). The cause of vascular spiders, palmar erythema, and hemangiomas is

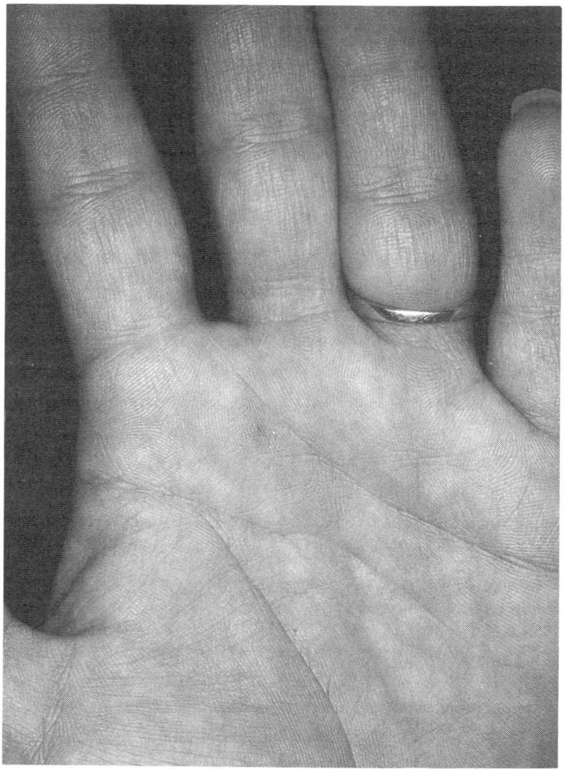

Figure 4 Spider angioma.

unknown, although elevated levels of circulating estrogens, high levels of angiogenesis factor(s), a marked rise in blood volume, increased blood flow, and a genetic predisposition are thought to be important (1,2,5,18,36,39,40).

Varicosities develop in up to 40% of pregnancies, primarily in the dependent portions of the body such as the anus (i.e., hemorrhoids), legs, and vulvar areas (Fig. 6) (1,2,4,5,21). Varicosities result from a combination of factors, including a familial tendency for increased elastic tissue fragility, increased venous pressures in femoral and pelvic vessels due to compression from an enlarging uterus, and increased vascular volume (1,2,4–6,17,19,21). Prolonged sitting, standing, and the use of elastic garters and panty girdles are exacerbating factors (1). Much regression of varicosities occurs postpartum (19).

Prevention and treatment of varicosities during pregnancy include frequent elevation of the legs, sleeping in a left lateral decubitus position, exercise, the use

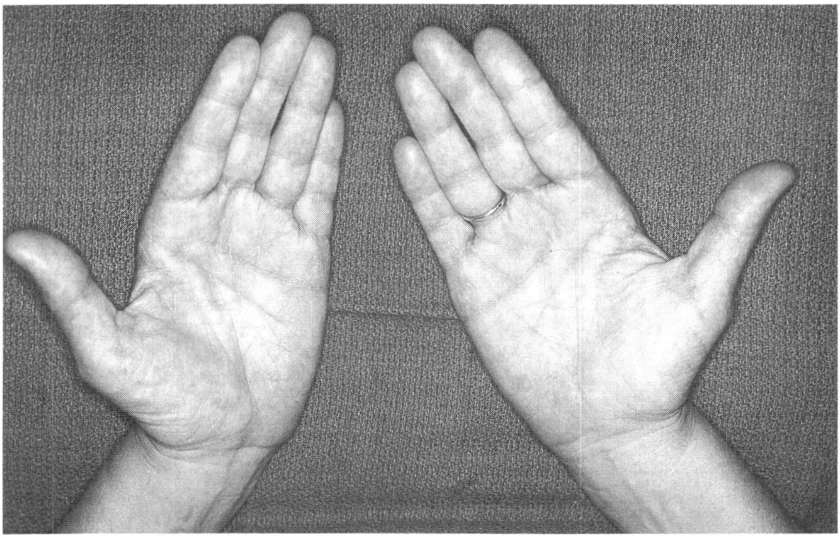

Figure 5 Palmar erythema.

of graded elasticized compression stockings with an open toe and closed heel, and avoidance of extended sitting and standing (1,2,41–44). Vulvar and vaginal varicosities (Jacquemier sign) occur early in pregnancy and frequently may be painful and difficult to treat (4,21). They can complicate a delivery (21). Supportive pantyhose and pressure pads can be helpful (1). Hemorrhoidal varicosities with pain or bleeding often respond to hot sitz baths, compresses, stool softeners, suppositories, and topical anesthetics (1,2). Severe and recalcitrant postpartum varicosities should be referred to the general surgeon (1,2).

Cutaneous hemangiomas occur in up to 5% of pregnancies, usually appearing by the beginning of the second trimester (19). I prefer to remove these lesions postpartum.

A brief discussion is in order here in regard to surgery during pregnancy. If possible, surgery in pregnant patients should be avoided, especially during the period of organogenesis (days 15–56) (45,46). The pregnant woman is susceptible to hypertensive and syncopal episodes and should be positioned on the left side during surgery (47). Local lidocaine, systemic penicillin, and oral erythromycin should be safe during pregnancy (47). Acetaminophen is recommended for analgesic and fever control (47).

Cutis marmorata (livedo reticularis) of the legs, presenting as a transitory bluish reticulated pattern on cold exposure, purpura, and pigmented purpura (capillaritis) of the legs (Fig. 7) can occur during pregnancy (1,2,17,19,20). The cause is

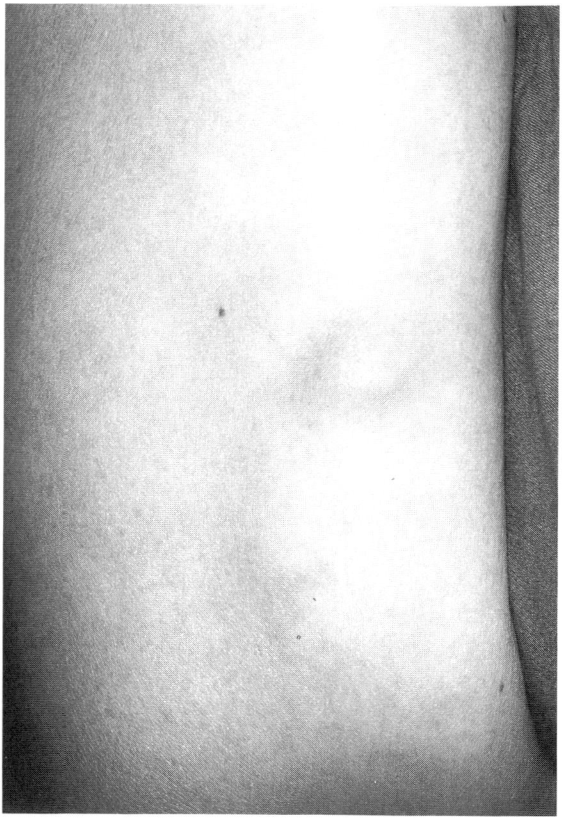

Figure 6 Varicosities on the legs.

unknown, although vasomotor instability as a contributing factor to cutis marmorata, and increased capillary fragility, elevated hydrostatic pressure, and increased permeability as contributing factors to purpura have been postulated (1,2,4,17,19, 20).

IV. CUTANEOUS TUMORS

The pyogenic granuloma of pregnancy (granuloma gravidarum, pregnancy tumor) is usually seen as a lesion of the gums that appears during the first half of pregnancy. It occurs in up to 2% of pregnant women. This tumor is microscopically identical to the pyogenic granuloma. The classic presentation of the lesion is an isolated, protruding, fluctuant, shiny red or red-purple mass with a mulberrylike surface.

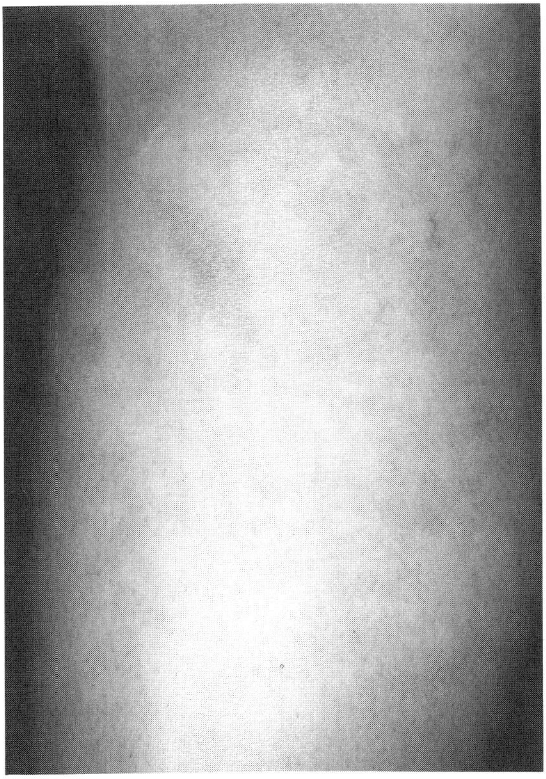

Figure 7 Pigmented purpura (capillaritis) of the legs.

The pregnancy tumor usually arises from the interdental papillae, but it may arise anywhere on the gingivae. It may bleed or ulcerate with trauma. Teeth adjacent to the tumor may undergo migration and become more mobile. Generally, the lesion will regress somewhat following pregnancy, but surgical extirpation is often required for complete resolution. Unless there is excessive pain, bleeding, or interference with chewing, surgery should be delayed until after pregnancy. Excision during pregnancy can sometimes be followed by a quick recurrence. Prior to parturition, if possible, scaling and root planing, along with oral hygiene instructions, is recommended to reduce local irritative factors such as plaque and calculus. The cause of granuloma gravidarum may be secondary to the hormonally modified tissue response to trauma (1,2,6,17,48–51).

Skin tags (acrochordons, molluscum fibrosum gravidarum) occur during the second half of pregnancy and are seen on the sides of the face and neck, chest, axillae (Fig. 8), and inframammary areas. These flesh-colored or slightly pigmented pedunculated fleshy papules can reach up to 7–8 mm in size. They may not regress postpartum, but they may easily be treated with liquid nitrogen, light electrodesiccation, or surface-level shave (1,2,6,17–19,37).

V. STRETCH MARKS

Stretch marks (striae distensae, striae gravidarum) are seen in up to 90% of pregnant women during the third trimester and are most common in white women. There may be a familial tendency. These linear pink to violaceous atrophic lines

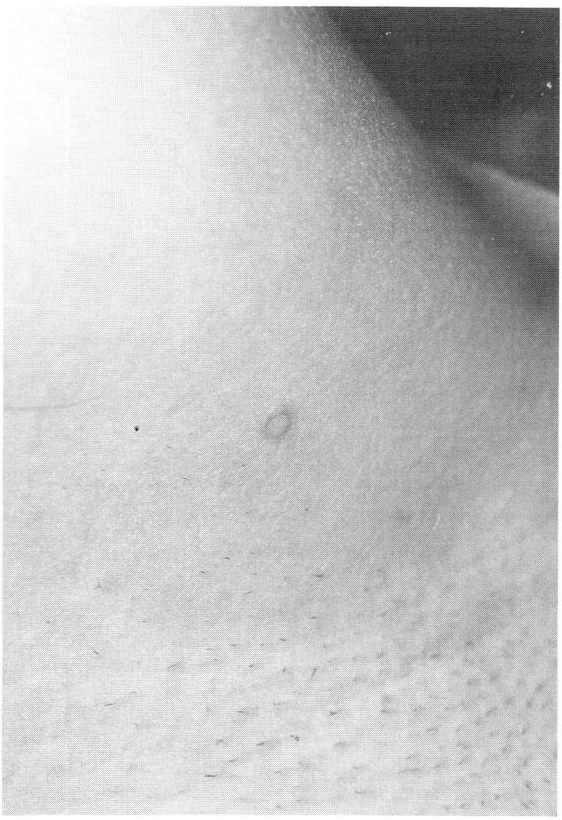

Figure 8 Acrochordons.

develop opposite to the skin tension lines on the abdomen (Fig. 9), breasts, and/or thighs; when extensive, striae can include the upper arms, lower back, and buttocks. Striae tend to be more extensive in heavier or obese mothers. Although the cause of stretch marks is uncertain, they will improve greatly postpartum and become less noticeable (1,2,6,17,18,20,30,37). Topical olive oil has been advocated as a preventive during pregnancy, and topical tretinoin has been advocated as therapy postpartum in non–breast-feeding mothers. Their effectiveness is still in debate (52–54).

VI. GLANDULAR ACTIVITY

Eccrine sweating increases near the end of pregnancy and may lead to hyperhidrosis, miliaria, and dyshidrotic eczema. The cause is unknown. A 20% solution of aluminum chloride hexahydrate in ethyl alcohol applied for several nights on dry skin and then as necessary can be effective (1–3,5,6,19,21,50,55). Apocrine gland activity decreases during pregnancy, but there may be a rebound postpartum (1–3,5,6,17,21,37,56). There is no consistent change in sebaceous gland activity during pregnancy, but complaints of greasy skin are common, and acne occasionally develops initially or worsens during pregnancy (1,2,6,17,21). Pruritic follicu-

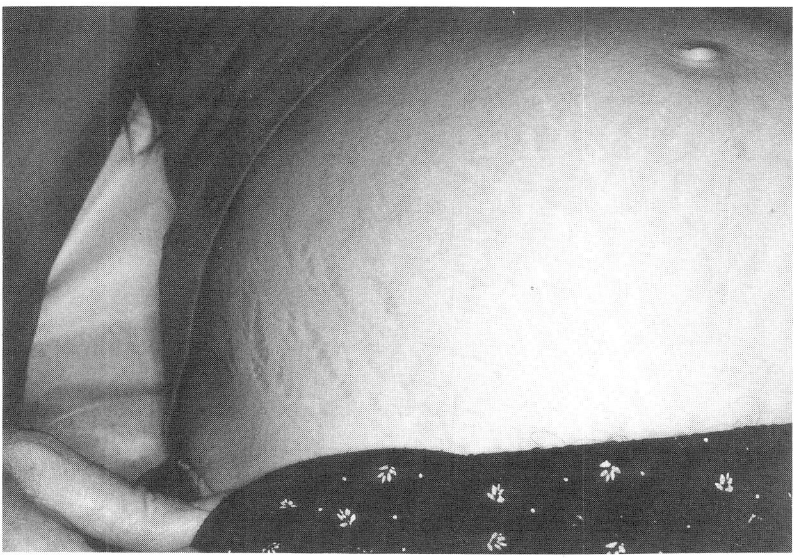

Figure 9 Stretch marks from a previous pregnancy.

litis of pregnancy has been described in six patients as a generalized eruption of pruritic, excoriated, erythematous 3–5 mm follicular papules that usually resolve by 2 weeks postpartum (3,4,14). These cases have been described as a hormonally induced acne, and the condition is apparently harmless to both mother and fetus (4,5,15,16). Treatment with a cream containing 10% benzoyl peroxide and 1% hydrocortisone has been reported to be helpful (10).

Breast changes during pregnancy are numerous, including enlargement, tenderness, erect nipples, hyperpigmentation of nipples and areolae (see Fig. 1), secondary pinkish areolae (weblike darkening surrounding the areolae), venous prominence, striae, and Montgomery tubercles (hypertrophied sebaceous glands associated with lactiferous ducts on the areolae appearing as small brown papules (see Fig. 1). Montgomery tubercles occur in 30–50% of pregnant women and tend to regress postpartum (1–3,5,6). The cause of all these glandular changes is unknown.

VII. NONPITTING EDEMA

Nonpitting edema is common in healthy women late in pregnancy. This occurs on the eyelids and face during 50% of pregnancies and on the ankles and feet in over 70%. Edema of the hands also occurs. The edema decreases during the day with activity (1,2,6,17,19,37,42). The sodium and fluid retention is due to increased capillary permeability and increased hydrostatic blood pressure as a result of an enlarging uterus impairing blood return from the lower extremities by obstructing the inferior vena cava (1,2,19,42,44). Treatment for the legs is similar to that for varicosities. The edema may be further managed with salt restriction and, occasionally, diuretics. Resolution usually occurs postpartum (1,2,44,56).

VIII. PRURITUS

Pruritus, with or without skin lesions, can be frustrating to treat and more so in pregnancy, since one has to be more cautious in prescribing medications. Pruritus is common in pregnancy, especially of the abdominal skin, and affects up to 20% of pregnant women, usually during the third trimester (1,2,17). Pruritus gravidarum, drug reaction, scabies, atopic dermatitis, xerosis, and neurodermatitis need to be considered in the differential diagnosis and ruled out (1,57). Dermographism and urticaria can also occur in pregnancy (1,2). Pruritus invariably clears postpartum. Therapy for idiopathic pruritus includes avoiding anxiety, hot weather, fatigue, and irritating clothing. Oatmeal baths, topical corticosteroids, and oral antihistamines (diphenhydramine, tripelennamine, pheniramine, and chlorpheniramine are thought to be safe, but the most current literature references need to be checked for any recent changes in recommendation) may be helpful. Nonerythemogenic doses of ultraviolet B radiation 3–5 days a week are sometimes successful

(1,2,58,60). Localized pruritus such as pruritus ani, pruritus vulvae, and scalp pruritus also occur in pregnancy (16).

IX. HAIR AND NAIL CHANGES

During pregnancy, most women develop some degree of hirsutism, starting early in pregnancy, and is more profuse in women with abundant body hair or dark hair (1,2,5,6,17,37). Hirsutism is most pronounced on the face, but the arms, legs, back, and suprapubic areas can be involved (1,2,17,20). Most of the excess fine lanugo hairs disappear postpartum but the coarse terminal hairs usually remain (1,2). Before pregnancy, individual hairs are in different phases of growth and the shedding of hair is unnoticed. During the course of pregnancy, there is a prolongation of hair cycles, possibly due to high levels of estradiol and progesterone, and so the percentage of anagen hairs (growing hairs) increases. After delivery, a reverse process occurs: The percentage of anagen hairs decreases below the values recorded during the first trimester (3,6,18,60,61). Primiparas show more striking trichological changes than multiparas (60). Electrolysis is an option postpartum for hirsutism; otherwise, reassurance is key to patient management.

Telogen effluvium (a rapid shedding of hairs) commonly occurs 1–5 months after delivery when there is a rapid conversion of anagen hairs to telogen hairs (resting hairs). Hair loss can continue for several months, and complete hair regrowth may take up to 15 months. The hair may not be as abundant as it was before gestation. The causes of telogen effluvium include the stress of delivery (fever, surgical stress, blood loss) and changes in the hormone balance (1,2,5–7,14–20,61,62). Reassurance is in order.

A mild degree of male-pattern frontoparietal recession and diffuse thinning out of the hair can occur late in pregnancy (Fig. 10). There is usually complete reversion postpartum. The cause is unknown (1,2,5,17,19,20). Topical minoxidil may be helpful in persistent cases.

During pregnancy, the rate of nail growth increases. Nail changes such as transverse grooving, increased brittleness and softening, distal onycholysis, and subungual keratosis can occur early in pregnancy. Transverse grooving, also known as Beau lines, may develop after delivery. The causes of these changes are unknown. Nails should be trimmed, trauma avoided, and external sensitizers (nail polish, artificial nails) eliminated if nail changes occur (1–3,5,6,17,37).

X. MUCOUS MEMBRANES

Pregnancy gingivitis has been reported to occur in most pregnant women but with varying degrees of severity (50). It is histologically similar to normal chronic gingivitis with an inflammatory cell infiltrate and formation of new blood vessels and connective tissue. Pregnancy gingivitis is most likely to have its onset during

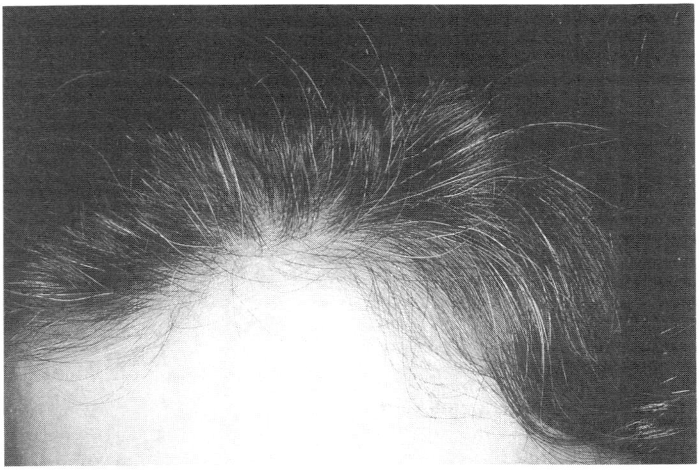

Figure 10 Diffuse thinning of the frontal scalp.

the first trimester. It increases in severity until the eighth month; after delivery, full regression may take months. This condition presents as an increase in size of the interdental papillae with blunting. The papillae and marginal gingiva become edematous, glassy, and smooth. The color will be pink to red to raspberry with loss of stippling. There is a higher tendency toward bleeding, pain, and ulceration. Two percent of the cases develop a pregnancy tumor that can attain a size of 3 cm in diameter (1,2,5,18,19,37,49–51,63,64).

The cause of pregnancy gingivitis is unknown. A variety of factors has been suggested as causative: local irritative factors, poor oral hygiene (presence of plaque and calculus), alterations in the composition of the subgingival plaque (an increase in the proportions of *Prevotella intermedia*), changes in the maternal immunoresponsiveness, and nutritional deficiencies (1,2,5,37,49,50,65,66). Treatment includes proper dental hygiene (plaque and calculus removal), avoidance of trauma, use of mouthwashes, and topical applications of folate (49–51,62,63,67).

Pelvic organs show changes during pregnancy. Early in pregnancy, a bluish or purplish hue to the vagina due to an increased blood supply is called the Chadwick sign, and a bluish discoloration of the cervix due to increasing vascularity is called the Goodell sign (1).

REFERENCES

1. R. C. Wong and C. N. Ellis. Physiologic skin changes in pregnancy, *J. Am. Acad. Dermatol. 10*:929 (1984).

2. R. C. Wong and C. N. Ellis. Physiologic skin changes in pregnancy, *Semin. Dermatol. 8*:7 (1989).
3. J. P. Callen. Pregnancy's effects on the skin, *Postgrad. Med. 75*:138 (1984).
4. J. C. Murray. Pregnancy and the skin, *Dermatol. Clin. 8*:327 (1990).
5. A. G. Martin and S. Leal-Khouri. Physiologic skin changes associated with pregnancy, *Int. J. Dermatol. 31*:375 (1992).
6. F. Powell and B. Powell. Cutaneous changes during pregnancy, *Ir. Med. J. 80*:50 (1987).
7. G. B. Winton, Dermatoses of pregnancy. *J. Assoc. Mil. Dermatol. 7*:20 (1981).
8. J. Alcalay. Skin diseases unique to the pregnant woman, *Dermatol. Nurs.* 2:148 (1990).
9. J. V. Dacus and D. Muram. Pruritus in pregnancy, *South. Med. J. 80*:614 (1987).
10. M. M. Black, Prurigo of pregnancy, papular dermatitis of pregnancy, and pruritic folliculitis of pregnancy. *Semin. Dermatol. 8*:23 (1989).
11. W. D. James, M. S. Meltzer, M. A. Guill, T. G. Berger, and O. G. Rodman, Pigmentary demarcation lines associated with pregnancy, *Cutis 11*:438 (1984).
12. M. Vazquez, M. I. Ibanez, and J. L. Sanchez. Pigmentary demarcation lines during pregnancy, *Cutis 38*:263 (1986).
13. J. M. Fryer and V. P. Werth. Pregnancy-associated hyperpigmentation: Longitudinal melanonychia, *J. Am. Acad. Dermatol. 26*:493 (1992).
14. E. Zoberman and E. Farmer. Pruritic folliculitis of pregnancy, *Arch. Dermatol. 112*:1534 (1976).
15. R. C. Holmes and M. M. Black. The specific dermatoses of pregnancy, *J. Am. Acad. Dermatol. 8*:405 (1989).
16. J. V. Dacus. Pruritus in pregnancy, *Clin. Obstet. Gynecol. 33*:738 (1990).
17. G. B. Winton and C. W. Lewis. Dermatoses of pregnancy, *J. Am. Acad. Dermatol. 6*:977 (1982).
18. T. R. Wade, S. L. Wade, and H. E. Jones. Skin changes and diseases associated with pregnancy. *Obstet. Gynecol. 52*:233 (1978).
19. P. D. Hellreich. The skin changes of pregnancy, *Cutis 13*:82 (1974).
20. A. W. McKenzie. Skin Disorders in pregnancy, *Practitioner 206*:773 (1971).
21. T. Parmley and T. J. O'Brien. Skin changes during pregnancy, *Clin. Obstet. Gynecol. 331*:713 (1990).
22. J. L. Sanchez, L. D. Figueroa, and E. Rodriguez. Behavior of melanocytic nevi during pregnancy, *Am. J. Dermatopathol. 6*(Suppl):89 (1984).
23. D. L. Ellis and R. G. Wheeland. Increased nevus estrogen and progesterone ligand binding related to oral contraceptives or pregnancy, *J. Am. Acad. Dermatol. 14*:25 (1986).
24. E. Foucar, T. J. Bentley, D. W. Laube, et al. A histopathologic evaluation of nevocellular nevi in pregnancy, *Arch. Dermatol. 121*:350 (1985).
25. K. Shizume and A. B. Lerner. Determination of melanocyte-stimulating hormone in urine and blood, *J. Clin. Endocrinol. 14*:1491 (1954).
26. B. C. G. Dahlberg. Melanocyte stimulating substances in the urine of pregnant women, *Acta Endocrinol (Kbh) 38 (Suppl. 60)*:1 (1961).
27. B. W. McGuinness. Melanocyte-stimulating hormone: A clinical and laboratory study, *Ann. N.Y. Acad. Sci. 100*:640 (1963).

28. A. J. Thody, N. A. Plummer, and J. L. Burton. Plasma beta-melanocyte-stimulating hormone levels in pregnancy, *J. Obstet. Gynaecol. Br. Commonw. 81*:875 (1974).
29. D. Clark, A. J. Thody, S. Shuster, and H. Bowers. Immunoreactive alpha-MSH in human plasma in pregnancy, *Nature 273*:163 (1978).
30. R. S. Snell and P. G. Bischitz. The effect of large doses of estrogen and progesterone on melanin pigmentation, *J. Invest. Dermatol. 35*:73 (1960).
31. N. P. Sanchez, M. A. Pathak, S. Sato, et al. Melasma: A clinical, light microscopic, ultrastructural, and immunofluorescence study, *J. Am. Acad. Dermatol. 4*:698 (1981).
32. M. A. Pathak, F. C. Riley, and T. B. Fitzpatrick. Melanogenesis in human skin following exposure to long-wave ultraviolet and visible light, *J. Invest. Dermatol. 39*:435 (1962).
33. A. G. Smith, S. Shuster, A. J. Thody, et al. Chloasma, oral contraceptives, and plasma immunoreactive beta-melanocyte-stimulating hormone, *J. Invest. Dermatol. 68*:169 (1977).
34. A. M. Kligman and I. Willis. A new formula for depigmenting human skin, *Arch. Dermatol. 111*:40 (1975).
35. L. M. Balina and K. Graupe. The treatment of melasma: 20% azelaic acid versus 4% hydroquinone cream, *Int. J. Dermatol. 30*:893 (1991).
36. W. B. Bean, R. Cogswell, M. Dexter, and J. F. Embick. Vascular changes of the skin in pregnancy, *Surg. Gynecol. Obstet. 88*:739 (1949).
37. K. Cummings and V. J. Derbes. Dermatoses associated with pregnancy, *Cutis 3*:120 (1967).
38. R. S. Barnhill and J. E. Wolf, Sr. Angiogenesis and the skin, *J. Am. Acad. Dermatol. 16*:1226 (1987).
39. S. Spetz. Peripheral circulation during normal pregnancy, *Acta Obstet. Gynaecol. Scand. 43*:309 (1964).
40. R. C. Wong and C. N. Ellis. Reply. *J. Am. Acad. Dermatol. 12*:372 (1985).
41. E. A. Husni, J. O. C. Ximenes, and F. G. Hamilton. Pressure bandaging of the lower extremity, *JAMA 206*:2715 (1968).
42. G. J. Kerbleski and J. W. Moore. Management of pedal changes encountered with pregnancy, *J. Am. Pod. Med. Assoc. 70*:340 (1989).
43. J. W. Downing and L. T. Bees. The influence of lateral tilt on limb blood flow in advanced pregnancy, *S. Afr. Med. J. 50*:728 (1976).
44. M. K. Jacobs, K. L. McCance, and M. L. Stewart. External pneumatic intermittent compression for treatment of dependent pregnancy edema, *Nurs. Res. 31*:159 (1982).
45. H. Pedersen and M. Finster. Anesthetic risk in the pregnant surgical patient, *Anesthesiology 51*:439 (1979).
46. *Drug Evaluations*, 6th ed. Chicago, American Medical Association, 1986, pp. 41–52.
47. D. E. Gormley. Cutaneous surgery and the pregnant patient, *J. Am. Acad. Dermatol. 23*:269 (1990).
48. S. B. Sydney. Treating pregnancy related gingival problems: A case report, *Dent. Surv. 56*:46 (1980).
49. M. A. Lynch, *Burket's Oral Medicine*, Lippincott, Philadelphia, 1977, p. 443.
50. H. S. Goldman and M. Z. Marder. *Physician's Guide to the Diseases of the Oral Cavity*, Medical Economics, Oradell, NJ, 1982, p. 118.

51. R. A. Colby, D. A. Kern, and H. B. G. Robinson. *Color Atlas of Oral Pathology*, Lippincott, Philadelphia, 1971, pp. 79, 90.
52. C. M. H. Davey. Factors associated with the occurrence of striae gravidarum, *J. Obstet. Gynaecol. Br. Commonw. 79*:1113 (1972).
53. M. L. Elson. Treatment of striae distensae with topical tretinoin, *J. Dermatol. Surg. Oncol. 16*:267 (1990).
54. L. O. S. Poidevin. Striae gravidarum—their relation to adrenal cortical hyperfunction, *Lancet 2*:436 (1959).
55. P. C. B. MacKinnon and I. L. MacKinnon. Palmar sweating in pregnancy, *J. Obstet. Gynaecol. Br. Commonw. 62*:298 (1955).
56. T. Cornbleet. Pregnancy and apocrine diseases: hidradenitis, Fox-Fordyce disease, *Arch. Dermatol. Syph. 65*:12 (1952).
57. D. Sasseville, R. D. Wilkinson, and J. Y. Schrader. Dermatoses of pregnancy, *Int. J. Dermatol. 20*:223 (1981).
58. P. Greenberger and R. Patterson. Safety of therapy for allergic symptoms during pregnancy, *Ann. Intern. Med. 89*:234 (1978).
59. W. Jurecka and W. Gebhart. Drug prescribing during pregnancy, *Semin. Dermatol. 8*:30 (1989).
60. L. Bartosová, A. Werkmannová, S. Smolan, and H. Fingerová. Trichological alterations in women during pregnancy and after delivery, *Acta Univ. Palacki. Olomuc. Fac. Med. 117*:225 (1987).
61. Y. L. Lynfield. Effect of pregnancy on the human hair cycle, *J. Invest. Dermatol. 35*:323 (1960).
62. B. Schiff and A. B. Kern. Study of postpartum alopecia, *Arch. Dermatol 87*:609 (1963).
63. B. J. Martin and R. M. Reeb. Oral health during pregnancy: A neglected nursing area, *Am. J. Mat. Child Nurs. 7*:391 (1982).
64. A. R. C. Pack and M. E. Thomson. Effects of topical and systemic folic acid supplementation on gingivitis in pregnancy, *J. Clin. Periodontol. 7*:402 (1980).
65. R. P. Levin. Pregnancy gingivitis, *J. Maryland State Dent. Assoc. 30*:27 (1987).
66. J. E. Raber-Durlacher, W. Leene, C. C. R. Palmer-Bouva, et al. Experimental gingivitis during pregnancy and postpartum: Immunohistochemical aspects, *J. Periodont. 64*:211 (1993).
67. M. E. Thomson and A. R. C. Pack. Effects of extended systemic and topical folate supplementation on gingivitis of pregnancy, *J. Clin. Periodontol. 9*:75 (1982).

3

Skin Diseases Specifically Associated with Pregnancy

Robert Charles-Holmes
Warwick Hospital, Warwickshire, England

I. INTRODUCTION

Over the past 15 years, there has a been a considerable advance in our understanding of the dermatoses of pregnancy. Fundamental to this was a reappraisal of the classification of the dermatoses of pregnancy (1). The terminology suggested in Table 1 is now widely accepted and the synonyms for the disorders are gradually falling out of use.

The two most clearly defined disorders are pruritic urticarial papules and plaques of pregnancy (PUPPP) and pemphigoid gestationis (PG). The clinical features of these two disorders have been described in detail in large studies and their separate identities established. PUPPP has been shown to be a surprisingly common disorder with a very varied morphology. There is no doubt that this eruption, with its variable morphology, has been the source of much of the confusion that has surrounded the classification of pregnancy dermatoses. Fortunately, PUPPP resolves spontaneously and does not have any serious adverse effects on the maternal or fetal prognoses. Before PUPPP became well recognized, patients frequently suffered prolonged discomfort through inappropriate treatment, and they also experienced unnecessary anxiety related to the fetal prognosis.

Although investigations of PUPPP have tended to concentrate on its clinical features, the studies of PG have looked beyond its clinical aspects into the

Table 1 Classification of the Dermatoses of Pregnancy

Suggested terminology	Synonyms
Pruritic urticarial papules and plaques of pregnancy	Polymorphic eruption of pregnancy Toxic erythema of pregnancy Late-onset prurigo of pregnancy Toxemic rash of pregnancy
Pemphigoid gestationis	Herpes gestationis
Poorly defined disorders of uncertain significance	
Prurigo of pregnancy	Prurigo gestationis of Besnier Early-onset prurigo of pregnancy
Pustular psoriasis of pregnancy	Impetigo herpetiformis
Pruritic folliculitis of pregnancy	
Autoimmune progesterone dermatitis of pregnancy	
Linear IgM dermatosis of pregnancy	
Papular dermatitis of pregnancy	

underlying etiological mechanisms. PG has proved to be a useful disease in which to unravel autoimmune processes, and it has been suggested that it may represent a unique model of autoimmunity (2).

Although PUPPP and PG are now clearly defined, the significance of the other eruptions which have been classified as "pregnancy dermatoses" remains in doubt. As our criteria for classifying diseases improve, we may well find that the list of genuine pregnancy dermatoses diminishes.

II. THE DERMATOSES OF PREGNANCY

A. Pruritic Urticarial Papules and Plaques of Pregnancy

It is not at all uncommon for women to develop a pruritic urticarial eruption in the last trimester of pregnancy or immediately postpartum. The first detailed description of the eruption was made in 1962 when it was termed toxemic rash of pregnancy (8); however, this name was misleading, as there was no association with toxemia (preeclampsia). Since then various descriptive terms have been used, including late-onset prurigo of pregnancy (9), pruritic urticarial papules and plaques of pregnancy (PUPPP) (5), toxic erythema of pregnancy (3), and polymorphic eruption of pregnancy (1,10). In the interests of consensus and understanding, it had been proposed that a single name should be used (11) and PUPPP is the natural choice, as it is the most widely used term.

1. *Etiology*

PUPPP is an inflammatory dermatoses that appears to occur solely in association with pregnancy; apart from this, its etiology is uncertain. Unlike pemphigoid gestationis, there is no evidence to suggest that PUPPP is an autoimmune disease. The frequency of autoantibodies is not increased (12), and the frequency of HLA antigens is normal (4). Immunofluorescence studies are generally negative (3,5).

Hormonal investigations, including serum beta human chorionic gonadotropin (β-hCG), estradiol, cortisol, and urinary estriol, have all been normal (12,13). Unlike pemphigoid gestationis, the eruption has not been described with the reestablishment of menstruation or in association with the oral contraceptive. Intradermal testing with aqueous preparations of estradiol and progesterone have been negative (14).

One striking clinical feature of PUPPP which may give a clue to its etiology is the association with striae. The eruption frequently begins in and around striae on the abdomen and thighs (3–5). It usually affects first pregnancies, in which striae are more common, and it has also been associated with twin pregnancies, in which striae can be particularly florid (15,16). There have been conflicting reports as to whether PUPPP is associated with an increase in maternal weight gain and fetal weight (15,17). Such an association might account for the relationship with striae. In a report which did note an increase in maternal weight gain, it was suggested that excessive abdominal distension or a reaction to it may play a role in the development of PUPPP (15).

Pregnancy is associated with an increase in circulating immune complexes. The possibility that these might be involved in the etiology of PUPPP has been explored. No abnormalities were detected in the levels of circulating immune complexes by the C1q binding or polyethylene glycol precipitation techniques in PUPPP. However, small- to medium-sized immune complexes detected by a rheumatoid factor–binding assay were found to be significantly reduced during the acute stage of PUPPP (6). It was suggested that PUPPP might develop following the perivascular accumulation of small-sized circulating immune complexes which had leaked through dilated upper dermal vessels (6). In accord with this, one immunopathological study of PUPPP showed perivascular deposition of immunoreactants in 25% of patients (18).

Recently, PUPPP was described occurring in sisters (19); however, apart from this, familial cases have not been described. As the eruption is so common, these familial cases could have occurred by chance.

2. *Histopathology*

The histopathology of PUPPP varies depending on the stage of the eruption (20). The early urticarial lesions demonstrate epidermal and upper dermal edema with a perivascular lymphohistiocytic infiltrate. Eosinophils are prominent in the infiltrate in approximately a quarter of the biopsies, and eosinophilic spongiosis has also been noted. The histopathology of vesicular lesions usually shows intense focal spongiosis (Fig. 1), although occasionally small subepidermal vesicles may have been seen (21). As the lesions resolve, there is patchy acanthosis and parakeratosis. Several reports have shown the varied histopathological features of PUPPP (5,22, 23). Although vasculitis does not appear to be a feature of PUPPP, four cases have been described with perivascular nuclear dust (24).

3. *Immunopathology*

Immunofluorescence studies are almost always entirely negative in PUPPP (3,5). In contrast to pemphigoid gestationis, there is no evidence of significant C3 or immunoglobulin G (IgG) deposition at the basement membrane zone in PUPPP. In view of the large number of patients with PUPPP that have now been studied, it is not surprising that occasional aberrant results have been described, including C3 deposition at the basement membrane zone (14,18,25), perivascular deposition of IgM, C3 and IgA (18), and an antiepidermal cell IgG (26). These are exceptional findings of very doubtful significance. Immunoelectron microscopy, which is more sensitive than immunofluorescence, has confirmed an absence of C3 and IgG at the basement membrane zone in PUPPP (27).

There has been considerable debate as to whether direct immunofluorescence studies should be performed routinely in PUPPP. One view is that this is the only

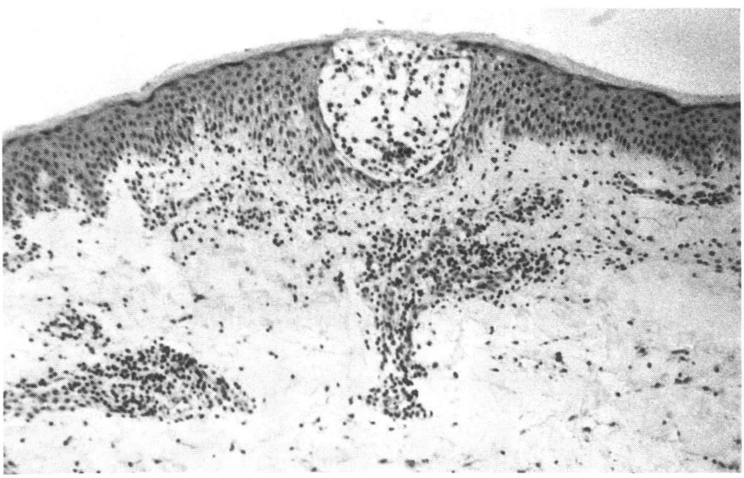

Figure 1 Histopathology of PUPPP showing an intraepidermal vesicle.

way to differentiate between two rare disorders (28,29). The opposing view is that PUPPP is not at all uncommon, and the regular subjection of these patients to immunofluorescence studies would be unnecessarily expensive (30,31). Perhaps the answer to this matter is for the individual clinician to use immunofluorescence studies if their personal clinical experience of pregnancy dermatoses is insufficient for them to confidently differentiate between PUPPP and pemphigoid gestationis.

Cell maker studies in PUPPP have shown that the majority of cells in the infiltrate are T lymphocytes (32).

4. *Clinical Features*

a. Incidence. PUPPP is by far the most common of the pregnancy dermatoses. A detailed prospective study over 2 years revealed an incidence of 1 in 160 pregnancies (4). In order to achieve an accurate assessment of the incidence of PUPPP, it was necessary to establish very close communication with the obstetricians and midwives, with almost daily visits to their wards and out-patient clinics. It was clear that under ordinary circumstances many patients would never have come to the attention of the dermatology department. This would explain the views of some investigators that the condition is rare (33).

b. Onset. The majority of patients who develop PUPPP do so in the last month of pregnancy or immediately postpartum. The average time of onset is at 36 weeks of gestation (4). It is most unusual for the eruption to begin before the third trimester; however, a patient has been reported with an onset of PUPPP in the fourth week of pregnancy (15).

c. Duration. The average duration of PUPPP is 6 weeks; however, the eruption is not usually severe for more than 1 week (4). Postpartum exacerbations may occur in PUPPP, but these are less common than in pemphigoid gestationis (3).

d. Morphology. The eruption of PUPPP begins with urticarial papules (Fig. 2) which frequently coalesce to produce urticarial plaques. If the patients are reexamined, as the eruption evolves, target lesions or polycyclic wheals are found in 20% of patients (Fig. 3) and vesicles in 40% (Fig. 4). The vesicles are usually no bigger than pinhead sized and do not develop into bullae. As the eruption resolves, there is usually fine scaling and crusting, producing an eczematous appearance (4).

e. Distribution. The initial lesions of PUPPP frequently develop in and around striae on the lower abdomen and thighs (see Fig. 2). The periumbilical skin is usually relatively spared. As the eruption develops, it often becomes widely distributed on the trunk and limbs (Fig. 5). Although the hands and feet are affected in approximately 25% of cases of PUPPP (Fig. 6), the palms and soles are rarely

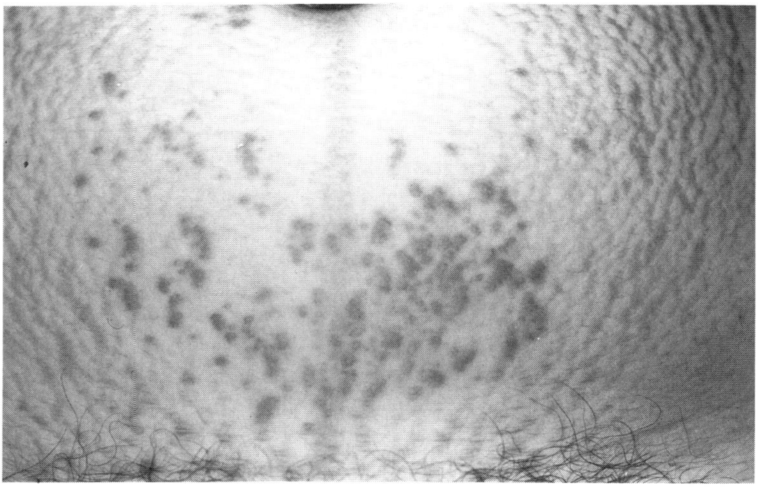

Figure 2 PUPPP—urticarial papules on the abdomen in association with striae. (Courtesy of Churchill Livingstone. R. C. Holmes. Pregnancy Dermatoses. In *Modern Management of Common Skin Diseases*, edited by C. F. H. Vickers, 1986.)

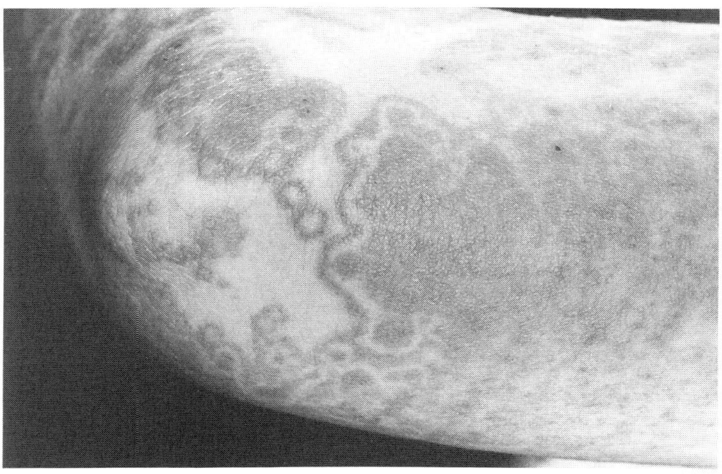

Figure 3 PUPPP—target lesions on the elbow. (From Ref. 3.)

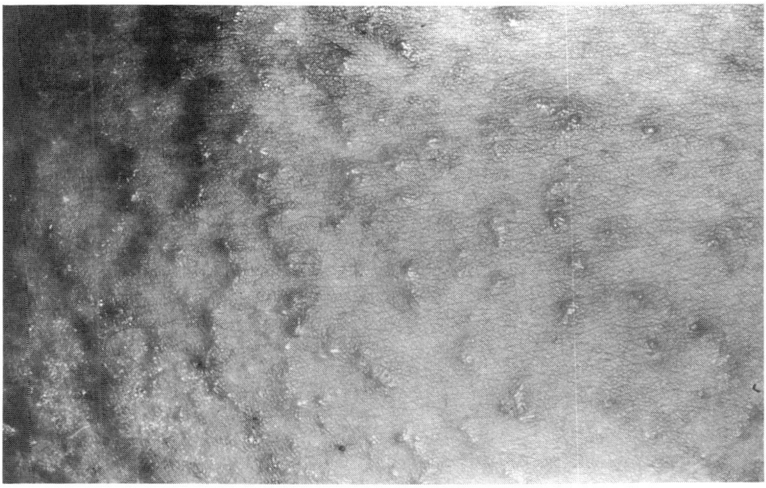

Figure 4 PUPPP—small vesicles in association with striae.

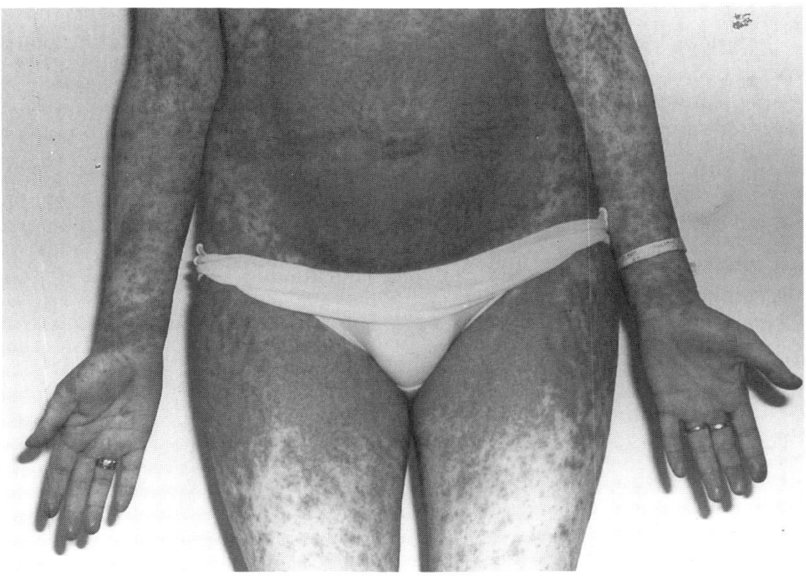

Figure 5 PUPPP—diffuse erythematous eruption on the trunk and limbs.

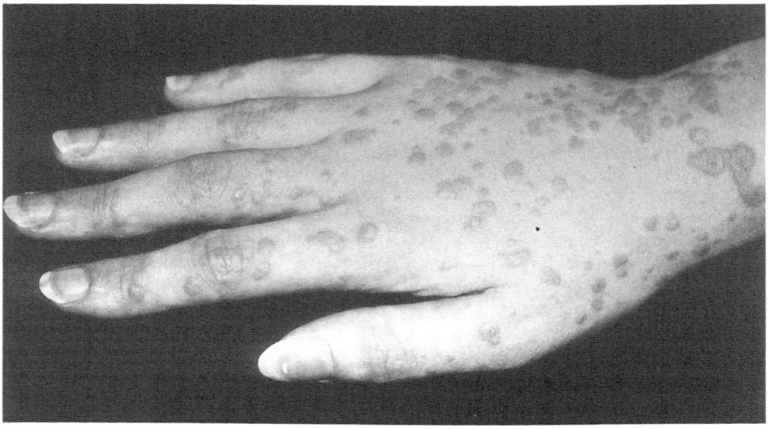

Figure 6 PUPPP—erythematous papules on the dorsum of the hand.

involved. It is most unusual for the face to be affected (4,34). In fact, involvement of the face is so unusual that when it does occur it has been suggested that an alternative diagnosis, such as contact dermatitis, should be carefully considered (7). Involvement of the mucous membranes and the scalp has not been described in PUPPP.

f. Differential Diagnosis. In view of the varied morphology of PUPPP, it is not surprising that it may easily be misdiagnosed. The intense pruritus not infrequently leads to an erroneous diagnosis of scabies, particularly in the presence of acral lesions. When the eruption is widespread, it may be mistaken for a drug eruption. The presence of target lesions may lead to PUPPP being misdiagnosed as erythema multiforme. When vesicles are a prominent feature, the diagnosis of pemphigoid gestationis needs to be considered. The differential diagnosis will vary depending on the stage of the eruption. In the resolving phase of PUPPP, it often has an "eczematous" appearance. PUPPP may be exacerbated at the site of an adhesive plaster, such as epidural sites. This can produce an eruption in the shape of a plaster and therefore mimic contact dermatitis.

When the diagnosis of PUPPP is in doubt, it is particularly helpful to establish the precise location of the initial lesions. If these were on the abdomen and thighs in association with striae, then the diagnosis is likely to be PUPPP.

5. *Prognosis*

a. Maternal. Apart from the severe discomfort of the eruption of PUPPP, the maternal prognosis is normal (4). PUPPP appears to be unlikely to recur in subsequent pregnancies. A very mild urticarial eruption has been described in subsequent pregnancies in a few patients, but this is of doubtful significance (4). It has been suggested that the eruption may be more severe in twin pregnancies (16).

b. Fetal. There is no increase in fetal mortality or morbidity in PUPPP (4). An increase in fetal birth weight has been described (15). The frequency of twin pregnancies appears to be increased in PUPPP (15). Despite the very common occurrence of PUPPP, only one isolated case has been described in which the infant appeared to have a similar eruption (35). In view of the nonspecific features of the infant's eruption, it seems likely that this was a coincidental problem rather than a case of infantile PUPPP.

6. Treatment

As the maternal and fetal long-term prognoses in PUPPP are normal, the treatment is symptomatic. Fortunately, adequate relief of the pruritus can usually be achieved with a moderately potent topical corticosteroid cream. More severely affected patients have been treated with systemic corticosteroids with apparent benefit (5,16, 36). Some patients have been delivered early with the expectation that this will terminate the PUPPP (37). Although this has appeared to have been the outcome in some cases (16), it has been pointed out that the resolution of PUPPP is usually unrelated to delivery. Therefore, treating PUPPP by early delivery should be discouraged, as it is unlikely to be followed by immediate resolution of the eruption (38).

7. Summary

PUPPP is a particularly common disorder affecting approximately 1 in 200 pregnancies (3,4). Numerous studies have clearly demonstrated that it is quite distinct from PG (3,5). Its etiology has not been established, but there is some evidence to suggest that leakage of small immune complexes through dilated upper dermal vessels may play a role in the pathogenesis of PUPPP (6). The eruption demonstrates the isomorphic phenomenon (Koebner phenomenon), being prominent in striae and other sites of injury (7). Patients are frequently primigravida, and the eruption usually begins in the last trimester or immediately postpartum (3,4). All patients develop urticarial papules and a proportion of patients will also develop urticarial plaques, vesicles, target lesions, and polycyclic wheals (3). As the eruption resolves, it is scaly and crusted with an "eczematous" appearance (4). The mean duration of PUPPP is 6 weeks, although it is rarely severe for more than 1 week (4). The fetal and maternal prognoses are normal (4).

B. Pemphigoid Gestationis (Herpes Gestationis)

Pemphigoid gestationis has been recognized for over 180 years (56). It was first termed herpes gestationis in 1872, because of the resemblance of the early lesions to herpetic vesicles (57). The term *herpes gestationis* tends to be misleading, particularly to midwives and patients, raising unnecessary anxiety about a herpes-virus infection. It is now known that "herpes gestationis" has a close clinical and pathological overlap with bullous pemphigoid. Therefore, in 1983, the name pemphigoid gestationis (PG) was proposed (1), and this has gained wide acceptance.

1. Etiology

Our knowledge of the etiology of PG provides us with useful insights into the mechanisms of immunobullous diseases. As PG occurs solely in association with pregnancy and the trophoblastic tumors, it was suggested that the eruption might develop as a result of an immune response to trophoblastic antigens and that this immune response could cross react with and damage an antigen at the basement membrane zone of skin (58). Since this hypothesis was proposed much laboratory evidence has accumulated in its support. The most fundamental step was demonstrating that trophoblastic basement membranes and skin basement membranes do indeed share common antigens (59,60). It has been shown that trophoblastic tissue expresses antigens which cross react with the skin basement zone from 22 weeks of gestation (60).

Evidence of an immune attack on the placenta in PG was demonstrated by immunohistological studies showing increased numbers of bone marrow–derived cells within the chorionic villi adjacent to the maternal decidua (61,62). At the same site, it was also noted that some trophoblastic cells were most unusual in that they were expressing class II major histocompatibility complex (MHC) antigens (61–63). The reason for this aberrant expression of class II MHC antigens remains unclear; however, by expressing these DR antigens, trophoblastic cells would be able to act as antigen-presenting cells and initiate an autoimmune response. A similar mechanism has been proposed for organ-specific autoimmune disorders such as thyroid disease (64).

More recently, an alternative hypothesis has been proposed for the induction of autoimmunity in PG. It was suggested that the paternally derived antigens in the trophoblast could evoke an allogeneic reaction rather than the trophoblastic cells acting as antigen-presenting cells (2). In support of this, it was noted that in PG the DP and DR subregions of the MHC class II antigens are consistently expressed, whereas the expression of DQ is absent or variable (62,63). Mononuclear cells which incompletely express class II molecules in this way are poor antigen-presenting cells but potent in provoking allogeneic reactions (65).

A further finding in PG which supports the possibility of an allogeneic reaction to trophoblasts relates to the immunogenetics found in skipped pregnancies. Patients were reported in which PG occurred in pregnancies in which there was HLA DR incompatibility between the mother and the fetus, but PG did not occur when the mother and fetus shared common HLA DR antigens (58). Where the paternally derived trophoblastic antigens are presented to the maternal immune system in the context of self MHC molecules, then tolerance to these antigens would be expected (66), and this may explain why PG did not occur in some pregnancies with fetomaternal HLA DR compatibility. There is certainly evidence in PG of an increase in maternal antibodies to paternally derived HLA antigens with alloreactivity to paternal MHC molecules in 85–100% of cases (67,68).

Finally, a most unusual case has been reported which may represent a fortuitous experimental model for the induction of a bullous eruption similar to PG. The patient was an 80-year-old man who was given intramuscular injections of placental extracts as a rejuvenating treatment. Subsequently, he developed a pemphigoid-like bullous eruption (69). This patient's eruption differed from PG in that immunoblotting showed the target antigen to be a 43-kD glycoprotein (70).

2. *Histopathology and Ultrastructure*

The histopathology of the urticarial lesions of PG demonstrates epidermal and papillary dermal edema with occasional foci of eosinophilic spongiosis. In the dermis, there is a perivascular infiltrate composed of lymphocytes, histiocytes, and frequently eosinophils. The bullous lesions demonstrate subepidermal bullae (Fig. 7),

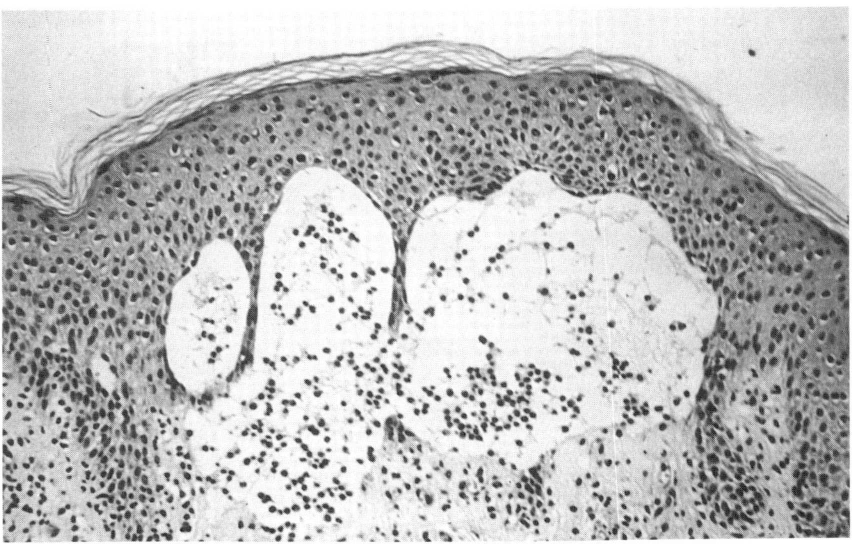

Figure 7 Histopathology of pemphigoid gestationis showing a subepidermal vesicle. (From Ref. 3.)

which invariably contain numerous eosinophils (20,71–73). Focal areas of basal cell necrosis have been described (72–74). Recently, a patient was reported in whom there were flame figures in the dermis similar to those which have been previously described in pemphigoid (75).

Ultrastructural studies of PG have demonstrated degenerative changes in the basal cells leading to necrosis (71,76). Blister formation occurs within the lamina lucida between the necrotic epidermal cells and the lamina densa (73,76). These findings are somewhat different than those which are usually seen in bullous pemphigoid where the blister formation appears to arise within the lamina lucida with intact basal cells (76).

3. *Immunopathology*

Standard immunofluorescence studies demonstrate that in all cases of PG there is deposition of C3 at the basement membrane zone of skin (Fig. 8), and in most cases a C3 binding factor (PG factor) can be demonstrated in the serum (78). Indirect immunofluorescence studies using split skin as a substrate reveal that the PG factor binds to the epidermal side of the split (60). The frequency of positive direct and indirect immunofluorescence findings for C3 and IgG are shown in Table 2.

The reason for the absence of IgG on direct and indirect tests in some cases is simply the lack of sensitivity of the technique. Using monoclonal antibodies to the

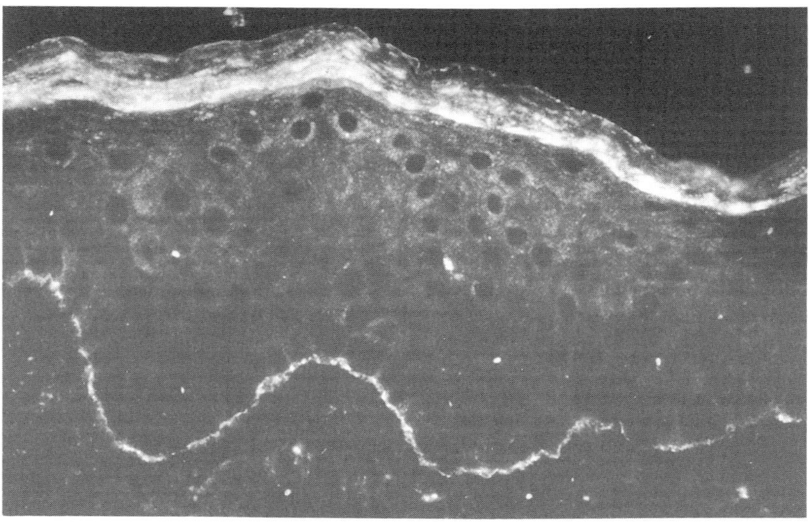

Figure 8 Direct immunofluorescence demonstrating C3 deposition at the BMZ in pemphigoid gestationis.

Table 2 Immunofluorescence Findings in PG

Direct	C3	100%
	IgG	27%
Indirect	C3	91%
	IgG	21%

Source: Data from Ref. 3.

IgG subclasses, all cases show evidence of deposition of an IgG1 on direct immunofluorescence (44). Immunoelectron microscopy studies have also shown the presence of IgG at the basement membrane zone where the immunofluorescence findings were negative (27,79).

Initially there were conflicting reports with regard to the precise localization of the deposits of IgG and C3 within the lamina lucida in PG. Some studies showed localization around hemidesmosomes (80,81), as in bullous pemphigoid, whereas another showed uniform deposition within the lamina lucida (76). Immunofluorescence studies on isolated basal cell keratinocytes show two patterns of staining in PG. There is either a polar fluorescence, as in bullous pemphigoid, or a uniform fluorescence around the periphery (82). This suggests that there may be heterogeneity of antigen recognition in PG which would account for the different patterns of immunoreactant localization which have been demonstrated by immunoelectron microscopy (76,80,81). An immunogold technique showed cleavage occurring at the level of the subbasal dense plate in association with the hemidesmosomes (83). These findings provide further support for the association of PG and bullous pemphigoid.

Immunoblotting has shown that the major target antigen in PG is a 180-kD glycoprotein (84,85), although some patients have been reported with antibodies to 220-kD and 240-kD glycoproteins (84,85). These findings highlight the overlap between PG and bullous pemphigoid. In bullous pemphigoid, the major target antigen is either a 220- or 240-kD glycoprotein, whereas some patients have an antibody to the 180-kD antigen (86). Bullous pemphigoid appears to be a heterogeneous disorder with PG constituting one or perhaps more subtypes. The 180-kD glycoprotein has been shown to be a hemidesmosomal polypeptide (45).

4. *Immunogenetics*

There is a strong genetic component determining susceptibility to PG. It has been shown that 61–80% of patients have DR3 (controls 22%), 52–53% have DR4 (controls 33%), and 43–50% have DR3/DR4 (controls 3%) (3,52). These genes have been associated with a number of autoimmune disorders and are thought to be markers of a nonspecific increase in immune responsiveness.

Recent analysis of complement component genetics in PG identified a significant association with C4 null alleles (53). Null alleles are recognized by a lack of expression for that particular complement component. PG was associated with C4 null alleles in 90% of patients compared with 43% in controls. There was a particular association with the C4 null allele (C4A*QO). In systemic lupus erythematosus, there appears to be a functional significance in the association between the disease and C4 null alleles (87); in PG, however, it remains unclear whether the association is of functional relevance or simply a manifestation of the high degree of linkage disequilibrium between C4A*QO and DR3.

An increased frequency of HLA DR2 was reported in the husbands of patients with PG (67), but this was not confirmed in a further study (58).

5. *Pathogenesis*

Our understanding of the pathogenesis of PG began in 1973 when Provost and Tomasi demonstrated the deposition of C3, C5, and properdin along the basement membrane zone of lesional skin (88). A factor was demonstrated in the serum which was capable of binding C3 to the basement membrane zone. This was termed the HG factor (PG factor). Although this was initially thought not to be an immunoglobulin, subsequent investigations into the character of the PG factor showed that it was an IgG (89–91). Recently, the PG factor has been shown to belong to the IgG1 subclass (44). This IgG activates complement via the classic pathway (89–91). There is also deposition of alternative pathway components, such as properdin and factor B, at the basement membrane zone. This probably occurs by activation of the C3 amplification loop. A patient has been described with the C3 nephritic factor (C3NF) (92). This is an IgG autoantibody to alternative pathway C3 convertase, which prolongs the half-life of this convertase and therefore enhances the alternative pathway. The presence of this factor could be the explanation for other patients in whom there has been significant alternative pathway activation.

Clinical evidence supporting the pathogenic role of the circulating PG factor comes from the occurrence of bullous lesions in neonates, where there will have been passive transfer of the autoantibody across the placenta (93–95). The clinical improvement that has beeen noted in patients following plasmapheresis also provides further support for a pathogenic role of the PG factor (91,96).

6. *Clinical Features*

a. Incidence. There have been various estimates of the incidence of PG ranging from 1 in 3000 (97) to 1 in 60,000 pregnancies (98). It is undoubtably very rare and a frequency of approximately 1 in 50,000 pregnancies is probably a reasonably accurate assessment (49). Most patients with PG have been white, although the condition has also been described in black patients of African origin (99).

b. Onset. The onset of PG may vary from the ninth week of gestation to 1 week postpartum; the average time of onset is 21 weeks of gestation (3). The eruption usually occurs earlier in subsequent pregnancies.

c. Duration. The activity of PG may diminish in the last few weeks of pregnancy, but there is usually a brisk flare immediately postpartum (3). The duration of the eruption postpartum is very variable. Patients have been described with the disease persisting for more than 10 years postpartum (46,47); however, in the majority of cases, the bullous lesions of PG resolve within 2 months of delivery and the urticarial lesions within 1 year (3).

d. Morphology. The initial lesions consist of intensely pruritic urticarial papules, target lesions, and annular wheals. Subsequently, large tense bullae develop within areas of urticated erythema (Fig. 9). The bullae usually contain straw-colored fluid, but they may be hemorrhagic. Occasionally, the bullae are grouped in an annular pattern. There may be an interval of 1 month after the onset of the eruption before bullous lesions develop (3). There have been very occasional reports of patients with PG in whom bullous lesions were absent. One case has been described in which there were prominent pustular lesions (100).

e. Distribution. The eruption of PG usually begins on the abdomen with a predilection for the periumbilical region (3). The palms and soles are also common

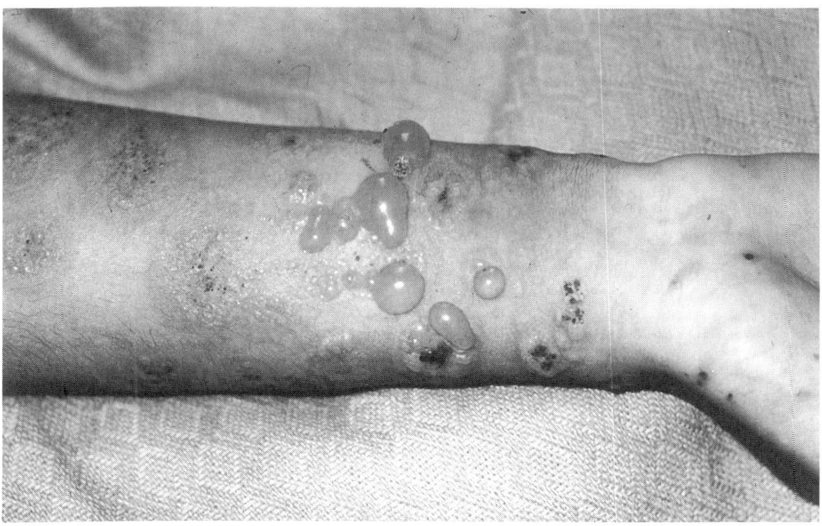

Figure 9 Pemphigoid gestationis—bullous lesions on the wrist.

presenting sites (48). Subsequently, the eruption becomes widespread with particular involvement of the abdomen, thighs, and forearms. Unlike PUPPP, facial lesions are not uncommon and the oral and vaginal mucous membranes may also be affected (48,74). There have been no reports of involvement of the ocular mucous membranes in PG.

f. Clinical Associations. PG has a strong association with the HLA antigens DR3 and DR4 (52,58). These genes are associated with an increased risk of autoimmune disease. In accord with this, PG has been described in association with Graves disease (54) and neonatal alloimmune thrombocytopenia (101). A review of secondary autoimmune diseases in PG revealed a frequency of Graves disease of 11%, whereas there is a prevalence of only 0.4% in the normal female population (55). The coexistence of PG and Graves disease was thought to be in excess of that expected simply as a result of the HLA DR3 association.

7. *Prognosis*

a. Maternal. PG is a severe disease which invariably requires hospital admission for its treatment. Most patients need systemic corticosteroids and are subject to the side effects of this treatment, which if the disease is protracted, includes Cushing's syndrome (102). In the majority of patients, the bullous lesions resolve within 2 months postpartum and the urticarial eruption within 1 year of delivery. However, cases have been reported that have persisted for more than 10 years postpartum (46,47).

PG invariably recurs in subsequent pregnancies, in which it tends to develop earlier, to be more severe, and to persist longer (47,48). Therefore, patients with PG need to consider whether sterilization would be appropriate. There have been exceptional cases in which subsequent pregnancies have been unaffected, sometimes in association with changed paternity (74). Recurrence of PG has occurred with the oral contraceptives (103–107) and in association with menstruation (58), suggesting that hormonal factors may modulate the disease activity.

In some autoimmune diseases, the severity appears to be greater in patients with the HLA antigen DR3; there is no evidence to suggest that this is the case in PG (108).

It has been suggested that prolactin may exacerbate PG. A patient with postpartum PG was reported who appeared to respond to treatment with the prolactin-inhibiting drug bromocriptine, and it was suggested that PG was more severe in women who breast-fed (109). However, a more detailed assessment suggested that women who breast-fed were, in fact, less severely affected (58).

b. Fetal. When the published data on PG consisted of collected case reports, the impression was given that there was a significant increase in fetal morbidity and mortality (110). However, cases with a serious outcome were more likely to have been reported. Recently more comprehensive studies of PG have recorded a much better fetal prognosis. An increase in small-for-dates babies has been noted which was attributed to slight impairment of placental function (50). Patients who were treated with oral corticosteroids were no more likely to have children that were small-for-dates (50,51). A recent large study of 126 affected pregnancies showed no increase in spontaneous abortions or stillbirths (51).

There has been a recent report of a fetal death in PG secondary to an umbilical cord knot. As such knots are more common with reduced fetal size, they might be slightly more likely to occur in PG than in normal pregnancy (111).

Infants may develop transient bullous lesions similar to those of their mother (94,95). This has been attributed to passive transfer of the anti–basement membrane zone antibody across the placenta.

Mothers with PG often ask whether their daughters are also likely to experience the same bullous eruption when they in turn become pregnant. They may be reassured that, as yet, no familial cases have been described.

8. *Treatment*

If the eruption in PG is particularly mild, then it may be possible to control the condition adequately with a potent topical corticosteroid. However, PG generally requires treatment with systemic corticosteroids. Most investigators advocate commencing treatment with prednisolone 40 mg daily (1,48,49) and then adjusting the dose depending on the response (108). If the eruption resolves well, it is worthwhile to reduce the dose of prednisolone, as some patients respond to doses of prednisolone as low as 5–10 mg daily. A temporary increase in prednisolone treatment is required if the eruption flares immediately postpartum. Fortunately, the administration of systemic corticosteroids in the second and third trimesters of pregnancy does not appear to confer any significant risk to the fetus. The duration of postpartum treatment will depend on the persistence of the eruption.

If steroid treatment proves unsuccessful or is contraindicated, then plasmapheresis should be considered. This has been used successfully for PG during pregnancy (96) and also postpartum (91). Other treatments that have been reported include sulfonamides and pyridoxine, although these drugs are not consistently helpful (108). More recently, a patient was reported in whom severe PG resolved following the prevention of premature labor with ritodrine (112). This is a β-adrenergic drug with predominantly a β_2 receptor agonist activity. There has been some support for the suggestion that this may be a useful treatment in PG (113).

9. *Summary*

PG is a severe bullous eruption which develops in association with either pregnancy or the trophoblastic tumors—hydatidiform mole or choriocarcinoma (39–43). It is characterized by the production of a complement-fixing IgG 1 autoantibody (44) to a component of the hemidesmosome (45). The eruption usually begins in the mid trimester and settles within 1 year postpartum (3). However, patients have been described with blistering that has persisted for more than 10 years postpartum (46,47). PG tends to recur in subsequent pregnancies, when it is usually more severe with an earlier onset (48). Treatment with oral corticosteroids is usually effective (49). There is an increased frequency of small-for-dates infants, but apart from this the fetal prognosis is normal (50,51). PG is associated with the HLA antigens DR3, DR4, and a C4 null allele (3,52,53). There is an increased frequency of Graves disease associated with PG (54,55).

III. DIFFERENTIATING PRURITIC URTICARIAL PAPULES AND PLAQUES OF PREGNANCY AND PEMPHIGOID GESTATIONIS

PUPPP is a very common disorder and therefore one which dermatologists and obstetricians are likely to be familiar with. However, in contrast, PG is exceedingly rare and many clinicians will have no personal experience of it. Fortunately, there is usually no difficulty in distinguishing PUPPP and PG clinically. Helpful differentiating features are listed in Table 3. The site of onset of the eruption is particularly important. In PG, the initial lesions are frequently in the periumbilical area or on the palms and soles, whereas in PUPPP, the eruption usually starts in association with prominent striae on the abdomen or thighs. The most important

Table 3 A Comparison of Pruritic Urticarial Papules and PUPP and PG

	PUPPP	PG
Urticarial papules	100%	100%
Vesicles	44%	95%
Target lesions	19%	95%
Bullae	0%	95%
Primigravida	76%	30%
Onset (mean gestation)	35 weeks	21 weeks[a]
Postpartum exacerbations	15%	75%
Striae	90%	21%
Periumbilical lesions	10%	84%
Palmoplantar lesions	4%	41%
Immunofluorescence (BMZ C3)		
Direct	0%	100%
Indirect	0%	91%

[a]First affected pregnancies.
Source: Data from Refs. 3 and 4.

clinical feature which will indicate a diagnosis of PG is the development of large bullous lesions, as bullae of this size are never encountered in PUPPP. It may take several weeks for the bullous lesions to develop in PG, and therefore clinical differentiation may be facilitated by the lapse of time.

One situation that might possibly create diagnostic confusion is where PG occurs without the development of bullous lesions. This has been reported (3,74) but is exceptionally rare. In these "mild" cases of PG, the value of establishing the diagnosis would be in predicting a likely recurrence in subsequent pregnancies with increased severity. Where there is any clinical doubt about the diagnosis, the matter may be resolved by taking a skin biopsy for direct immunofluorescence. This will demonstrate C3 deposition at the basement membrane zone in all cases of PG but an absence of C3 deposition in PUPPP. Other investigations such as skin biopsies for histology or serum for indirect immunofluorescence studies do not always differentiate the disorders so clearly.

There has been a lively debate as to whether direct immunofluorescence studies should be performed in all cases of PUPPP to exclude the possibility of "nonbullous" PG (28–31). PUPPP is so common and nonbullous PG so exceptionally rare that it would seem inappropriate to advocate routine direct immunofluorescence studies in all cases of PUPPP. Direct immunofluorescence should certainly be performed it there is any doubt about the diagnosis, and it is understandable that this investigation would be performed in academic centers that are making a special study of pregnancy dermatoses.

IV. POORLY DEFINED DISORDERS OF UNCERTAIN SIGNIFICANCE

A. Prurigo of Pregnancy

Prurigo of pregnancy has been described in as many as 1 in 300 pregnancies (9). In 1968, the distinction was drawn between this eruption, which consisted of firm papules developing early in pregnancy (early-onset prurigo), and an urticarial eruption developing later in pregnancy (late-onset prurigo) (9). The eruption which was termed late-onset prurigo of pregnancy is now generally referred to as PUPPP. As the terms *early-onset* and *late-onset prurigo of pregnancy* are no longer in common use, it is easier to refer to early-onset prurigo of pregnancy simply as prurigo of pregnancy.

1. *Etiology*

It has been suggested that prurigo of pregnancy may not be specifically related to pregnancy but the result of pruritus gravidarum occurring in latent atopics (1). Atopics have a strong propensity to develop prurigo lesions, and this would be especially likely if they developed the intractable pruritus which is frequently associated with pregnancy.

2. *Pathology*

In prurigo of pregnancy, there is parakeratosis and acanthosis which may be accompanied by excoriation. In the dermis, there is a perivascular lymphocytic infiltrate with occasional areas of fibroplasia. Direct and indirect immunofluorescence studies are negative in prurigo of pregnancy (1).

3. *Clinical Features*

a. Onset. The eruption of prurigo of pregnancy develops between 25 and 30 weeks of gestation.

b. Duration. The eruption of prurigo of pregnancy may persist for up to 3 months postpartum.

c. Morphology. The lesions of prurigo of pregnancy consist of firm papules which are frequently excoriated.

d. Distribution. The lesions of prurigo of pregnancy may be grouped on the extensor surfaces of the limbs, the abdomen, and the shoulders or they may be widespread (Fig. 10).

4. *Prognosis*

The maternal and fetal prognoses in prurigo of pregnancy appear to be normal.

5. *Differential Diagnosis*

In view of the marked pruritus and the nonspecific features of the eruption of prurigo of pregnancy, the patient's liver function tests should be checked to investigate the possibility of cholestasis of pregnancy.

6. *Treatment*

Prurigo of pregnancy does appear to be particularly resistant to symptomatic treatment; however, emollients and a mild topical corticosteroid cream may provide some relief of the pruritus.

B. Pustular Psoriasis of Pregnancy (Impetigo Herpetiformis)

The term *herpes impetiginiformis* was first introduced in 1872 to describe a severe pustular eruption occurring in association with pregnancy (114). Subse-

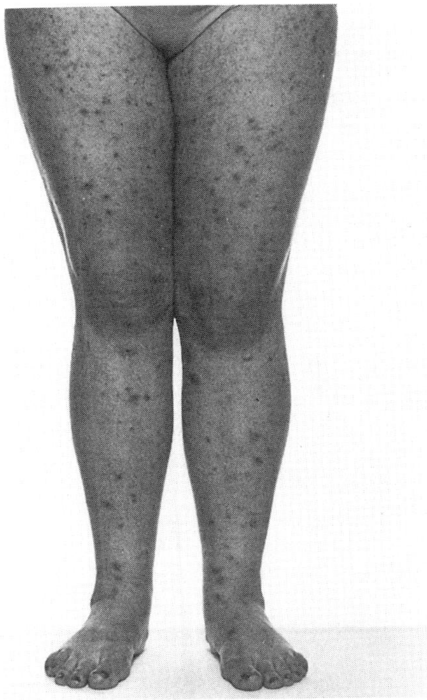

Figure 10 Prurigo of pregnancy.

quently, a similar eruption was reported in men, children, and nonpregnant women (115). As the histopathology shows spongiform pustulation similar to that seen in pustular psoriasis, the eruption is generally regarded as a form of pustular psoriasis precipitated by hormonal changes rather than a dermatosis specifically related to pregnancy (116,117). Investigators who think that impetigo herpetiformis is a distinct disorder cite differences in the morphology of impetigo herpetiformis and pustular psoriasis, the frequent absence of a past history of psoriasis, and the fact that the eruption resolves with conclusion of pregnancy (118–120).

1. Etiology

Hypocalcemia has been implicated as a precipitating factor of pustular psoriasis of pregnancy (121). Progesterone may also play a role in the etiology, as patients have been reported in which the eruption developed after the administration of progestogens (122,123).

2. *Pathology*

The histopathology of the lesions of pustular psoriasis of pregnancy generally shows spongiform pustules as seen in psoriasis (124). Some patients have been described in which there were unusual mononuclear cells within the pustules and dermal infiltrate. These contained abundant cytoplasm and large irregularly shaped nuclei (118). However, these findings have not been confirmed in subsequent reports (120). Microbiological studies show that the pustules do not contain any significant pathogens.

3. *Clinical Features*

a. Onset. The onset of pustular psoriasis of pregnancy is usually in the third trimester.

b. Morphology. The lesions of pustular psoriasis of pregnancy consist of grouped pustules developing on an intensely erythematous base. They are often annular or polycyclic with concentric rings of pustules (Fig. 11). Coalescing lesions producing lakes of pus occur less commonly than in typical pustular psoriasis.

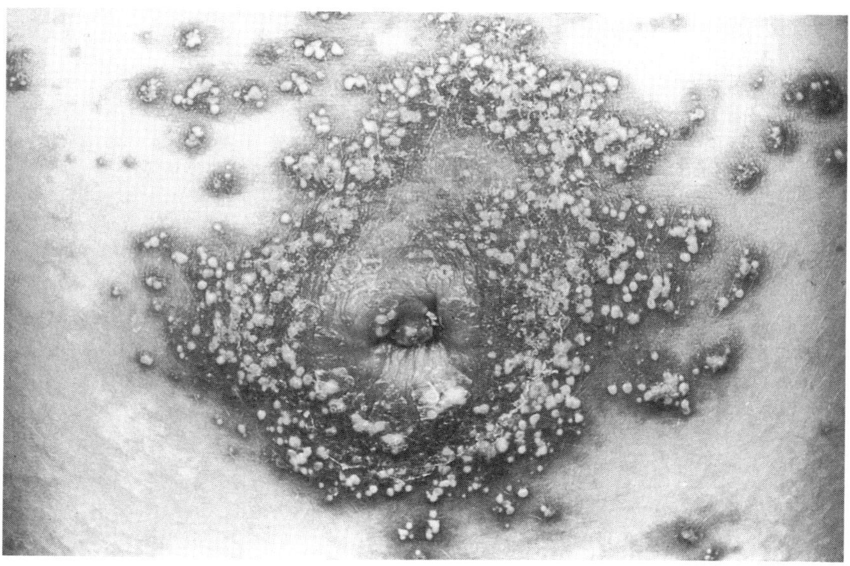

Figure 11 Pustular psoriasis. (Courtesy of Drs. J. Hughes and A. C. Pembroke, King's College Hospital, London.)

c. Distribution. The eruption of pustular psoriasis of pregnancy may be distributed widely on the trunk and limbs with a predilection for the flexures.

d. Systemic Features. Patients with pustular psoriasis of pregnancy are generally systemically unwell with malaise, anorexia, fever, and rigors. Patients may also have hypocalcemia.

4. *Differential Diagnosis*

There is usually no difficulty in distinguishing between pustular psoriasis of pregnancy and pemphigoid gestationis. However, a case of PG has been described in which there was a predominance of pustular lesions (100). Also, it is important to note that immunofluorescence tests may not provide an unequivocal answer as a patient with so-called pustular psoriasis was described in which direct immunofluorescence showed deposition of C3 at the basement membrane zone (122).

5. *Prognosis*

a. Maternal. The maternal prognosis in pustular psoriasis of pregnancy was initially considered to be very poor with a high maternal mortality (114); however, some recent case reports have had a more favorable outcome (117–125), suggesting that current management may have improved the prognosis. The eruption usually settles promptly postpartum, but recurrences have been described with subsequent pregnancies (119,123,125), with the use of oral contraceptives (123), and with menstruation (126). The eruption tends to be more severe with each subsequent pregnancy (119,123,124).

b. Fetal. Impaired placental function (125), stillbirths (125) and neonatal deaths (123) have been described in association with this pustular psoriasis of pregnancy. However, the rarity of the this disorder has made it difficult to assess the frequency of fetal mortality.

6. *Treatment*

Systemic corticosteroids are generally prescribed in pustular psoriasis of pregnancy, usually at an initial dose of prednisolone 80 mg daily. The response to treatment is very variable, with some patients appearing to derive little benefit (117,120,123,125,127–129). If hypocalcemia is present, it should be corrected. As there is an increased risk to the fetus, placental function must be carefully monitored and early delivery may be required. In view of the severity of the eruption and the likelihood of recurrence in subsequent pregnancies, sterilization should be considered.

The eruption usually resolves promptly after delivery; however, a recent report described persistence of the eruption until retained placental tissue was removed

(120). Therefore, meticulous care should be taken at delivery to ensure complete removal of the placenta and chorioamniotic membranes.

C. Pruritic Folliculitis of Pregnancy

Pruritic folliculitis of pregnancy was first described in 1981 (130). Since that time only a very small number of patients have been described (1,131). During pregnancy, women do appear to be more susceptible to infection with *Pityrosporum*, as demonstrated by the florid examples of pityriasis versicolor that may occur. As a widespread folliculitis has been described as a result of *Pityrosporum* infection (132), this etiology should be considered as a possible explanation for pruritic folliculitis of pregnancy. A further suggestion is that pruritic folliculitis of pregnancy may be a form of hormonally induced acne (1).

1. Etiology

The etiology of pruritic folliculitis of pregnancy is unknown.

2. Pathology

In pruritic folliculitis of pregnancy, there is an acute folliculitis with focal spongiosis and exocytosis of polymorphonuclear cells and mononuclear cells. In the dermis, there is edema with a perivascular infiltrate of variable intensity. Direct immunofluorescence studies have been negative in this condition (130).

3. Clinical Features

a. Morphology. The lesions of pruritic folliculitis of pregnancy consist of follicular erythematous papules (Fig. 12).

b. Distribution. The eruption in pruritic folliculitis of pregnancy is usually widespread, but it may be localized to the abdomen and arms.

c. Onset. The onset of pruritic folliculitis of pregnancy occurs between 4 and 9 months of gestation.

d. Resolution. The eruption of pruritic folliculitis of pregnancy may resolve during pregnancy. If it does persist postpartum, it will usually have resolved within 2 weeks. Recurrences have been described in two patients in succeeding pregnancies (130).

4. Prognosis

The maternal and fetal prognoses in pruritic folliculitis of pregnancy are normal.

5. Treatment

In some patients, treatment with topical benzoyl peroxide has proved helpful in the treatment of pruritic folliculitis of pregnancy (1).

Figure 12 Pruritic folliculitis of pregnancy—erythematous follicular papules on the back. (Courtesy of Churchill Livingstone. R. C. Holmes. Pregnancy Dermatoses. In *Modern Management of Common Skin Diseases*, edited by C. F. H. Vickers, 1986.)

D. Autoimmune Progesterone Dermatitis of Pregnancy

The term *autoimmune progesterone dermatitis* was introduced in 1964 when a patient was described with a pruritic vesicobullous eruption which began postpartum following two consecutive pregnancies (133). Subsequent reports have largely related to dermatoses demonstrating premenstrual exacerbations rather than having any specific relationship to pregnancy (134–136). There has been only one report that attributes autoimmune progesterone dermatitis to pregnancy itself (137). There have, in fact, been two reports in which the condition resolved during pregnancy (135,138), and in the original account, the eruption was in remission during pregnancy and flared postpartum (133). The apparent inactivity of autoimmune progesterone dermatitis during pregnancy is surprising in view of the fact that this is a time when progesterone levels are at their highest.

1. Etiology

Autoimmunity to progesterone was proposed as the eruption occurs when progesterone levels are elevated premenstrually and also following the administration of progestogens. The suppression of ovulation and oophorectomy, which will prevent rises in progesterone, have resulted in resolution of the eruption. Positive skin tests to progesterone, both of an immediate (135) and a delayed type (134,136), have been reported. In vitro studies have shown evidence of circulating antiprogesterone antibodies (135,136). It has been noted that some of the patients had taken synthetic progesterone prior to the development of the eruption. Therefore, it has been proposed that the problem may begin with an immune reaction to synthetic progesterone which subsequently cross reacts with endogenous progesterone (136).

2. *Clinical Features*

The patient with an eruption associated with pregnancy had acneiform pustules distributed on the arms, legs, and buttocks (137). The eruption occurred in two successive pregnancies developing on each occasion within the first 2 weeks of pregnancy. Both pregnancies ended in spontaneous abortion at 3 and 4 months of gestation, respectively. The eruption resolved immediately following the abortion in the first pregnancy but persisted after the second pregnancy.

Patients with autoimmune progesterone dermatitis unrelated to pregnancy have been described with a variety of lesions, including vesicles, bullae, and target lesions.

In view of the paucity of evidence associating autoimmune progesterone dermatitis with pregnancy, it does not seem appropriate to include this disorder as a dermatosis of pregnancy.

E. Linear IgM Dermatosis of Pregnancy

The term *linear IgM dermatosis of pregnancy* was introduced in 1988 to describe a patient who was thought to have a unique dermatosis (139). The eruption consisted of firm erythematous papules and some pustules which were distributed on the abdomen and limbs. The onset was at 37 weeks of gestation and resolution occurred at 6 weeks postpartum. The histopathology of the lesions demonstrated acanthosis, a perivascular infiltrate, and some dermal fibrosis. Direct immunofluorescence revealed linear deposition of IgM at the basement membrane zone, whereas indirect immunofluorescence was negative.

Subsequently, five patients were described in whom there was a circulating anti–basement membrane zone IgM antibody, but direct immunofluorescence was negative (140). The clinical features were similar to the original report in that the onset of the eruption was in the last trimester in four of the five patients and the lesions consisted of erythematous macules and papules distributed on the abdomen, limbs, and breasts. In one case, the eruption was atypical in that it started much earlier in pregnancy, at 11 weeks of gestation, and the lesions included vesicles. In this patient, there was a history of atopy.

A large study of immunofluorescence results showed that linear IgM deposition at the basement membrane zone can occur as a nonspecific finding with no apparent pathological significance (141). Therefore, it seems likely that the patients that have been described with this immunofluorescence finding, by direct or indirect immunofluorescence, do not constitute a specific entity.

F. Papular Dermatitis of Pregnancy

Papular dermatitis of pregnancy is one of the most controversial of the "pregnancy dermatoses." There is considerable doubt as to whether it is a distinct entity, and the original investigators' conclusions regarding the prognosis and treatment have also been questioned (1,10,142).

The term *papular dermatitis of pregnancy* was first introduced in 1962 (143). It was claimed that the disorder had characteristic clinical and biochemical features which made it distinct from other pruritic papular dermatoses of pregnancy. The clinical feature which was cited as distinctive was the widespread distribution of the papules rather than localized grouping. However, patients with prurigo of pregnancy and PUPPP may also have widespread lesions. The biochemical parameters which were proposed as features of papular dermatitis of pregnancy were raised urinary hCG, reduced plasma cortisol, and reduced urinary estriol (143,144). The assay of hCG which was used was a frog bioassay devised in 1949. Such assays were notoriously nonspecific, and therefore these results would have been most unreliable. The cortisol findings are also of doubtful significance in view of the type of assay used and the fact that they were probably random estimations of a parameter with a marked diurnal variation.

It was claimed that papular dermatitis of pregnancy was associated with a fetal mortality of 27%; however, some of the fetal deaths which were included in the study occurred in previous pregnancies unaffected by papular dermatitis of pregnancy (143). The fetal loss which was actually associated with papular dermatitis of pregnancy was 12.5%. Also within "fetal deaths" they included spontaneous abortions, which occur with a frequency of up to 15% in a normal population (145). Therefore, the "fetal mortality" appears to have been certainly overestimated and its true significance of some doubt.

The treatment which was proposed for papular dermatitis of pregnancy consisted of either prednisolone up to a dosage of 200 mg daily or diethylstilbestrol. It was claimed that these treatments reduced the fetal mortality. Subsequently, it became apparent that the administration of diethylstilbestrol during pregnancy could damage the fetal reproductive tract (146,147). The incidence of vaginal and cervical clear-cell adenocarcinoma is also increased (147). The original investigators acknowledged that treatment with diethylstilbestrol would certainly no longer be appropriate (148). The indication for prednisolone treatment is also very questionable in view of the unreliability of the mortality data for papular dermatitis of pregnancy.

Despite several centers making a special study of pregnancy dermatoses (3,12, 25), none has reported cases of papular dermatitis of pregnancy. If papular dermatitis of pregnancy were a genuine entity with a significant fetal loss, then one would have expected a series of patients to have been reported by another investigator at some stage over the 32 years since the original report. In the few cases that have been designated as papular dermatitis of pregnancy, the clinical and biochemical findings have produced insufficient evidence to establish papular dermatitis of pregnancy as a definite entity (149–151).

REFERENCES

1. R. C. Holmes and M. M. Black. The specific dermatoses of pregnancy, *J. Am. Acad. Dermatol.* *8*:405 (1983).
2. S. E. Kelly, M. M. Black, and S. Fleming. Pemphigoid gestationis: A unique mechanism of initiation of an autoimmune response by MHC Class II molecules? *J. Pathol.* *158*:81 (1989).
3. R. C. Holmes, M. M. Black, J. Dann, D. C. O. James, and B. Bhogal. A comparative study of toxic erythema of pregnancy and herpes gestationis, *Br. J. Dermatol.* *106*:499 (1982).
4. R. Charles-Holmes, Polymorphic eruption of pregnancy, *Semin. Dermatol.* *8*:18 (1989).
5. T. J. Lawley, K. C. Hertz, T. R. Wade, A. B. Ackerman and S. I. Katz. Pruritic urticarial papules and plaques of pregnancy, *JAMA* *241*:1696 (1979).
6. E. Kasp-Grochowska, J. Beck, R. C. Holmes, M. M. Black, and D. Timlin. The role of circulating immune complexes in the aetiology of polymorphic eruption of pregnancy, *Arch. Dermatol. Res.* *276*:71 (1984).
7. A. Carruthers. Facial involvement in PUPPP, *J. Am. Acad. Dermatol.* *17*:302 (1987).
8. G. Bourne. Toxaemic rash of pregnancy, *Proc. R. Soc. Med.* *55*:462 (1962).
9. D. S. Nurse. Prurigo of pregnancy, *Aust. J. Dermatol.* *9*:258 (1968).
10. R. C. Holmes and M. M. Black. The specific dermatoses of pregnancy: A reappraisal with special emphasis on a proposed simplified clinical classification, *Clin. Exp. Dermatol.* *7*:65 (1982).
11. J. Alcalay and J. E. Wolfe. Pruritic urticarial papules and plaques of pregnancy: the enigma and confusion, *J. Am. Acad. Dermatol.* *19*:1115 (1988).
12. J. Alcalay, A. Ingber, and B. Kafri. Hormonal evaluation and autoimmune background in pruritic urticarial papules and plaques of pregnancy, *Am. J. Obstet. Gynecol.* *158*:417 (1988).
13. J. Alcalay, A. Ingber, M. David, B. Hazaz, and M. Sandbank. PUPPP: A review of 21 cases, *J. Reprod. Med.* *32*:315 (1987).
14. W. R. Faber, Th. van Joost, R. Hausman, and G. H. Weenink. Late prurigo of pregnancy, *Br. J. Dermatol.* *106*:511 (1982).
15. L. M. Cohen, E. L. Capeless, P. A. Krusinski, and M. E. Maloney. Pruritic urticarial papules and plaques of pregnancy and its relationship to maternal-fetal weight gain and twin pregnancy, *Arch. Dermatol.* *125*:1534 (1989).
16. C. B. Bunker, K. Erskine, M. H. A. Rustin, and J. J. H. Gilkes. Severe polymorphic eruption of pregnancy occurring in twin pregnancies, *Clin. Exp. Dermatol.* *15*:228 (1990).
17. D. Roger, L. Vaillant, and G. Lorette. Pruritic urticarial papules and plaques of

pregnancy are not related to maternal or fetal weight gain, *Arch. Dermatol. 126*:1517 (1990).
18. I. K. Aronson, S. Vomvouras, V. C. Fiedler, and S. Bond. Immunopathology of pruritic urticarial papules and plaques of pregnancy, *J. Invest. Dermatol. 94*:504 (1990).
19. R. Weiss and P. Hull. Familial occurrence of pruritic urticarial papules and plaques of pregnancy, *J. Am. Acad. Dermatol. 26*:715 (1992).
20. R. C. Holmes, W. Jurecka, and M. M. Black. A comparative histopathological study of polymorphic eruption of pregnancy and herpes gestationis, *Clin. Exp. Dermatol. 8*:523 (1983).
21. R. C. Holmes, D. H. McGibbon, and M. M. Black. Polymorphic eruption of pregnancy with subepidermal vesicles, *J. R. Soc. Med. 77*:22 (1984).
22. A. R. Ahmed and R. Kaplan. Pruritic urticarial papules and plaques of pregnancy, *J. Am. Acad. Dermatol. 4*:679 (1981).
23. R. A. Schwartz, R. C. Hansen, and P. J. Lynch. Pruritic urticarial papules and plaques of pregnancy, *Cutis 27*:425 (1981).
24. J. P. Callen and R. Hanno. Pruritic urticarial papules and plaques of pregnancy (PUPPP). A clinicopathologic study, *J. Am. Acad. Dermatol. 5*:401 (1981).
25. K. B. Yancey, R. P. Hall, and T. J. Lawley. Pruritic urticarial papules and plaques of pregnancy: Clinical experience in twenty-four patients, *J. Am. Acad. Dermatol. 10*:473 (1984).
26. A. Trattner, A. Ingber, and M. Sandbank. Anti-epidermal cell surface antibodies in a patient with PUPPP, *J. Am. Acad. Dermatol. 24*:306 (1991).
27. W. Jurecka, R. C. Holmes, M. M. Black, P. McKee, A. K. Das, and B. Bhogal. An immunoelectron microscopy study of polymorphic eruption of pregnancy and herpes gestationis, *Br. J. Dermatol. 108*:147 (1983).
28. J.-H. Saurat. Immunofluorescence biopsy for pruritic urticarial papules and plaques of pregnancy, *J. Am. Acad. Dermatol. 20*:711 (1989).
29. J. K. Shornick. Routine immunofluorescence for pruritic urticarial papules and plaques of pregnancy, *J. Am. Acad. Dermatol. 18*:1146 (1988).
30. J. Goodall. Routine immunofluorescence for pruritic urticarial papules and plaques of pregnancy, *J. Am. Acad. Dermatol. 18*:1146 (1988).
31. J. Goodall. Immunofluorescence biopsy for pruritic urticarial papules and plaques of pregnancy, *J. Am. Acad. Dermatol. 22*:322 (1990).
32. R. Rand, T. J. Harrist, A. K. Bhan, K. Reed, and M. C. Mihm. The immunopathology of pruritic urticarial papules and plaques of pregnancy (PUPPP syndrome), *Clin. Res. 31*:597 (1983).
33. M. Nilles, W. Weyers, and K. Grunder. Pruritic urticarial papules and plaques of pregnancy. *Hautarzt 40*:586 (1989).
34. J. Alcalay, M. David, and M. Sandbank. Facial involvement in PUPPP, *J. Am. Acad. Dermatol. 15*:1048 (1986).
35. S. R. Uhlin. Pruritic urticarial papules and plaques of pregnancy. Involvement in mother and infant, *Arch. Dermatol. 117*:238 (1981).
36. H. E. Stoller. Pruritic urticarial papules and plaques of pregnancy, *JAMA 243*:2156 (1980).
37. V. P. Beltrani and V. S. Beltrani. Pruritic urticarial papules and plaques of pregnancy:

A severe case requiring early delivery for relief of symptoms, *J. Am. Acad. Dermatol.* *26*:266 (1992).
38. A. Carruthers. Pruritic urticarial papules and plaques of pregnancy, *J. Am. Acad. Dermatol.* *29*:125 (1993).
39. J. A. Elliott. Bullous dermatoses of toxic origin: report of a case involving association with choriocarcinoma, *Arch. Dermatol. Syph.* *37*:219 (1938).
40. W. G. Tillman. Herpes gestationis with hydatidiform mole and chorionepithelioma, *Br. Med. J.* *1*:1471 (1950).
41. C. Dupont. Herpes gestationis with hydatidiform mole, *Trans. St. Johns Dermatol.* *60*:103. (1974).
42. J. G. Tindall, T. H. Rea, I. Shulman, and F. P. Quismorio. Herpes gestationis in association with hydatidiform mole, *Arch. Dermatol.* *117*:510 (1981).
43. L. Slazinski and S. Degefu. Herpes gestationis associated with choriocarcinoma, *Arch. Dermatol.* *118*:425 (1982).
44. S. Kelly, R. Cerio, B. S. Bhogal, and M. M. Black. The distribution of IgG subclasses in pemphigoid gestationis: PG factor is an IgG1 autoantibody, *J. Invest. Dermatol.* *92*:695 (1989).
45. L. A. Diaz, H. Rattie, and W. S. Saunders. Isolation of a human epidermal cDNA corresponding to the 180Kd antigen recognised by bullous pemphigoid and herpes gestationis sera: Immunolocalisation of this protein to the hemidesmosome, *J. Clin. Invest.* *86*:1088 (1990).
46. J. D. Fine and E. F. Omura. Herpes gestationis. Persistent disease activity 11 years postpartum, *Arch. Dermatol.* *121*:924 (1985).
47. R. C. Holmes, M. M. Black, and D. M. Williamson. Herpes gestationis persisting for 12 years postpartum, *Arch. Dermatol.* *122*:375 (1986).
48. R. C. Holmes and M. M. Black. Herpes gestationis, *Dermatol. Clin.* *1*:195 (1983).
49. J. K. Shornick. Herpes gestationis. *J. Am. Acad. Dermatol.* *17*:539 (1987).
50. R. C. Holmes and M. M. Black. The fetal prognosis in pemphigoid gestationis (herpes gestationis), *Br. J. Dermatol.* *110*:67 (1984).
51. J. K. Shornick and M. M. Black. Fetal risks in herpes gestationis, *J. Am. Acad. Dermatol.* *26*:63 (1992).
52. J. K. Shornick, P. Stastny, and J. N. Gilliam. High frequency of histocompatibility antigens HLA DR3 and DR4 in herpes gestationis, *J. Clin. Invest.* *68*:553 (1981).
53. J. K. Shornick, C. M. Artlett, R. E. Jenkins, D. C. Briggs, K. I. Welsh, M. P. Garvey, S. E. Kelly, and M. M. Black. Complement polymorphism in HG: Association with C4 null allele, *J. Am. Acad. Dermatol.* *29*:545 (1993).
54. R. C. Holmes and M. M. Black. Herpes gestationis: A possible association with autoimmune thyrotoxicosis (Graves' disease), *J. Am. Acad. Dermatol.* *3*:474 (1980).
55. J. Shornick and M. M. Black. Secondary autoimmune disease in herpes gestationis (pemphigoid gestationis), *J. Am. Acad. Dermatol.* *26*:563 (1992).
56. J. B. H. Bunel. Essai sur le pemphigus, National Library of Medicine, Surgeon General's Catalogue, First series, 2, Paris (1811).
57. J. L. Milton. *The Pathology and Treatment of Diseases of the Skin.* Robert Hardwick, London. 1872, p. 205.
58. R. C. Holmes, M. M. Black, W. Jurecka, J. Dann, D. C. O. James, D. Timlin, and B.

Bhogal. Clues to the aetiology and pathogenesis of herpes gestationis, *Br. J. Dermatol. 109*:131 (1983).
59. J.-P. Ortoune, B.-L. Hsi, P. Verrando, F. Bernerd, G. Pautrat, A. Pisani, and C.-J. G. Yeh. Herpes gestationis factor reacts with the amniotic epithelial basement membrane, *Br. J. Dermatol. 117*:147 (1987).
60. S. E. Kelly, B. Bhogal, F. Wojnarowska, and M. M. Black. Expression of a pemphigoid gestationis related antigen by human placenta, *Br. J. Dermatol. 118*:605 (1988).
61. G. M. Borthwick, C. A. Sunderland, R. C. Holmes, M. M. Black, and G. M. Stirrat. Abnormal expression of HLA-DR antigen in the placenta of a patient with pemphigoid gestationis, *J. Reprod. Immunol. 6*:393 (1984).
62. G. M. Borthwick, R. C. Holmes, and G. M. Stirrat. Abnormal expression of Class II MHC antigens in placenta from patients with pemphigoid gestationis: analysis of Class II MHC sub-region product expression, *Placenta 9*:81 (1988).
63. S. E. Kelly, S. Fleming, B. S. Bhogal, F. Wojnarowska, and M. M. Black. Immunopathology of the placenta in pemphigoid gestationis and linear IgA disease, *Br. J. Dermatol. 120*:735 (1989).
64. T. Hanafusa, R. Pujol-Borrell, R. Chiovata, R. C. G. Russell, D. Doniach, and G. F. Bottazo. Aberrant expression of HLA-DR antigen on thyrocytesin Graves' disease: Relevance for autoimmunity, *Lancet 2*:1111 (1983).
65. T. A. Gonwa, J. J. Picker, H. N. Raff, S. M. Gayert, J. Silver, and J. D. Stoker. Antigen presenting capabilities of human monocytes correlates with their expression of HLA-DS, an 1a determinant distinct from HLA-DR, *J. Immunol. 130*:706 (1983).
66. P. Matzinger, P. Zamoyska, and H. Waldmann. Self tolerance is H-2 restricted, *Nature 308*:738 (1984).
67. J. K. Shornick, P. Stastny, and J. N. Gilliam. Paternal histocompatibility (HLA) antigens and maternal anti-HLA antibodies in herpes gestationis, *J. Invest. Dermatol. 81*:407 (1983).
68. R. E. Jenkins, K. I. Welsh, and M. M. Black. Anti-HLA antibodies in pemphigoid gestationis and polymorphic eruption of pregnancy, *Br. J. Dermatol. 129*:27 (1993).
69. C. Fournier, L. Didierjean, P. Carraux, D. Salomon, Y. Merot, and J. H. Saurat. Placental-pemphigoid: A bullous pemphigoid-like dermatosis after injections of placental extracts in a man. Detection of antibodies to cutaneo-placental antigens, *J. Invest. Dermatol. 87*:140 (1986).
70. J.-H. Saurat, L. Didierjean, Y. Merot, and D. Salomon. Blistering skin disease in a man after injections of human placental extracts, *Br. Med. J. 297*:775 (1988).
71. G. Schaumburg-Lever, O. E. Saffold, C. E. Orfanos, and W. F. Lever. Herpes gestationis: Histology and ultrastructure, *Arch. Dermatol. 107*:888 (1973).
72. K. C. Hertz, S. I. Katz, J. Maize, and A. B. Ackerman. Herpes gestationis: A clinicopathologic study. *Arch. Dermatol. 112*:1543 (1976).
73. A. Kint, M. L. Goerts, B. Vanneste, and C. De Cuyper. Herpes gestationis. Etude histologique et ultrastructurale, *Ann. Dermatol. Venereol. 107*:113 (1980).
74. J. K. Shornick, J. L. Bangert, R. G. Freeman, and J. N. Gilliam. Herpes gestationis: Clinical and histological features of twenty-eight cases, *J. Am. Acad. Dermatol. 8*:214 (1983).
75. N. P. Burrows and R. Russell Jones. Unusual histopathological findings in herpes gestationis, *Br. J. Dermatol. 125*:96 (1991).

76. H. Yaoita, M. Gullino, and S. I. Katz. Herpes gestationis. Ultrastructure and ultrastructural localisation of in vivo bound complement, *J. Invest. Dermatol. 66*:383 (1976).
77. J. Pierard, M. Thiery, and A. Kint. Histologie et ultrastructure de l'herpes gestationis, *Arch. Belg. Dermatol. Syphil. 25*:321 (1969).
78. J. A. Carruthers, M. M. Black, and N. Ramnarain. Immunopathological studies in herpes gestationis, *Br. J. Dermatol. 96*:35 (1977).
79. K. Holubar, K. Konrad, and G. Stingl. Detection by immunoelectron microscopy of immunoglobulin deposits in skin of immunofluorescence negative herpes gestationis, *Br. J. Dermatol. 96*:569 (1977).
80. H. Honigsman, G. Stingl K. Holubar, and K. Wolff. Herpes gestationis: fine structural pattern of immunoglobulin deposits in the skin in vivo, *J. Invest. Dermatol. 66*:389 (1976).
81. C. I. Harrington and S. S. Bleehen. Herpes gestationis: immunopathological and ultrastructural studies, *Br. J. Dermatol. 100*:389 (1979).
82. S. E. Kelly, E. McVittie, M. M. Black, and S. Fleming. Isolated basal keratinocytes express pemphigoid gestationis antigen, *Br. J. Dermatol. 126*:42 (1992).
83. S. Karpati, W. Stolz, M. Meurer, O. Braun-Falco, and T. Krieg. Herpes gestationis: Ultrastructural identification of the extracellular antigenic sites in diseases skin using immunogold technique, *Br. J. Dermatol. 125*:17 (1991).
84. L. H. Morrison, R. S. Labib, J. J. Zone, L. A. Diaz, and G. J. Anhalt. Herpes gestationis autoantibodies recognise a 180KD human epidermal antigen, *J. Clin. Invest. 81*:2023 (1988).
85. S. E. Kelly, B. S. Bhogal, F. Wojnarowska, P. Whitehead, I. M. Leigh, and M. M. Black. Western blot analysis of the antigen in pemphigoid gestationis, *Br. J. Dermatol. 122*:445 (1990).
86. R. S. G. J. Labib, H. P. Anhalt, D. F. M. Patel, and L. A. Diaz. Molecular heterogeneity of the bullous pemphigoid antigen as detected by immunoblotting, *J. Immunol. 136*:1231 (1986).
87. A. H. L. Fielder, M. J. Walport, J. R. Batchelor, R. I. Rynes, C. M. Black, I. A. Dodi, and G. R. V. Hughes. Family study of the major histocompatibility complex in patients with systemic lupus erythematosus: importance of null alleles of C4A and C4B in determining disease susceptibility, *Br. Med. J. 286*:425 (1983).
88. T. T. Provost and T. B. Tomasi. Evidence of complement activation via the alternative pathway in skin diseases. I. Herpes gestationis, systemic lupus erythematosus and bullous pemphigoid, *J. Clin. Invest. 52*:1779 (1973).
89. R. E. Jordan, K. G. Heine, G. Tappeiner, L. L. Bushkell, and T. T. Provost. The immunopathology of herpes gestationis: Immunofluorescence studies and characterisation 'HG factor,' *J. Clin. Invest. 57*:1426 (1976).
90. S. I. Katz, K. Hertz, and H. Yaoita. Herpes gestationis. Immunopathology and characterisation of the HG factor, *J. Clin. Invest. 57*:1434 (1976).
91. J. A. Carruthers and A. R. Ewins. Herpes gestationis: studies on the binding characteristics, activity and pathogenetic significance of the complement-fixing factor, *Clin. Exp. Immunol. 31*:38 (1978).
92. R. Grimwood, C. M. Arroyave, W. L. Weston, and J. L. Aeling. Herpes gestationis associated with the C3 nephritic factor, *Arch. Dermatol. 116*:1045 (1980).

93. P. Rimbaud, R. Jean, H. Bonnet, J. Meynadier, D. Rieu, and J. Guilhon. Herpes gestationis. Eruption bulleuse chez le nouveau-ne, *Bull. Soc. Fr. Derm. Syph. 78*:419 (1971).
94. T. P. Chorzelski, S. Jablonska, E. H. Beutner, E. Marciejowska, and M. Jarzabek-Chorzelska. Herpes gestationis with identical lesions in the newborn, *Arch. Dermatol. 112*:1129 (1976).
95. A. Katz, O. J. Minta, J. W. P. Toole, and W. Medwidsky. Immunopathologic study of herpes gestationis in mother and infant, *Arch. Dermatol. 113*:1069 (1977).
96. A. van de Wiel, H. Ch. Hart, J. Flinterman, J. A. M. Kerckhaert, J. A. Du Boeuff, and J. W. Imhof. Plasma exchange in herpes gestationis, *Br. Med. J. 2*:1041 (1980).
97. B. Russell and N. A. Thorne. Herpes gestationis, *Br. J. Dermatol. 69*:339 (1957).
98. R. C. Kolodny. Herpes gestationis. A new assessment of incidence, diagnosis and fetal prognosis, *Am. J. Obstet. Gynecol. 104*:39 (1969).
99. J. K. Shornick, T. J. Meek, L. T. Nesbitt, and J. N. Gilliam. Herpes gestationis in blacks, *Arch. Dermatol. 120*:511 (1984).
100. L. Bercovitch, H. A. Bogaars, and D. O. Murray. Pustular herpes gestationis, *Arch. Dermatol. 119*:91 (1983).
101. B. Adraans, H. Pullon, and A du Vivier. Pemphigoid gestationis and neonatal alloimmune thrombocytopenia, *Clin. Exp. Dermatol. 15*:134 (1990).
102. R. Holmes, M. M. Black. D. M. Williamson, and R. W. B. Scutt. Herpes gestationis and bullous pemphigoid: a disease spectrum, *Br. J. Dermatol. 103*:535 (1980).
103. F. W. Lynch and R. J. Albrecht. Hormonal factors in herpes gestationis, *Arch. Dermatol. 93*:446 (1966).
104. D. M. Mitchell. Herpes gestationis and "the pill," *Br. Med. J. 2*:1324 (1966).
105. B. Gordon. Herpes gestationis and the 'pill,' *Br. Med. J. 1*:51 (1967).
106. C. Dupont. Herpes gestationis and the 'pill,' *Br. Med. J. 2*:699 (1968).
107. J. K. Morgan. Herpes gestationis influenced by an oral contraceptive, *Br. J. Dermatol. 80*:456 (1968).
108. R. Charles-Holmes and M. M. Black. Herpes gestationis, *Management of Blistering Diseases* (F. Wojnarowska and R. A. Briggaman, eds.). Chapman and Hall, London, 1990, p. 93.
109. J. Bazex, A. Boubes, J. Peyrot, F. Oksman, M. Parant, C. Boulard, and A. Bazex. Herpes gestationis et prolactine. *Ann. Dermatol., Venerol. 108*:173 (1981).
110. T. J. Lawley, G. Stingl, and S. I. Katz. Fetal and maternal risk factors in herpes gestationis, *Arch. Dermatol. 114*:552 (1978).
111. A. Frumkin. Herpes gestationis, umbilical cord knot and fetal death, *J. Am. Acad. Dermatol. 21:*812 (1989).
112. K. J. S. Macdonald and E. J. Raffle. Ritodrine therapy associated with remission of pemphigoid gestationis, *Br. J. Dermatol. 111*:630 (1984).
113. R. L. Dobson. Herpes gestationis and ritodrine, *J. Am. Acad. Dermatol. 18*:1145 (1988).
114. F. Hebra. Herpes impetiginiformis, *Lancet 1*:339 (1872).
115. L. von Zumbusch. Psoriasis and pustular exanthem, *Arch. Derm. Syph. Berlin 99*:335 (1910).
116. H. Baker and T. J. Ryan. Generalised pustular psoriasis—A clinical and epidemiological study of 104 cases, *Br. J. Dermatol. 80*:771 (1968).

117. R. J. Oosterling, R. E. Nobrega, J. A. Du Boeuff, and J. B. van der Meer. Impetigo herpetiformis or generalised pustular psoriasis? *Arch. Dermatol. 114*:1527 (1978).
118. G. E. Pierard, C. Pierard-Franchinont, and M. de la Brassinne. Impetigo herpetiformis and pustular psoriasis during pregnancy, *Am. J. Dermatopathol. 5*:215 (1983).
119. I. Katzenellenbogen and E. J. Feuerman. Psoriasis pustulosa and impetigo herpetiformis: single or dual entity? *Acta Derm. Venereol 46*:86 (1966).
120. M. Lotem, V. Katzenelson, A. Rotem, M. Hod, and M. Sandbank. Impetigo herpetiformis: A variant of pustular psoriasis or a separate entity? *J. Am. Acad. Dermatol. 20*:338 (1989).
121. C. H. Beek. On Impetigo Herpetiformis, *Dermatologica 102*:145 (1951).
122. F. R. Murphy and L. P. Stolman. Generalised pustular psoriasis, *Arch. Dermatol. 115*:1215 (1979).
123. O. Y. Oumeinish, S. E. Farraj, and A. S. Bataineh. Some aspects of impetigo herpetiformis. *Arch. Dermatol. 118*:103 (1982).
124. F. Kogoj. Die spungiforme (schwammartige) pustel, *Derm. Wochen 107*:1485 (1938).
125. G. W. Beveridge, R. A. Harkness, and J. R. B. Livingstone. Impetigo herpetiformis in two successive pregnancies. *Br. J. Dermatol. 78*:106 (1966).
126. E. Hvidberg. Impetigo herpetiformis, *Dermatologica 114*:337 (1957).
127. A. K. Bajaj, V. Swarup, O. P. Gupta, and S. C. Gupta. Impetigo herpetiformis. *Dermatologica 155*:292 (1977)
128. G. C. Sauer and B. J. Geha. Impetigo herpetiformis. Report of a case treated with corticosteroids—review of the literature, *Arch. Dermatol. 83*:119 (1961).
129. M. Gligora and Z. Kolacio. Hormonal treatment of impetigo herpetiformis, *Br. J. Dermatol. 107*:253 (1982).
130. E. Zoberman and E. R. Farmer. Pruritic folliculitis of pregnancy. *Arch. Dermatol. 117*:20 (1981).
131. E. Esteve, L. Vaillant, Y. Bacq, P. Descamps, M. C. Grangeponte, and G. Lorette. Pruritic folliculitis of pregnancy: role of associated intrahepatic cholestasis, *Ann. Dermatol. Venereol. 119*:37 (1992).
132. O. Back and J. Faergemann. Pityrosporum folliculitis: A common disease of the young and middle-aged, *J. Am. Acad. Dermatol. 12*:56 (1985).
133. W. B. Shelley, R. W. Preucel, and S. S. Spoont. Autoimmune progesterone dermatitis: cure by oophorectomy, *JAMA 190*:35 (1964).
134. W. N. Jones and V. H. Gordon. Autoimmune progesterone eczema: An endogenous progesterone hypersensitivity, *Arch. Dermatol. 99*:57 (1969).
135. F. S. Farah and Z. Shbaklu. Autoimmune progesterone urticaria, *J. Am. Clin. Immunol. 48*:257 (1971).
136. R. Hart. Autoimmune progesterone dermatitis, *Arch. Dermatol. 113*:426 (1977).
137. S. M. Bierman. Autoimmune progesterone dermatitis of pregnancy, *Arch. Dermatol. 107*:896 (1973).
138. D. H. McGibbon, M. W. Greaves, and G. M. Besser. Post-ovulation dermatosis, *Br. J. Dermatol. 101*(Suppl. 17):65 (1979).
139. J. Alcalay, A. Ingber, B. Hazaz, M. David, and M. Sandbank. Linear IgM dermatosis of pregnancy, *J. Am. Acad. Dermatol. 18*:412 (1988).
140. A. Zurn, C. R. Celebi, P. Bernard, L. Didierjean, and J.-H. Saurat. A prospective immunofluorescence study of 111 cases of pruritic dermatoses of pregnancy: IgM

anti-basement membrane zone antibodies as a novel finding, *Br. J. Dermatol. 126*:474 (1992).

141. P. J. Velthuis, M. C. J. M. de Jong, and M. H. Kruis. Is there a linear IgM dermatosis? Significance of linear IgM junctional staining in cutaneous immunopathology, *Acta Derm. Venereol. (Stockh.) 68*:8 (1988).
142. W. N. Otterson. Diethylstilbestrol in management of papular dermatitis of pregnancy, *Am. J. Obstet. and Gynecol. 113*:570 (1972).
143. A. S. Spangler, W. Reddy, W. A. Bardawil, C. C. Roby, and K. Emerson. Papular dermatitis of pregnancy, *JAMA 181*:577 (1962).
144. A. S. Spangler and K. Emerson. Estrogen levels and estrogen therapy in papular dermatitis of pregnancy, *Am. J. Obstet. Gynecol. 110*:534 (1971).
145. D. B. Roth. The frequency of spontaneous abortions, *Int. J. Fertil. 8*:431 (1963).
146. A. L. Herbst, H. Ulfelder, and D. C. Poskanzer. Adenocarcinoma of the vagina. Association of Maternal Stilbestrol Therapy with Tumour Appearance in Young Women, *N. Engl. J. Med. 284*:878 (1971).
147. A. L. Herbst, P. Cole, T. Cotton, S. J. Robboy, and R. E. Scully. Age-incidence and risk of diethylstilbestrol-related clear cell adenocarcinoma of the vagina and cervix, *Am. J. Obstet. Gynecol. 128*:43 (1977).
148. A. S. Spangler and K. Emerson. Diethylstilbestrol in management of papular dermatitis of pregnancy. A reply to the editor, *Am. J. Obstet. Gynecol. 113*:571 (1972).
149. K. A. Pruett and R. Kim. Papular dermatitis of pregnancy, Obstet. *Gynecol. 55*(3):38 (1980).
150. R. M. Michaud, D. Jacobson, and M. V. Dahl. Papular dermatitis of pregnancy, *Arch. Dermatol. 118*:1003 (1982).
151. L. Q. Nguyen and O. R. Sarmini. Papular dermatitis of pregnancy: A case report, *J. Am. Acad. Dermatol. 22*:690 (1990).

4

Impact of Pregnancy on Skin Diseases

Wolfgang Jurecka
University of Vienna, Vienna, Austria

I. INTRODUCTION

Pregnancy is a time of profound endocrine and metabolic changes in the female body. The skin may be affected in various ways by these changes leading to amelioration or aggravation of certain preexisting skin diseases. Although fundamental mechanisms are not yet understood, the estrogens and the progesterones mainly are considered responsible for these phenomena.

For example, in heritable connective tissue disorders such as the Ehlers-Danlos syndrome or pseudoxanthoma elasticum which show impairment of the mechanical properties of the connective tissue, it is evident that the increasing body weight of the pregnant woman and especially of the growing fetus may aggravate the symptoms or even may have impact on the outcome of pregnancy. There are other diseases such as Fox-Fordyce disease, acne vulgaris, or hidradenitis suppurativa which are thought to be hormonally modulated, and it can be assumed that these entities are influenced by pregnancy. However, surprisingly, these entities show only little or unpredictable response to the hormonal changes during pregnancy. In contrast, other conditions such as the metabolic and nutritional disorders are much more affected by the hormonal changes or by the increased requirements of essential nutrients during pregnancy.

There is increasing evidence that the hormonal changes during pregnancy directly influence the immune system. The immune system responds to both estrogens and androgens and also progesterone, prolactin, and other hormones may be involved (1,2). In general, estrogens stimulate T-cell response and increase immunoglobulins, whereas progesterone and androgens suppress T-cell response and decrease immunoglobulins. These changes probably protect the growing fetus from being rejected by the immune system of the mother and may also be of relevance in diseases with altered immunity. Again surprisingly, few influences can be seen in clinical practice regarding, for example, the impact of pregnancy on the course of lupus erythematosus. Of more practical importance, this mechanism seems to occur in some infectious disease, such as leprosy, for example, where pregnancy may lead to severe aggravation of the disease.

In the following six sections, the impact of pregnancy on infectious diseases, diseases of altered immunity, metabolic and nutritional disorders, heritable connective tissue disorders, benign and malignant tumors, and miscellaneous skin conditions will be discussed by reviewing the literature. In recent years, several excellent articles have been published on physiological and pathological skin changes during pregnancy (3–7). In contrast to some of these articles, no attempt will be made to classify these disorders in two broad categories of disorders which will be ameliorated or aggravated during pregnancy. The reason is simple, as in some of these disorders the impact of pregnancy is unpredictable and in others, such as, for example, in lupus erythematosus or melanoma, the opinion about the influence of pregnancy on their course has changed fundamentally within recent years. This also may occur in other disorders when more controlled studies will become available.

II. INFECTIOUS DISEASES

There is nowadays increasing evidence that sex hormones (estrogen, testosterone, and others) have a significant influence on the immune system. Obviously estrogens are the natural stimulants of the defense system and androgens and progesterone have an immunosuppressant activity. Thus, it is not surprising that the female immune system is more competent than that of males. However, during pregnancy, especially the cell-mediated immunity as measured by a variety of tests such as lymphocyte transformation, cytotoxic function, helper-suppressor ratios, and others is altered in the general direction of immunosuppression (8,9,10). Therefore, certain infectious diseases, where the infectious agent survives mainly intracellularly or which are controlled mainly by the cell-mediated immune system, may appear for the first time, may occur more frequently, or may become more severe during pregnancy (9–12).

A. Candidiasis

Candidiasis is a common infection mainly of the skin, nails, and mucous membranes caused by *Candida albicans* and occasionally by other yeasts of the genus

Candida. Candida albicans has a predilection for colonizing moist, macerated folds of skin; thus intertriginous or occluded areas are mostly affected. Several factors are associated with increased rates of colonization with *Candida.* These include diabetes mellitus, oral contraceptives, and pregnancy. The incidence of vulvovaginal candidiasis has been reported to be 10–20 times higher in pregnant women than in nonpregnant women (13,14); data about increased skin manifestations of *Candida* infection during pregnancy are not available. The rarity of vulvovaginal *Candida* isolation in girls before menarche and the lower prevalence of candidal vaginitis after menopause emphasize the hormonal dependence of this infection. Elevated estrogen and/or progesterone levels have been considered responsible for the higher incidence of candidal infections during pregnancy (15,16).

Acute vulvitis is frequently accompanied with candidal vaginitis during pregnancy presenting with itching, burning, soreness, and painful micturition. The disease may spread onto the perineum, perianal region, gluteal folds, and inguinal region. The diagnosis is established by clinical signs and potassium hydroxide microscopic examination.

Treatment consists of topical antimycotics. Systemic treatment should be avoided, and ketoconazole is contraindicated during pregnancy.

B. Pityrosporum Folliculitis

Tinea (pityriasis) versicolor is the most common disease caused by the fungus *Malassezia furfur.* It is a superficial chronic fungal infection of the stratum corneum characterized by scaly hypopigmented and hyperpigmented, irregular macules most often occurring on the trunk and proximal extremities. It also has been put forth that *M. furfur* contributes to the pathogenesis of seborrhoic dermatitis (17).

Pityrosporum folliculitis is a well-recognized and often misdiagnosed clinical entity. It is characterized by asymptomatic or slightly pruritic, monomorphic follicular papules or pustules distributed on the trunk, upper extremities, or face (18).

Factors predisposing to the appearance of the eruption are diabetes mellitus or prior antibiotic, corticosteroid, or immunosuppressant therapy (19–21). The disorder is frequently diagnosed as an acneiform eruption.

There are only two case reports showing an association of pityrosporum folliculitis with prior administration of oral contraceptives (21) and pregnancy (22). An association with the hormonal changes or impaired cell-mediated immunity during pregnancy has been discussed. Owing to its acneiform and asymptomatic appearance, it might be possible that pityrosporum folliculitis during pregnancy is an underrecognized disease. Topical antifungal preparations should be safe and effective treatment for pityrosporum folliculitis.

C. Leprosy

Leprosy (Hansen disease) is a chronical progressive, contagious infectious disease caused by *Mycobacterium leprae.* This microorganism is a small, bent, gram-positive, acid-fast rod, 0.5–1.5 μm long. The exact mode of transmission of *M. leprae* from person to person is not known. A significant number of cases of the disease occur through long direct contact with infected persons. Insect vectors such as flies and fleas may possibly also play a role. Sites of predilection for leprosy are the skin, mucous membranes, upper respiratory tract, and peripheral nerves, although involvement of other organs has been described.

On the basis of clinical, bacteriological, histological, and immunological findings, leprosy is classified along a spectrum of infectious and immunological symptoms into five broad categories: the principal, or polar, types of the two ends of the spectrum are the pathogen-rich anergic lepromatous leprosy (LL) with numerous skin lesions and the pathogen-poor allergic tuberculoid leprosy (TL) with only single skin lesion. Between these two stable, polar forms the unstable forms of borderline lepromatous (BL), midborderline (BB), and borderline tuberculoid (BT) are defined in the spectrum.

Of clinical importance are the adverse immunological reactions which have been described in leprosy. These are acute episodic exacerbations of the disease which can occur spontaneously or in connection with lepromin testing or therapy.

Two types of reactions have been described: the type 1 reaction, also called upgrading or hypersensitivity reaction, occurs in all forms of leprosy and shows acute exacerbation of existing skin lesions due to increase in cell-mediated immunity; and the type 2 reaction, or immune-complex reaction, occurs typically in LL and BL. The type 2 reaction is also called erythema nodosum leprosum. Besides erythema nodosum–like skin lesions, this reaction is characterized by severe systemic illness. For further information about the clinical spectrum of the disease, immunological reactions, and therapy, the reader is referred to two excellent reviews (23,24).

The adverse effects of pregnancy on leprosy have recently been reviewed extensively (25). New overt leprosy, reactivation, or relapse was recorded in nearly 50% of pregnancies most commonly during the third trimester, or within 1 year after pregnancy (26). This is the time when cell-mediated immunity is maximally suppressed. Interestingly, patients from the whole spectrum of classification of leprosy are affected (26,27) even if they are under effective chemotherapy (27). Thus, leprosy formerly under good control with chemotherapy may relapse and subclinical disease may first become apparent during gestation.

Both adverse reactions of leprosy may be induced by pregnancy. The type 1 reaction may show exacerbation of skin and nerve lesions during pregnancy, whereas reaction in nerves alone is more a feature of the lactation period (25,27).

However, especially in type 2 reaction, the erythema nodosum leprosum may be a problem of pregnancy. In a prospective study, nearly 40% of lepromatous patients developed erythema nodosum leprosum during pregnancy with a peak incidence in the third trimester (26). Furthermore, neuritis with loss of sensation and motor function is likely to occur during pregnancy; also without clinical features of type 1 or 2 reaction. To prevent permanent nerve damage, patients should be treated immediately (25).

In conclusion, pregnancy may have severe adverse effects on leprosy. Whenever possible, patients should be informed before they become pregnant, so that pregnancies can be planned to occur when leprosy is under good control.

D. Condylomata Acuminata

About 65 different human papillomaviruses (HPVs) types have been described within the past two decades (28). These viruses may induce growth of benign epithelial proliferations on the skin or mucous membranes which are mainly called warts or verrucae, condylomata acuminata, or papillomas. A subset of these viruses is also associated with the development of epithelial malignancies.

Warts in the anogenital area are called condylomata acuminata; they also can be seen in the mucous membranes of the mouth. These lesions are epidermal and dermal papules or nodules on the perineum, genitalia, in crural folds, and the anus. They vary in size and can form large, exophytic—cauliflowerlike—tumors. Condylomata accuminata may extend into the urethra, vagina, or rectum.

Pregnancy may stimulate the growth and enlargement of condylomata acuminata producing large excrescences which even may block the birth canal (5,13,29). Also, marked regression in size during the postpartum period has been described.

At present there are at least 15 types of HPVs identified in the human genitalia, each carrying with it a low, intermediate, or high risk for the development of cancer. In a recent study, it could be demonstrated that the intermediate-risk types (HPV-31, HPV-33, and HPV-35) and the high-risk types (HPV-16 and HPV-18) are also present in a high percentage of pregnant women with or without clinical symptoms (30). The low-risk HPV types 6 and 11 have been shown to be associated with juvenile respiratory papillomas, which may cause severe medical problems during early childhood. It is assumed that transmission occurs during vaginal delivery (13,29,31). Whether the intermediate-risk and high-risk types also can be transmitted by vaginal delivery and whether these types are responsible for any adverse effects in the growing infant are not yet known.

None of the common topical preparations which are normally used in the treatment of condylomata acuminata should be used during pregnancy or only used with extreme care. Podophyllin may cause systemic toxicity and is associated with fetal death. 5-Fluorouracil, bleomycin, and trichloroacetic acid are also contraindicated in pregnancy. Although interferon therapy may be helpful in the treatment of condylomata acuminata, there are no reliable data on its use in pregnancy. Thus, mainly surgical procedures such as electrodesiccation, cryotherapy, or laser treatment can be recommended.

E. Herpes Simplex

Herpes simplex is a recurrent disease caused by two closely related viruses: herpes simplex virus type 1 (HSV-1) and herpes simplex virus type 2 (HSV-2). Following a primary infection, the virus enters a latent state. Recurrent disease is caused by reactivation of the dormant virus, which then travels down the nerve fiber to establish a new skin infection.

Primary infection in herpes simplex occurs by direct mucocutaneous contact with another infected individual. Primary infection is defined as the first infection with herpes simplex virus in a seronegative unprotected patient. It may present with gingivostomatitis or with herpetic lesions in other mucocutaneous locations accompanied by fever, enlarged lymph nodes, and visceral disease.

Recurrent infection is usually milder and of shorter duration than the primary infection. Certain triggering events such as exposure to sunlight, severe stress, and other factors will reactivate the latent virus to express its genome. Between episodes there is no evidence of viral particles, proteins, or nucleic acids in the skin at the affected site.

During pregnancy primary herpes simplex or recurrent herpes simplex may occur. Both may lead to severe complications in the pregnant mother and in the fetus. Here only the adverse effects on the mother will be discussed, whereas the complications on the offspring such as intrauterine growth retardation, congenital infections, and neonatal infections will be discussed elsewhere in this book (32,33).

Some animal models suggest that the clinical course of primary herpes virus infection in pregnancy is more severe than in nonpregnant animals (34,35), but no reports on human studies are available. Severe mucocutaneous infections and visceral disease characteristically occur in immunoincompetent hosts who are immunosuppressed owing to, for example, organ transplantation, steroid use, burn, lymphoma, or HIV infection. A recent study compares the data of 23 pregnancies complicated by disseminated herpes simplex virus infection and shows a high mortality rate (36). The major disease manifestations appear to be hepatitis and encephalitis accompanied by fever, malaise, chills, myalgia, vomiting, and abdominal pain.

Although recurrent genital herpes simplex infection is not specifically exacerbated by pregnancy, its relation to fetal morbidity and mortality is of critical interest, especially if a recurence occurs in the perinatal time with possible infection of the neonate.

Although there is still an official recommendation not to use acyclovir during pregnancy, there are numerous publications on the safety of this drug during pregnancy in humans. Despite the potential risks, there are several circumstances in which the benefits of acyclovir therapy in pregnancy appear to outweigh possible fetal harm. These certainly include disseminated primary HSV infections (37–40).

F. Varicella-Zoster

Varicella and herpes zoster are two distinct clinical entities caused by the same member of the herpesvirus family, the varicella-zoster virus (VZV). The differences between these two diseases are due to differences in the immunological situation of the host. Varicella is the clinical manifestation of the primary exogenous VZV infection, whereas herpes zoster is the result of reactivation of a latent endogenous infection that has persisted within sensory ganglia following an earlier infection with VZV. Similar to herpes simplex, after infection with VZV, the primary infection with its generalized illness is more harmful to a pregnant mother and her growing fetus.

In general, varicella infection is more severe in adults than in children. There are no sufficient data as to whether it is even more severe in pregnant women. In adults, fever and constitutional symptoms are more prominent and prolonged. The rash is more profuse, and complications are more frequent.

Primary varicella pneumonia is the major complication of adult varicella. Pneumonia generally appears 1–6 days after onset of the rash, and the degree of pulmonary involvement correlates best with the severity of the cutaneous eruption. Only a few large series of pregnant women with varicella have been studied. In one study, 43 pregnancies complicated by varicella were published, showing 4 women suffering from pneumonia, 1 of whom died subsequent to severe illness (41). In another study, 24 of 118 cases developed pneumonia and 11 of them died (42). Thus, primary maternal chickenpox infection appears to be abnormally severe, presumably due to depressed cellular immunity in pregnancy.

Fortunately, herpes zoster infections, which are far more common in adults than is varicella, do not seem to cause complications during pregnancy even if they appear in the perigenital region just before term.

Besides the possible fatal consequences for the mother, varicella infection during pregnancy may also have a severe impact on the fetus. Maternal viremia may result in intrauterine VZV infection leading to congenital varicella syndrome or congenital herpes zoster (43–47). These effects will be discussed in another chapter.

G. Acquired Immunodeficiency Syndrome

Acquired immunodeficiency syndrome (AIDS) is caused by a lymphotropic retrovirus, the human immunodeficiency virus (HIV). One might anticipate that the physiological mild immunosuppression of the cell-mediated immunity by normal pregnancies would place the pregnant HIV-positive women at a much increased risk for advanced disease. However, there are still insufficient data for such a conclusion.

A review of relevant published data indicates that among HIV-infected women adverse clinical outcomes of pregnancy are common. HIV-related complications in immunosuppressed (i.e., <300 $CD4^+$ cells/ml) pregnant women occur frequently, whereas in seropositive but not immunocompromised pregnant women, no adverse effects could be seen (48). Examining CD4 and CD8 counts during pregnancy and 1-year postpartum, it could be shown that the levels of CD4 cells fall during pregnancy and do not recover thereafter. The CD8 levels are consistently higher in seropositive women. The investigators concluded that the loss of CD4 cells was faster during pregnancy than in the postpartum period and speculated that pregnancy may accelerate HIV-induced depletion of CD4 cells and increase the risk of opportunistic infection (49,50).

It is not yet clear whether opportunistic infections in HIV-positive pregnant women run a more aggressive course. However, several case reports show a fatal outcome more frequently than in nonpregnant women, but probably the favorable cases are not reported (51–54).

Vertical transmission and infection of the fetus is a further concern of HIV infection in a pregnant woman. The adverse affects of HIV infection on the outcome of pregnancy are discussed in another chapter.

Zidovudine has been shown to prolong survival in patients with AIDS and to delay progression of the disease in HIV-positive patients. It interferes with the reversal transcriptase inhibiting HIV replication. Only recently has this drug been demonstrated to be effective in the prevention of HIV transmission from mother to infant (55,56).

III. DISEASES OF ALTERED IMMUNITY

Pregnancy is associated with fundamental changes in the immune system; it is generally accepted that mainly the cell-mediated immunity is impaired. Thus, it is not surprising that diseases of altered immunity are influenced in their course by pregnancy. In most of these disorders, the basic defect, etiology, and pathogenesis are still poorly understood, making it difficult to explain or predict the influence of pregnancy on the course of these disorders. In the following sections, some aspects of the so-called connective tissue disorders and pemphigus are discussed in relation to pregnancy.

A. Lupus Erythematosus

There are two principal forms of lupus erythematosus (LE): chronic discoid lupus erythematosus (CDLE) and systemic lupus erythematosus (SLE). Also, several rare special forms and an intermediary form, which has been termed subacute cutaneous lupus erythematosus (SCLE), have been described. Chronic discoid lupus erythematosus shows skin changes with a chronic course but no visceral involvement. The skin lesions mainly occur on the face but also can be widespread. They consist of sharply demarcated erythematokeratotic lesions which heal with atrophic scarring, and thus displaying three events—erythema, hyperkeratosis, and atrophy—following each other. Some type of cutaneous involvement is present in 85% of patients with SLE. The typical rash occurs on the face (butterfly erythema) and consists of erythematous papulovesicular lesions which heal without atrophy or scarring. In addition to systemic illness with arthritis, serositits, renal, neurological, hematological, and immunological disorders, a maculopapular rash on the trunk may occur.

SCLE is characterized by annular or psoriasiform lesions without atrophy and scarring in light-exposed areas. It also shows some signs of systemic involvement, most frequently anti-Ro or anti-LA antibodies (57).

Pregnancy appears not to have a consistent effect on CDLE, although CDLE can disappear during pregnancy only to recur postpartum. There also is no evidence of fetal complications. On the other hand, the situation in SLE and SCLE is more complicated.

SLE and SCLE show a clear predisposition to occur most frequently in females of childbearing age (57,58). Furthermore, there is evidence that estrogens or oral contraceptives may unmask a lupus diathesis or may exacerbate preexisting LE (59–62). However, to date there are no prospective clinical studies available evaluating the effects of estrogen or progesterone in patients with SLE and SCLE. Thus, it seems prudent to avoid estrogen-containing medications whenever it is possible (63).

Early studies suggest an aggravating effect of pregnancy on the course of SLE (64–67). However, it is difficult to identify clinical abnormalities such as proteinuria, thrombocytopenia, erythema, alopecia, fatigue, musculoskeletal aching, and anemia as lupus related or as pregnancy related (68). Flare of SLE during pregnancy can be diagnosed with confidence only in the face of a rising anti-DNA antibody titer or the occurrence of inflammatory rash, fever, lymphadenopathy, and leukopenia. There is only one recent prospective study which concludes that flare of lupus during pregnancy is common and occurs significantly more frequently than does flare in nonpregnant patients with SLE or in the same patients after pregnancy (69). Most of the other recent reports contradict these views (70–73). It is assumed that exacerbation of SLE during pregnancy is dependent on the activity of the disease at the time of conception following its natural course and is not aggravated by pregnancy. Further large studies will be necessary to clarify this important question.

Fetal complications tend to be much more common than maternal ones. The neonatal lupus syndrome is especially common in newborns from mothers with antibodies to the Ro antigens and LA antigens. This illness consists of rash, thrombocytopenia, and congenital heart block singly or in combination (57,68). Fetal losses also have been attributed to antiphospholipid antibody and/or lupus anticoagulant in women suffering from SCLE or the newly recognized anti-phospholipid antibody syndrome (74,75).

Therapy of SLE during pregnancy should concentrate on drugs with a high benefit to risk ratio. In most cases, chloroquine or corticosteroids can be used, whereas other drugs effective in SLE are contraindicated during pregnancy (76).

B. Polymyositis/Dermatomyositis

Polymyositis and dermatomyositis have been considered to be essentially the same disease except for the presence or absence of a rash. The diseases are characterized by proximal symmetrical muscle weakness that progresses over a period of weeks to months, elevated serum levels of muscle-related enzymes, an abnormal electromyogram, an abnormal muscle biopsy, and the presence of cutaneous changes typical of dermatomyositis such as heliotrope rash and Gottron papules (77).

There are few reports in the literature of dermatomyositits in pregnancy. Twenty-six pregnancies have been reported in 21 patients with dermatomyositis (78,79). In 12 patients, the disease was diagnosed previous to pregnancy, whereas in 9 patients, it started during pregnancy. About 15% of the cases show clinical exacerbation of the disease during pregnancy. Fetal prognosis seems to parallel the activity of maternal disease; fetal loss reached 50% when the disease started during pregnancy (78). Thus, pregnancies associated with polymyositis/dermatomyositis should be considered high-risk pregnancies. Patients should be treated with steroids according to disease activity.

C. Rheumatoid Arthritis

Dermatologists are frequently concerned with the diagnosis and management of several types of skin lesions which are associated with the complex illness of rheumatoid arthritis (RA), which also presents symptoms in several other organs. The main dermatological presentations of RA are rheumatoid nodules, linear subcutaneous bands, vascular lesions, leg ulcers, transparent skin in association with osteoporosis, sclerotic changes on the hands, ulcerating panniculitis, and others (80,81).

Rheumatoid arthritis has a strong hormonal basis, which is documented by the fact that the female to male incidence ratio is between 2 and 3:1. It has been well known for more than 100 years that pregnancy ameliorates RA, and this has also been documented by numerous studies in recent years (82). It is assumed that the global immunosuppression of pregnancy offers ideal conditions for development of immunotolerance toward different antigens potentially involved in the triggering of RA. It has been shown that estrogens and/or oral contraceptives may mitigate or postpone the onset of RA slightly but that they are not able to alleviate the symptoms of RA (83). Thus, other mechanisms also must be involved. One mechanism could be that the maternal immune response to fetal HLA antigens may influence RA activity during gestation (84). It also has been speculated that low androgen concentrations are a cause of rheumatoid arthritis and that this is responsible for a number of established features of the disease (85).

Unfortunately, remission of RA is short lived during pregnancy, and over 80% of patients will relapse within 3 months of delivery and reach a degree of activity similar to that seen before pregnancy.

D. Systemic Sclerosis

Scleroderma may present in a localized and a systemic form. Whereas the localized form only shows skin symptoms, systemic sclerosis is a multisystem disorder with cutaneous changes and changes in various organs such as the esophagus, lungs, heart, and kidneys. Additionally, the Raynaud phenomenon is frequent.

Numerous case reports have been published about pregnancies complicated by systemic sclerosis. The main problem which developed was renal failure with signs of preeclampsia in the third trimester. Frequently, a fulminant clinical course led to maternal death within days (86,87). Both pregnancies with preexisting renal involvement and those with renal involvement during pregnancy were affected.

Obviously, case reports are likely to be biased to such severe outcomes. On the other hand, surprisingly few series containing unselected cases are available. In two series with 105 pregnancies of women with scleroderma, only one death occurred (88,89). One of these studies also compared the frequency of renal crisis occurring in pregnant and nonpregnant patients suffering from systemic sclerosis. The data showed no significant difference between both groups (89). Thus, it is not justified to state that scleroderma and concomitant pregnancy are associated with a high risk for maternal mortality. Other studies also show that there is no increase in spontaneous abortion, whereas the number of low birth weight babies is increased. This seems to be a consequence of small-for-gestational-age infants than of prematurity (90).

E. Pemphigus

Pemphigus vulgaris, foliaceus, or vegetans in pregnancy is extremely rare. The activity of the disease seems not to be altered by pregnancy. The main concern of pemphigus during pregnancy is transplacental transfer of the pemphigus IgG antibody from the mother to the fetus. This may lead to stillbirth or to neonatal pemphigus vulgaris lasting for approximately 3 weeks. Disease-free live babies also have been reported to have been born of affected mothers (91–94). Endemic pemphigus foliaceus (fogo selvagem) is also an autoimmune disease mediated by autoantibodies. In contrast to pemphigus vulgaris, neonatal skin disease does not appear to occur in babies born to mothers suffering from endemic pemphigus foliaceus (95).

IV. METABOLIC AND NUTRITIONAL DISORDERS

The metabolic and nutritional disorders which may show skin symptoms include a broad spectrum of several disorders such as the porphyrias, xanthomas, and abnormalities of lipid metabolism, mucinoses, amyloidoses, gout, metabolic storage disorders as a result of inherited defects of enzymes (e.g., mucopolysaccharidoses, Fabry disease, Farber disease, phenylketonuria), hypo- and hypervitaminoses, and the lack of other essential nutrients due to insufficient intake of food, malabsorption, or diarrhea.

In most of these disorders, little is known about the influence of pregnancy on their course. However, in general, it can be assumed that in nutritional disorders due to a lack in vitamins, minerals, or elements, the increased metabolic requirement in pregnancy leads to an aggravation of symptoms.

Diabetes mellitus may be severely influenced by pregnancy as high plasma estrogens, progesterone, free cortisol, and human chorionic somatomammotropin increase peripheral resistance to insulin. Among women with diabetes prior to pregnancy, almost all require increased insulin dosage as pregnancy advances, and those with easily managed diabetes will frequently become labile. In most cases, insulin requirements return to prepregnancy levels after delivery. Cutaneous side effects of diabetes mellitus in pregnant women are not reported to be increased in number, although at least cutaneous infections and pruritus should be more frequent, whereas more chronic symptoms such as microangiopathy or neuropathy with mal perforans are more likely to occur in other age groups.

In the following sections, the porphyrias, xanthomas and abnormalities of lipid metabolism, and zinc deficiency syndrome are discussed.

A. Porphyrias

The porphyrias are a group of rare inborn or acquired diseases related to disorders in heme biosynthesis. These defects lead to elevated contents of certain porphyrins or their precursors in tissues (liver), urine, or stool. The porphyrins are hepatotoxic and light-sensitizing (phototoxic) substances, and disorders related to the porphyrias result in phototoxic symptoms in skin areas exposed to light. The pathophysiology of the development of cutaneous lesions in the porphyrias is explained by absorption of radiant energy leading to photoexcited states of porphyrins reacting with molecular oxygen, inflammatory cells, and the release of soluble mediators (96). The porphyrias are classified by most investigators according to the primary site of expression of the specific enzymatic defect and the abnormal porphyrin profile of patients in three groups with several distinct entities (96–100). Alcoholism, intoxication with heavy metals or pesticides (hexachlorobenzene), liver or hematological diseases, intake of several drugs (e.g., sedatives, antibiotics, griseofulvin, chloroquine, estrogens), chronic dialysis, and pregnancy are associated with manifestation or worsening of some of the porphyrias.

1. Porphyria Cutanea Tarda

Porphyria cutanea tarda (PCT) is the most frequent disorder of the porphyrias and is either acquired or inherited. It shows vesicular, bullous, and ulcerative lesions primarily on light-exposed skin, increased skin fragility to mechanical trauma, scarring alopecia, milia on fingers and hands, hyperpigmentation, and hypertrichosis (96). Deficiency of uroporphyrinogen decarboxylase in the liver or red blood cells leads to accumulation of several porphyrins in plasma, urine, and feces.

PCT is known to be adversly influenced by estrogen, iron, and alcohol intake; therefore an adverse effect of pregnancy on the disease also might be expected. Estrogens are able to increase the synthesis of porphyrins in liver cell culture (101). In animal models, estrogens inhibit uroporphyrinogen decarboxylase in the liver and lead to increased porphyrinuria (102,103). Thus, it is assumed that a genetically determined deficiency of uroporphyrinogen decarboxylase together with the intake of estrogens may lead to manifestation of PCT (101). This also has been documented in several patients suffering from carcinoma of the prostate who were treated with estrogens and developed porphyria cutanea tarda (104,105).

Divergent reports exist about the influence of pregnancy on PCT. Case reports showing no exacerbation during pregnancy have led to speculation that endogenous estrogens are not harmful or that estrogen effects on PCT have been overestimated (106–108). Contrasted are reports by others (106–111) showing a clear worsening of disease activity during pregnancy. Possibly the maternal loss of iron to the fetus (106), a lesser porphyrinogenic effect of endogenous estrogens (107), or the limited time of pregnancy is responsible for this discrepancy. Later in pregnancy, when blood volume increases and fetal iron requirements rise leading to a fall in serum iron and hemoglobin, skin symptoms improve. Phlebotomy with careful monitoring of the hematocrit can be recommended for treatment of PCT during pregnancy.

2. Acute Intermittent Porphyria

Although acute intermittent porphyria (AIP) does not show cutaneous lesions, this disorder is discussed briefly. The defect in AIP is attributed to an insufficient quantity of the enzyme porphobilinogen deaminase. Drugs that induce the enzyme aminolevulinic acid synthase lead to an increase in the quantity of δ-aminolevulinic acid and porphobilinogen, substances which are not photosensitizers (96). The disease is characterized by episodic attacks of abdominal pain, vomiting, personality change, and occasionally seizures. Attacks seem to be stimulated by a variety of drugs and hormones. Cyclic menstrual attacks are common, and exogenous estrogens or oral contraceptives are involved. Also, pregnancy may result in more frequent attacks of AIP (112–116).

B. Xanthomas and Abnormalities of Lipid Metabolism

Xanthomas can be classified by their clinical and morphological aspects as xanthelasma palpebrarum, xanthoma planum diffusum, xanthoma tuberosum, xanthoma eruptivum, xanthoma palmare striatum and xanthoma palmare papulosum, and xanthoma tendinosum et articulare. They are reactive yellowish tumors caused by extravasation of serum lipoproteins through the vascular walls and through local ingestion and receptor-mediated endocytosis by macrophages. As a result of incorporation of lipoproteins, the cells change into richly vacuolated foam cells. Some xanthomas are reversible (117).

The classification of lipoprotein disturbances which may be associated with xanthomas was introduced by Fredrickson and coworkers (118). Now it is clear that the patterns they describe are not specific diseases but may be symptoms of various monogenetic, polygenetic, or other metabolic diseases.

Severe hypertriglyceridemia has been documented in association with exogenous estrogen (oral contraceptives) and endogenous estrogen (pregnancy) (119–122). In one pregnant woman, a corneal arcus developed and preexisting tendinous xanthomas increased in size (117). Only one patient has been described who developed eruptive xanthomas during pregnancy. This patient suffered from familial hyperlipidemia, which usually causes only a modest elevation in plasma lipid levels. It is assumed that with the added stimulus of estrogens during pregnancy hypertriglyceridemia and secondary complications such as xanthomas developed (123). Whether eruptive xanthomas during pregnancy are an underrecognized condition is not yet clear and awaits further clarification.

C. Acrodermatitis Enteropathica

The term *acrodermatitis enteropathica* is currently used for the zinc deficiency syndrome whether it is of a hereditary or nonhereditary basis. Hereditary acrodermatitis is believed to be transmitted as an autosomal recessive trait and is caused by a specific absorptive defect. Usually it begins within a few days or weeks after birth in infants who are bottle-fed or soon after weaning from the breast.

The clinical picture presents with a typical triad of acral dermatitis, alopecia, and diarrhea. The dermatitis begins slowly with dry, scaly, eczematous plaques on the face, scalp, and anogenital areas. Diarrhea is often present. Growth is stunted, and there is a decreased resistance to infections. Wound healing is poor.

Several conditions such as gastrointestinal disorders, dietary factors (e.g., alcoholism), burns, malignancies, infections, renal disorders, certain drugs, and pregnancy or lactation may cause secondary zinc deficiency (124) or induce manifestation of primary acrodermatitis enteropathica. Oral treatment with zinc sulfate has been successful in hereditary and nonhereditary acrodermatitis enteropathica (125). This rapidly eliminates all the symptoms. Acrodermatitis enteropathica may flare during pregnancy, and this may sometimes lead to the primary diagnosis of the disorder in these patients (126). The skin disease appears late in the first or early in the second trimester with progressive worsening until delivery and parallelly due to increased demand for zinc. Postpartum rapid spontaneous clearing is normal. A fall in zinc levels and aggravation of acrodermatitis have also been reported after intake of oral contraceptives; therefore, estrogens also seem to be involved in modulation of disease activity. Anencephaly (127) and achondroplastic dwarfism with neonatal death (128) of the offsprings have been associated with untreated maternal acrodermatitis enteropathica. Furthermore, animal models have shown the teratogenic effects of zinc deficiency. Thus, zinc supplementation must be recommended in pregnant patients with acrodermatitis enteropathica to prevent such undesirable effects (129).

V. HERITABLE CONNECTIVE TISSUE DISORDERS

Besides skin changes, heritable connective tissue disorders may show a variety of symptoms in other organs such as skeletal abnormalities, joint hypermobility, and vascular and ocular changes. All of these are inherited in a simple mendelian manner. They are due to mutations in the genes for components of connective tissue or in enzymes of their biochemical pathway. Of these disorders, three syndromes, the Ehlers-Danlos syndrome, pseudoxanthoma elasticum, and the Marfan syndrome are discussed in relation to pregnancy in the following sections.

A. Ehlers-Danlos Syndrome

The Ehlers-Danlos syndrome comprises a group of inherited disorders of collagen metabolism with at least 10 distinct clinical subtypes. The clinical features of this syndrome include fragility of the skin and blood vessels, hyperelasticity of the skin, and hypermobility of the joints (130). Additionally, the eye, gastrointestinal tract, bronchopulmonary tree, and cardiovascular system may be affected.

Although favorable outcomes of pregnancies should be expected in mild forms of the Ehlers-Danlos syndrome, only few reports exist about successful management of pregnancy and parturition (131–133). Severe complications are common during pregnancy in Ehlers-Danlos syndrome types I and IV, and they are also increased in number in types II and III (134).

Ehlers-Danlos syndrome type I, the gravis, or classic type, is characterized by soft, hyperextensible, fragile skin, severe hypermobility of joints, poor wound healing, cardiac defects, and rupture of large arteries.

Type IV, the arterial type, is very similar to type I with a lesser degree of skin and joint extensibility, whereas rupture of large intestine, uterus, or medium-sized arteries is more common. In type I, during pregnancy affected mothers may develop abdominal wall, inguinal, umbilical, and femoral hernias or varicosities of leg and vulval veins (135). Other severe complications include rupture of great vessel walls and severe postpartum hemorrhage with bleeding from episiotomy sites (136).

In type IV, complications are reported more often and included rupture of bowel, aorta, vena cava, or uterus. The overall risk of death in these patients approaches 25% (137,138).

Pregnancies frequently terminate prematurely and management of delivery may be difficult. Complications are likely to occur during labor or in the first day postpartum. Cesarean section should be considered, although it is not yet clear whether this results in fewer complications (138). Early termination of pregnancy may be advisable, and the risks and benefits should be discussed with the pregnant woman.

B. Pseudoxanthoma Elasticum

Pseudoxanthoma elasticum (PXE) is characterized by progressive aberrant calcification of elastic tissue. The skin, retina, and cardiovascular system are involved. Yellowish papules arise mainly in flexual areas of the skin during youth. During life the entire skin may be involved by progression. The skin may become lax and hang in folds. Angioid streaks are the characteristic ocular lesions of PXE. They result from breaks in the Bruch membrane owing to faulty elastic tissue in its outer portion. In the vascular system, calcification of the elastica media of blood vessels leading to proliferation of the intima and subsequently to claudication are the major problems. Angina pectoris or abdominal angina, hypertension, and gastrointestinal hemorrhage are common.

Besides the classic type of PXE in which there are skin, eye, and cardiovascular involvement, patients have been described with ocular and histopathological manifestations of PXE but without skin lesions. This led to a new classification of PXE in a consensus conference (139).

Regarding the implication of pregnancy on PXE, only few data are available. Uncomplicated pregnancies with normal fetuses have been described in several reports (140–143). From the few case reports and two larger studies reviewing respectively 8 women with 25 pregnancies and 20 women with 54 pregnancies (142,143), it can be concluded that pregnancy may particularly aggravate the vascular effects of the disease.

Intrauterine growth retardation of the fetuses has been attributed to vascular compromise leading to uteroplacental insufficiency (144,145). Hypertension seems to be frequent in patients with PXE during pregnancy, and this may lead to pre-eclampsia (141) or to gastrointestinal bleeding with severe hematemesis (142, 143). Because of the risk of cerebral and gastrointestinal hemorrhage, a careful reduction of the elevated blood pressure seems to be particularly important (141, 142).

There also seems to be an increased risk of first trimester miscarriage associated with PXE, which is possibly due to cervical incompetence (143). Prominent abdominal striae develop in nearly all patients, the severity of which correlates with weight gain and number of pregnancies. Such striae may lead to cosmetic deterioration of the abdominal skin (143).

C. Marfan Syndrome

Marfan syndrome (MS) is characterized by abnormalities in three organ systems: the cardiovascular system with aortic aneurysm and mitral valve redundancy; the skeletal system with excessive length of extremities, kyphoscoliosis, anterior chest deformity, and loose jointedness; and the eye with dislocation of the lens. In the skin, striae distensae are common and associated elastosis perforans serpiginosa is rare. The basic defect in MS is a defect in the long arm of the chromosome 15 causing a lack in fibrillin, a connective tissue protein associated with elastin in the involved tissues.

Pregnancy may adversely affect MS. The most severe cardiovascular complication in MS is cystic medial necrosis of the wall of the aorta which leads to aneurysm formation. Not surprisingly, aortic aneurysms complicated by dissection and rupture occur frequently during pregnancy (146–149), predominantly during the third trimester. It is unclear whether increased estrogen levels or increased cardiac output may play a role in the development of these severe complications. Additionally, an increase in hernias and massive striae gravidarum have been reported, but these are not cause for undue medical concern.

VI. BENIGN AND MALIGNANT TUMORS

A. Benign Tumors

1. *Vascular Tumors*

Vascular changes in the skin and mucous membranes are frequently seen during pregnancy and include proliferation of vessels, vasomotor instability, and congestion. Increased levels of estrogen, marked rise in blood volume, increased blood flow in pregnant women, genetic predisposition, and congestion alone or in combination with each other are possible causes for these changes. Vascular spiders and palmar erythema are so frequently observed during pregnancy that they are considered as physiological changes and are discussed elsewhere. Varicosities may affect as many as 40% of pregnant women (3) and may involve the saphenous system or small superficial vessels in the legs as well as the hemorrhoidal and vulvar networks. Increased venous pressure from the partial obstruction of venous return produced by the pressure of an enlarging uterus on the vena cava and other vessels and decreased soft tissue tone in the vascular wall and surrounding supporting tissue play a role in the development of varicose veins. Thrombosis is much more common in hemorrhoidal veins than in leg veins during pregnancy. Light exercise and elastic support should be recommended for varicose veins, sitting baths, laxatives, and local anesthetics may be helpful for hemorrhoids. Besides these changes, a number of true benign vascular tumors have been reported to be increased in number during pregnancy and some of these are discussed in detail in the following sections.

a. Pyogenic Granuloma of Pregnancy. Pyogenic granuloma of pregnancy, also called granuloma gravidarum or pregnancy tumor, occurs in up to 2% of pregnancies (150). Pyogenic granuloma is a rapidly enlarging lesion occurring in the skin or mucous membranes. The most common cutaneous location is on the fingers. More than three-fourths of mucosal lesions occur on the gingiva, and there have been some reports of lesions on the tongue and lips or nasal fossa (151,152). On the gingiva, the lesion is usually associated with extensive gingivitis during pregnancy. The etiology of pyogenic granuloma of pregnancy is unknown, but suggestions as to the cause range from minor trauma and irritation to hormonal factors associated with pregnancy.

Grossly, pyogenic granuloma of pregnancy is a red or purple tumor ranging from 1 mm to several centimeters in diameter. It arises from the gingival papilla between adjacent teeth or on the buccal or lingual surface of the marginal gingiva. Histologically, pyogenic granuloma of pregnancy is undistinguishable from pyogenic granuloma not associated with pregnancy. The lesion is composed of granulation tissue infiltrated with lymphocytes, plasma cells, and polymorphonuclear leukocytes and may be covered by stratified squamous epithelium or be ulcerated. Generally, the lesion requires no therapy during pregnancy and frequently shows spontaneous shrinkage postpartum. Treatment is conventional excision or laser excision or vaporation (153,154).

b. Hemangioma. During pregnancy preexisting hemangiomas may enlarge and new hemangiomas may spontaneously develop in as much as 5% of pregnant women. Usually, they appear at the end of the first trimester and slowly enlarge until delivery (4,5,155). After delivery, hemangiomas show a decrease in size or even regress. The high estrogen levels that occur during pregnancy are probably an etiological factor, and similar changes have also been described after change of oral contraceptives (156). Cutaneous hemangiomas rarely cause problems during pregnancy. Surgical removal is the treatment for lesions which persist postpartum. Large hemangiomas with arteriovenous shunting and subsequent high-output cardiac failure have been described (4). Hemangiomas may also arise on the oral mucosa (3) or in other organs, such as the liver, uterus, and spine, where they—although benign—may require treatment because of a dramatic increase in size under the effect of the gestational hormones (157–159).

c. Miscellaneous Tumors. Subcutaneous hemangioendotheliomas have been described around the eyes, breasts, and umbilical region. They present as exophytic, verrucous, highly vascular lesions with telangiectasias in the surrounding area (4). Also, glomangiomas are not uncommon during pregnancy (3). Only recently has acquired tufted angioma been described with recurrences associated with pregnancies (160). Although clear data are not available, all these conditions are believed to be related to changes associated with sex hormones during gestation, or, as in unilateral nevoid telangiectatic syndrome, to an increase in estrogen and progesterone receptors (161).

2. *Soft Tissue Tumors*

a. Molluscum Fibrosum Gravidarum. Molluscum fibrosum gravidarum (skin tag, acrochordon) is a small, usually 1–5 mm but sometimes larger, soft, pedunculated, fleshy, skin-colored or slightly pigmented tumor. Clinically, it is indistinguishable from a skin tag in a nonpregnant individual. Numerous such tumors often occur and are seen on the eyelids or sides of the face, neck, anterior portion of the chest, axillae, inframammary areas, and legs. These lesions appear during the later months of pregnancy. They may persist after delivery, and then they may present a cosmetic problem. The cause of the lesions is unclear, but endocrinological changes during pregnancy have been implicated. Histologically, molluscum fibrosum gravidarum consists of a core of normal dermal connective tissue covered with a thin epidermis.

Molluscum fibrosum gravidarum may be removed by simple snipping with curved scissors or by electrodesiccation (3,4,5,155).

b. Miscellaneous Soft Tissue Tumors. Several other types of soft tumors have been described during pregnancy, and sometimes it may be difficult to elucidate whether they are coincidential or really pregnancy related. However, it is generally believed that during pregnancy dermatofibromas commonly develop, leiomyomas may increase in size or become (more) painful, and keloids grow more rapidly (4,5).

c. Neurofibroma and Neurofibromatosis. Neurofibroma is a common benign nerve sheath tumor. It can be seen as a solitary lesion or in the context of neurofibromatosis. Although single neurofibromas may also show growth tendency during pregnancy or even new lesions may arise, they do not cause many problems during gestation compared with the severe impact which pregnancy may have on neurofibromatosis. Solitary lesions can easily be excised during pregnancy or after delivery.

Two types of neurofibromatosis have been described. Type I, which is more common, is known as von Recklinghausen disease, characterized by six or more café-au-lait spots, cutaneous and subcutaneous neurofibromas, and axillary freckling. Other features are Lisch nodules (iris hamartomas), macrocephaly, and short stature. Additionally, central nervous system and/or malignant tumors, endocrine tumors, and skeletal deformities may occur. Type I neurofibromatosis is caused by mutations affecting a gene mapped to chromosome 17q.

Type II neurofibromatosis, central neurofibromatosis, is rarer than type I. It is characterized by bilateral acoustic neurinomas and associated central nervous system tumors, and fewer cutaneous lesions. The gene defect in this type has been localized in gene 22q.

Most of the contemporary information on neurofibromatosis and pregnancy has been acquired from case reports, which mainly present the more outstanding and complicated cases. To date, only three large series of pregnancies in patients with neurofibromatosis have been published in the English literature (162–164). Neurofibromas increase in size during pregnancy, new tumors may appear, and some tumors also tend to regress after delivery (162).

Hemorrhage in large tumors may result in anemia, pain, or pressure symptoms (165). Hypertension, also a feature of neurofibromatosis, has been reported to be aggravated by pregnancy and may lead to eclampsia (162,166). Pheochromocytoma, which is also a frequent finding in patients suffering from neurofibromatosis, has been associated with an increased maternal mortality rate in pregnant women (167,168). Intrauterine growth retardation is possibly caused by a defect of placental vessels with an inability to supply adequate amounts of nutrients to the fetus (169,170). This may also be responsible for the higher rate of abortions and stillbirth in pregnant patients with neurofibromatosis (164,165).

Pregnancies in women suffering from neurofibromatosis should be regarded at risk. Frequent blood pressure monitoring is necessary. Skin lesions and pelvic tumors may grow during pregnancy, but conservative management should be the rule. Elective cesarean section should be considered in patients with pelvic deformities or extreme short stature. However, based on the complications described above and the autosomal dominant mode of transmission of the disease, therapeutic abortion and sterilization are frequently recommended to the patient.

3. Melanocytic Nevi

During pregnancy there may be increased growth or darkening of preexisting melanocytic nevi and also occasional production of new ones (4,5). Histologically, the melanocytes may be larger with increased melanization and more pronounced dendrites. Fortunately, most of the lesions are benign and do not require treatment. From these observations, it is clear that sex hormones affect melanocytic nevi. In a recent study, it was demonstrated that pregnancy and sex steroid hormones have effects on nevi of patients with the dysplastic nevus syndrome. Seventeen patients were studied during 22 pregnancies and compared with 31 patients who took oral contraceptives or hormone supplements. The study showed that the rate of dysplastic nevus changes increased during pregnancy or hormone supplementation (171).

B. Malignant Tumors

1. *Malignant Melanoma*

For a long time the impact of pregnancy on malignant melanoma has been regarded as being controversial. The concerns regarding the effects of pregnancy on melanoma have stemmed from observations that melanocytic nevi may grow or increase in number and hyperpigmentation occurs during pregnancy. Besides, the melanocyte-stimulating hormone estrogen has been considered to be responsible for this phenomenon and has been shown to increase melanocyte activity in animal studies. It has been presumed that hormonal changes of pregnancy accelerate melanocyte growth.

The possible role of exogenous estrogen in the etiology of melanoma has caused considerable controversy. It has been suggested that oral contraceptives increase the risk of developing melanoma (172). Although a link between oral contraceptive use and superficial melanoma has been suggested, overall results do not suggest a substantial effect of oral contraceptive use on the etiology of melanoma (173,174). Women with melanoma have a significantly better prognosis than men, which has been mainly attributed to differences in location and tumor thickness (175). On the other hand, women's better prognosis is interpreted as support for the argument that estrogens inhibit the growth of melanoma. Endogenous estrogens have an inhibitory effect on melanoma, which is emphasized by melanomas diagnosed in premenopausal women metastasizing years later in the postmenopausal period (176,177). A similar trend can be seen when patients taking exogenous estrogens either as oral contraceptives or for therapeutic reasons are analyzed. They present with significantly thinner tumors than women without hormone treatment (178). Additionally, in a recent study, it could be demonstrated that there are no detectable estrogen and progesterone receptors on melanoma cells (179). From all these studies, it can be concluded that exogenous estrogens play no role in the etiology of melanoma, that women have a survival advantage over men that could be due to an inhibitory effect of endogenous estrogens, and that exogenous estrogens do not promote progression of the disease in patients with melanoma. Women who have previously been treated for melanoma can safely use hormonal supplements (175).

Since 1951 there have been numerous reports that melanoma arising in pregnancy is associated with a poorer prognosis than melanoma arising independent of pregnancy. In one report, 14 of 32 pregnant patients died within 3 years or less because of their progressive disease (180). The investigators concluded that melanoma occurring during pregnancy was associated with rapid growth and metastasis. In 1954, two further cases were reported in which the investigators thought that the hormones of pregnancy influenced the growth and spread of the melanoma (181). They suggested that female patients with melanoma should be surgically sterilized to prevent metastatic disease.

On the other hand, in a group of 115 pregnant patients with melanoma in 1960, the 5- and 10-year survival rate was analyzed. The investigators found that the survival of pregnant patients with melanoma was not significantly different from that of the control group of 330 women (182). Another study reported 71 women with malignant melanoma, 30 of whom were diagnosed with melanoma from 1 year before and 5 years after pregnancy. There was no difference in survival or stage of the disease in patients with pregnancy-associated melanoma compared with those who were not pregnant (183). In a retrospective study, no statistically significant difference was seen in the survival of patients with stage I melanoma when nulliparous women were compared with multiparous women (184).

In a more recent study, 100 patients diagnosed with melanoma during pregnancy were followed for a mean of 6.8 years and compared with a nonpregnant female population. There was a significantly shorter disease-free interval for the pregnant group. Multivariant analysis demonstrated that pregnancy at diagnosis was significantly associated with the development of metastatic disease; however, it was not a risk factor for patient mortality (185). More or less similar results have been published in earlier studies, where investigators concluded that some factors associated with pregnancy favor the development of a malignant melanoma; however, once the diagnosis is made, the course of the melanoma does not differ from matched controls and that melanoma diagnosed before or during pregnancy does not appear to have a worse prognosis than melanoma not associated with pregnancy (186,187).

Within the last 10 years, at least five accurate controlled studies regarding the impact of pregnancy on malignant melanoma have been published (188–192). The conclusion which can be drawn from these studies is that there is no significant difference in survival rates between women who were diagnosed with stage I melanoma during pregnancy compared with those who were not pregnant. In two excellent recently published reviews, the investigators concentrated on the question if there is any difference in the prognosis of melanoma when it is diagnosed prior, during, or after pregnancy. On the basis of a limited number of controlled studies, they conclude that being pregnant before, after, or at the time of diagnosis of stage I melanoma does not influence the 5-year survival rate (193,194). However, women with melanoma diagnosed during pregnancy tend to have thicker melanomas, although this does not impair the prognosis compared with thick melanomas in nonpregnant women (194).

Today, on the basis of our current knowledge, women with stage I melanoma who wish to become pregnant should be informed that pregnancy does not appear to affect the prognosis. Since most recurrences of melanoma develop within 3 years after diagnosis, it seems advisable to recommend that patients avoid a subsequent pregnancy during this interval.

VII. MISCELLANEOUS CONDITIONS

A. Fox-Fordyce Disease

Fox-Fordyce disease is a chronic pruritic papular disease usually occurring in young women in areas of the body rich in apocrine sweat glands, especially in the axillae. The condition begins mainly at puberty and clears up spontaneously after the age of 50 years. In the axillae, and sometimes on the chest or perigenital area, one finds small, flat or conical, firm, skin-colored or yellowish papules. Affected individuals quite often have disturbances in menstruation or signs of virilization. The etiological factors responsible for these disturbances are unknown. Keratinous obstruction of the upper limits of the apocrine duct is followed by sweat retention and inflammatory changes. Endocrine factors, especially sex hormones, are thought to play a role in development of Fox-Fordyce disease because of their apparent but yet unidentified regulatory role in apocrine secretory physiology. Furthermore, Fox-Fordyce disease is clearly modulated by pregnancy showing improvement of the disease especially in the last trimester when endogenous estrogens and corticosteroid levels are highest (195). Levels of sex hormones are unchanged, suggesting the defect might be on the receptor side (196).

Estrogens and oral contraceptives have been used therapeutically in Fox-Fordyce disease with varying success. Oral contraceptives with antiandrogens, for example, cyproterone acetate, have been found to be of value (197), but they are contraindicated in pregnancy.

B. Acne Vulgaris

Acne is one of the most common diseases seen by dermatologists. That there is a hormonal influence in the development of acne is indicated by the fact that acne in normal individuals develops in puberty and regresses in early adulthood.

Furthermore, acne may be induced or aggravated by the administration of testosterone, anabolic agents, gonadotropins, corticosteroids, and adrenocorticotropin (198,199). The development of sebaceous gland acini and the extent of sebum production are controlled hormonally by androgens (testosterone and its metabolites). Sebaceous gland cells have receptors for androgens; for example for 5α-dihydrotestosterone. Estrogens inhibit sebum production, although only indirectly via the pituitary by the suppression of androgens (198). Despite high levels of estrogens during pregnancy, the effect of pregnancy on acne is variable (200). In many patients, the influence of pregnancy on acne is beneficial; others, however, may develop acne during pregnancy for the first time or have exacerbations of preexisting acne. Some women may even recurrently develop acne during pregnancy with subsequent clearing after parturition.

Tetracyclines should never be given to any pregnant woman for the treatment of acne, as severe adverse effects have been described. Isotretinoin, a systemic retinoid, is also strictly contraindicated during and before pregnancy. As these effective substances are frequently used for the treatment of severe acne, their withdrawal may result in a severe flare.

C. Hidradenitis Suppurativa

Hidradenitits suppurativa is a chronic, suppurative, and cicatritial disease of apocrine gland–bearing skin areas, especially the axillae and anogenital area. The term *acne inversa*, or apocrine acne, has been used to designate an association of extensive acne vulgaris with hidradenitis suppurativa. Whether the apocrine glandular apparatus or the hair follicles are primarily involved in the development of this condition is still a matter of discussion (195).

The disease does not occur before puberty, which indicates a hormonal influence on the development of this condition. Besides genetic factors, which may be involved in development of hidradenitis suppurativa (201), there is also strong evidence for an androgen dependency (202,203). This is supported by the observation that antiandrogens may be helpful at least in some patients (195). Similar as in acne, women suffering from hidradenitis suppurativa may benefit from pregnancy, showing a significant improvement of their disease. However, the course is unpredictable and also worsening may occur.

D. Psoriasis

Psoriasis is primarily an inherited inflammatory skin disease of acute exanthematic or chronic stationary course. The skin lesions are inflammatory, red, sharply demarcated plaques of various size and shape, with characteristic silvery scaling. Nail involvement is frequent. The disease can present in several other forms: psoriatic erythroderma with entire body involvement, pustular psoriasis either localized or generalized, or psoriatic arthropathy. Several provoking factors have been described, among them pregnancy and parturition. However, as a rule, pregnancy has a favorable influence on psoriasis. Localized forms are most refractory, whereas generalized forms tend to improve (204,205). Also, psoriatic arthritis normally shows improvement during pregnancy, as documented in a recent study showing that psoriatric arthritis improved in 80% of the pregnant patients (206).

Impetigo herpetiformis, also called generalized pustular psoriasis of pregnancy, is a rare, extremely serious inflammatory form of psoriasis that occurs during pregnancy. The onset is usually in the last trimester, but it has also been reported to develop at any stage of gestation. The eruption consists of urticated erythema which begins in the flexual areas, especially the inguinal region. Superficial sterile pustules form at the margins of the lesions, and the eruption may become widespread with involvement of mucous membranes. Fever, malaise, neutrophilia, hypocalcemia, and tetany are associated. The disease usually remits at delivery but may persist long afterward (207–209). The more severe and long standing the impetigo herpetiformis, the greater are the risks for mother and fetus with placental insufficiency leading to stillbirth, neonatal death, or fetal abnormalities (210). Management requires intensive medical care with fluid and electrolyte replacement and correction of hypocalcemia.

The treatment of choice for impetigo herpetiformis is administration of systemic corticosteroids. The condition recurs with severity in subsequent pregnancies and has therefore been classified by some investigators under the group of specific dermatoses of pregnancies (4,5). Exacerbation with menstruation and oral contraceptives has been described.

E. Erythema Nodosum

Erythema nodosum is a cutaneous reaction pattern consisting of inflammatory, spontaneously regressing, tender, nodular, painful lesions located primarily over the extensor surfaces of the lower extremities. The cause of this reaction is unknown. Erythema nodosum is associated with sarcoidosis, infections, enteropathies, malignant diseases, and drugs. Cases of repeated episodes of erythema nodosum in association with pregnancies and oral contraceptives have been described (211–214). In many of these reports, multiple episodes of erythema nodosum in association to exposure to female sex hormones (estrogens) and/or pregnancies have been documented (213,214). However, after reviewing all these cases, it is impossible to postulate a direct relation between pregnancies (female sex hormones) and erythema nodosum, although erythema nodosum is more common in women between menarche and menopause than in men.

As it is believed that the development of erythema nodosum is based on an immunological mechanism, it would be fascinating to speculate that either the female sex hormones are the antigenic stimulus or that they modulate the immune system in a yet unknown way. As there is increasing evidence that sex hormones influence the activity of the immune system, the latter hypothesis seems to be more likely, although the exact mechanisms await further clarification.

F. Erythema Multiforme

Erythema multiforme is thought to be an intolerance reaction of the skin which is precipitated by trigger factors that may remain undetected. Two main groups of such factors have been identified: infective agents (their toxins or metabolic products) and drugs. Furthermore, an association of erythema multiforme with several malignancies, physical factors, contact reactants, collagen diseases, and endocrine factors has been described. Additionally, pregnancy is a well-documented etiologic factor.

Clinically, the disease is characterized by acute onset with bright red, sharply demarcated lesions on the backs of the hands, extensor sides of the forearms, elbows, knees, backs of the feet, and sides of the face. Characteristically, the center of the lesion is flat, cyanotic, or hemorrhagic and frequently shows a blister formation, leading to the typical iris or target lesion. In addition to this minor form, a major form with severe changes on the mucous membranes has been described. The diagnosis is based on the typical clinical and histological findings.

A pregnant woman developing erythema multiforme may require a detailed work-up. Infections, drug administration, or illness for up to 3 weeks prior to the onset of the rash should be considered. Other skin diseases which also may present multiformelike (target) lesions such as figurate erythemas, the Sweet syndrome, lupus erythematosus, bullous pemphigoid, and herpes (pemphigoid) gestationis should be ruled out.

The treatment of erythema multiforme should be directed against the underlying cause regarding the safety recommendations for drugs during pregnancy. Short-term systemic corticosteroids may be necessary in some cases.

G. Hereditary Angioedema

Hereditary angioedema (HAE) is an autosomal dominant inherited disease marked by deficiency or dysfunction of the serum protein inhibitor of the first complement component (C1-INH).

Minor trauma or dental manipulation may lead to intermittent episodes of edema of the limbs, face, pharynx, vulva, and other sites. The activity of the disease is clearly hormonally modulated. In female patients, the frequency of attacks of HAE after puberty and during menstruation is increased. A synthetic androgenic steroid, danazol, has been shown to prevent attacks of HAE with good success.

In view of these data, it is not surprising that pregnancy also has an effect on HAE. With progressing pregnancy, significantly fewer or even no attacks are observed. Despite this beneficial effect of pregnancy on HAE, there seems to be some minimal risk in the peripartal area. So it might be advisable to administer 500 units C1 inactivator prophylactically before the expulsive phase of delivery (216–219).

VIII. CONCLUSIONS

In this chapter, an attempt has been made to give an overview of the present knowledge of the impact of pregnancy on the course of preexisting or simultaneously acquired skin diseases. Many readers will find this review incomplete and some even contradictory to their personal experience. This should not lead to disappointment but encourage all of us to contribute to the growing field of knowledge by case reports or prospective controlled studies to clarify the many open questions in relation to pregnancy and its influence on skin diseases.

REFERENCES

1. R. G. Lahita. The effects of sex hormones on the immune system in pregnancy, *Am. J. Reprod. Immunol. 28*:136–137 (1992).
2. I. Berczi. Prolactin, pregnancy and autoimmune disease, *J. Rheumatol. 20*:1095–1100 (1993).
3. R. C. Wong and C. N. Ellis. Physiologic skin changes in pregnancy, *J. Am. Acad. Dermatol. 10*:929–940 (1984).
4. G. B. Winton and C. W. Lewis. Dermatoses of pregnancy, *J. Am. Acad. Dermatol. 6*:977–998 (1982).
5. W. Dotz and B. Berman, Dermatologic problems of pregnancy, *Medical, Surgical, and Gynecologic Complications of Pregnancy* (S. H. Cherry, R. L. Berkowitz, and N. G. Kase, eds.). Williams & Wilkins, Baltimore, 1985, pp. 452–473.
6. S. F. Eudy and G. F. Baker. Dermatopathology for the obstetrician, *Clin. Obstet. Gynecol. 33*:728–737 (1990).
7. G. B. Winton. Skin diseases aggravated by pregnancy, *J. Am. Acad. Dermatol. 20*:1–13 (1989).
8. E. D. Weinberg. Pregnancy—associated depression of cell-mediated immunity, *Rev. Infect. Dis. 5*:814–831 (1984).
9. C. J. Grossmann. Regulation of the immune system by sex steroids, *Endocrine Rev. 5*:435–455 (1984).
10. A. H. W. M. Schuurs and H. A. M. Verheul. Effects of gender and sex steroids on the immune response, *J. Steroid. Biochem. 35*:157–172 (1990).
11. B. Styrt, B. Sugarman. Estrogens and infection, *Rev. Infect. Dis. 13*:1139–1150 (1991).
12. H. E. Müller. Das leistungsfähigere Abwehrsystem der Frau gegen Infektionserreger, *Wien. Med. Wochenschr. 17*:389–395 (1992).
13. C. Sullivan and L. G. Smith. Management of vulvovaginitis in pregnancy, *Clin. Obstet. Gynecol. 36*:195–205 (1993).
14. J. D. Sobel. Candidal vulvovaginitis, *Clin. Obstet. Gynecol. 36*:153–165 (1993).
15. P. S. Porter and J. S. Lyle. Yeast vulvovaginitis due to oral contraceptives, *Arch. Dermatol. 93*:402–403 (1966).
16. D. N. Danforth. *Obstetrics and Gynecology*, 3rd ed. Harper & Row, New York, 1977, p. 873.
17. M. C. Y. Heng, C. L. Henderson, and D. C. Barker. Correlation of pityrosporum ovale density with clinical severity of seborrhoeic dermatitis as assessed by a simplified technique, *J. Am. Acad. Dermatol. 23*:82–86 (1990).
18. L. K. Borton and R. A. Schwartz. Pityrosporum folliculitis: A common acneiform condition of middle age, *Ariz. Med. 38*:598–601 (1981).

19. P. E. Weary. Pityrosporum ovale, *Arch. Dermatol. 98*:408–422 (1968).
20. P. J. M. Berretty, H. A. M. Neumann, and H. J. Hulsebosch, Pityrosporum folliculitis: Is it a real entity?, *Br. J. Dermatol. 103*:565–568 (1980).
21. P. J. M. Berretty, H. A. M. Neumann, and H. J. Hulsebosch, Folliculitis door pityrosporum-organismen geinducerrd, *Ned. T. Geneesk. 124:* 1818–1821 (1980).
22. W. R. Heymann and D. J. Wolf, Malassezia (pityrosporum) folliculitis occurring during pregnancy, *Int. J. Dermatol. 25*:49–51 (1986).
23. A. C. McDougall and M. I. Ulrich. Mycobacterial disease: Leprosy, *Dermatology in General Medicine*, 4th ed. (T. B. Fitzpatrick, A. Z. Eisen, K. Wolff, I. M. Freedberg, and K. F. Austen, eds.), McGraw-Hill, New York, 1993, pp. 2395–2410.
24. W. H. Jopling and A. McDougall. *Handbook of Leprosy*, Heinemann, Oxford, U.K., 1988.
25. M. E. Duncan. A historical and clinical review of the interaction of leprosy and pregnancy: A cycle to be broken, *Soc. Sci. Med. 37*:457–472 (1993).
26. M. E. Duncan, R. Melsom, J. M. H. Pearson, and D. S. Ridley. The association of pregnancy and leprosy. New cases, relapse of cured patients and deterioration in patients on treatment during pregnancy and lactation—Results of a prospective study of 154 pregnancies in 147 Ethiopian women, *Lepr. Rev. 52*:245–263 (1981).
27. M. E. Duncan, J. M. H. Pearson, and D. S. Ridley. Pregnancy and leprosy: The consequences of alterations of cell-mediated and humoral immunity during pregnancy and lactation, *Int. J. Lepr. 50*:425–432 (1982).
28. E. De Villiers. Heterogeneity of the human papillomavirus group, *J. Virol. 63*:4898–4905 (1989).
29. M. D. Greenberg and L. H. Rutledge. Understanding human papillomarviral infections in women, *Semin. Dermatol. 11*:241–246 (1992).
30. P. A. Csango, J. Skuland, A. Nilsen, B. S. Pedersen, and G. Jagars. Papillomavirus infection among abortion applicants and patients out a sexually transmitted disease clinic, *Sex. Trans. Dis. 19*:149–153 (1992).
31. N. G. Osborne and M. D. Adelson. Herpes simplex and human papillomavirus genital infections: controversy over obstetric management, *Clin. Obstet. Gynecol. 33*:801–811 (1990).
32. C. G. Prober. Herpetic vaginitis in 1993, *Clin. Obstet. Gynecol. 36*:177–187 (1993).
33. M. Maccatto. Herpes in pregnancy, *Clin. Obstet. Gynecol. 36*:869–877 (1993).
34. J. E. Peacock and F. A. Sarubbi. Disseminated herpes simplex virus infection during pregnancy, *Obstet. Gynecol. 61*:135–185 (1983).
35. R. H. Kaufmann and S. Faro. Herpes genitalis: clinical features and treatment, *Clin. Obstet. Gynecol. 28*:152–163 (1985).
36. P. Mudida, G. S. Marshall, R. S. Howell, D. S. Schmid, S. Steger, and G. Adams. Disseminated herpes simplex virus infection during pregnancy, *J. Reprod. Med. 38*:964–968 (1993).
37. Z. A. Brown and D. A. Baker. Acyclovir therapy during pregnancy, *Obstet. Gynecol. 73*:526–531 (1989).
38. E. B. Andrews, B. C. Yankaskas, J. F. Cordero, K. Schoeffler, and S. Hampp. Acyclovir in pregnancy registry: Six years experience, *Obstet. Gynecol. 79*:7–13 (1992).
39. L. M. Frenkel, Z. A. Brown, Y. J. Bryson, L. Carey, J. D. Unedkof, P. A. Hensleigh,

A. M. Arvin, C. G. Prober, and J. D. Connor. Pharmacokinetics in acyclovir in the term human pregnancy and neonate, *Am. J. Obstet. Gynecol. 164*:569–576 (1991).

40. J. G. Spangler, J. K. Kirk, and M. P. Knudson. Uses and safety of acyclovir in pregnancy, *J. Fam. Pract. 38*:186–191 (1994).
41. S. G. Paryani and A. M. Arvin. Intrauterine infection with varicella-zoster virus after maternal varicella, *N. Engl. J. Med. 314*:1542–1546 (1986).
42. A. A. Gershon. Chicken pox, measles and mumps, *Infectious Diseases of the Fetus and Newborn Infant*, 3rd ed. (J. S. Remington and J. O. Klein, eds.). Saunders, Philadelphia, 1990, pp. 395–445.
43. P. A. Brunell. Varicella in pregnancy, the fetus and the newborn: Problems in management, *J. Infect. Dis. 166*(Suppl. 1):S42–47 (1992).
44. D. McIntosh and D. Isaacs. Varicella zoster virus infection in pregnancy, *Arch. Dis. Child. 68*:1–2 (1993).
45. K. L. Jones, K. A. Johnson, and C. A. Chambers. Offspring of women infected with varicella during pregnancy: A prospective study, *Teratology 49*:29–32 (1994).
46. A. L. Pastuszak, M. Levy, B. Schick, C. Zuber, M. Feldkamp, J. Gladstone, F. Bar-Levy, E. Jackson, A. Donnenfeld, W. Meschino, and G. Koren. Outcome after maternal varicella infection in the first 20 weeks of pregnancy, *N. Engl. J. Med. 330*:901–905 (1994).
47. J. Singh and J. M. Gibson. A case of presumed congenital herpes zoster ophthalmicus, *Br. J. Ophthalmol. 77*:459–461 (1993).
48. S. H. Vermund, M. A. Golbraith, S. C. Ebner, A. R. Sheon, and R. Kaslow. Human immunodeficiency virus/acquired immunodeficiency syndrome in pregnant women, *Ann. Epidemiol. 2*:773–803 (1992).
49. R. J. Biggar, S. Pahwa, and H. Minkoff. Immunosuppression in pregnant women infected with human immunodeficiency virus, *Am. J. Obstet. Gynecol. 161*:1239–1241 (1989).
50. M. K. Lindsay. Human immunodeficiency virus with obstetrician, *Clin. Obstet. Gynecol. 36*:821–831 (1993).
51. H. S. Gates and C. D. Barker. Pneumocystis carinii pneumonia in pregnancy, *J. Reprod. Med. 38*:483–486 (1993).
52. J. C. Glantz and D. J. Roberts. Pregnancy complicated by thrombocytopenia secondary to human immunodeficiency virus infection, *Obstet. Gynecol. 83*:825–827 (1994).
53. C. A. Hankins and M. A. Handley. HIV disease and AIDS in women: Current knowledge and a research agenda, *J. Acquir. Immune Defic. Syndr. 5*:957–971 (1992).
54. J. D. Moreno and H. Minkoff. Human immunodeficiency virus infection during pregnancy, *Clin. Obstet. Gynecol. 35*:813–820 (1992).
55. A. Rachlis and M. M. Fanning. Zidovudine toxicity, clinical features and management, *Drug Safety 8*:312–320 (1993).
56. Zidovudine for the prevention of HIV transmission from mother to infant, *MMWR 43*:285–287 (1994).
57. N. F. Rothfield. Lupus erythematosus, *Dermatology in General Medicine,* 4th ed. (T. B. Fitzpatrick, A. Z. Eisen, K. Wolff, I. M. Freedberg, and K. F. Austen, eds.). McGraw-Hill, New York, 1993, pp. 2137–2148.
58. P. B. Beeson. Age and sex association of 40 autoimmune diseases, *Am. J. Med. 96*:457–462 (1994).

59. P. Jungers, M. Dougados, C. Pelissier, F. Kuttenn, F. Tron, P. Lesavre, and J. F. Bach. Influence of oral contraceptive therapy on the activity of systemic lupus erythematosus. *Arthritis Rheum. 25*:618–623 (1982).
60. R. L. Travers and G. R. V. Hughes. Oral contraceptive therapy and systemic lupus erythematosus, *J. Rheumatol. 5*:448–451 (1978).
61. M. Garovich, C. Agudelo, and E. Pisko. Oral contraceptives and systemic lupus erythematosus, *Arthritis Rheum. 23*:1396–1398 (1980).
62. B. J. Tarzy, C. R. Garcia, and E. E. Wallach. Rheumatic disease, abnormal serology, and oral contraceptives, *Lancet 2*:501–503 (1972).
63. J. A. Yell and S. M. Burge. The effect of hormonal changes on cutaneous disease in lupus erythematosus, *Br. J. Dermatol. 129*:18–22 (1993).
64. A. S. Cohen, W. E. Reynolds, and E. C. Franklin. Erythematosus, *Bull. Rheum. Dis. 21*:643–648 (1971).
65. D. Estes and D. L. Larson. Systemic lupus erythematosus and pregnancy, *Clin. Obstet. Gynecol. 8*:307–321 (1965).
66. M. Garsenstein, V. E. Pollak, and R. M. Kark. Systemic lupus erythematosus and pregnancy, *N. Engl. J. Med. 267*:165–169 (1962).
67. M. Siegel, N. Gwon, and S. L. Lee. Survivorship in systemic lupus erythematosus: Relationship to race and pregnancy, *Arthritis Rheum. 12*:117–120 (1969).
68. M. D. Lockshin. Overview of lupus pregnancies, *Am. J. Reprod. Immunol. 28*:181–182 (1992).
69. M. Petri, D. Howard, and J. Repke. Frequency of lupus flare in pregnancy. The Hopkins lupus pregnancy center experience, *Arthritis Rheum. 34*:1538–1545 (1991).
70. L. D. Devoe and G. L. Loy. Serum complement levels and perinatal outcome in pregnancies complicated by systemic lupus erythematosus. *Obstet. Gynecol. 63*:796–800 (1984).
71. M. D. Lockshin. Pregnancy does not cause systemic lupus erythematosus to worsen, *Arthritis Rheum. 32*:665–670 (1989).
72. G. Mintz, J. Niz, G. Gutierrez, A. Garcia-Alonso, and S. Karchmer. Prospective study of pregnancy in systemic lupus erythematosus: Results of a multidisciplinary approach, *J. Rheumatol. 13*:732–739 (1986).
73. K. L. Wong and F. Y. Chan. Outcome of pregnancy in patients with systemic lupus erythematosus: A prospective study, *Arch. Intern. Med. 151*:269–273 (1991).
74. W. W. Piette. The antiphospholipid antibody syndrome, *Current Opinions in Dermatology*, 1st ed. (M. V. Dahl and P. J. Lynch, eds.). Current Science, Philadelphia, 1993, pp. 119–122.
75. R. A. Asherson and R. Cervera. Antiphospholipid syndrome, *J. Invest. Dermatol. 100*:21S–27S (1993).
76. G. M. Horrowitz and G. D. V. Hawkins. Cutaneous manifestations of collagen vascular disease in pregnancy, *Clin. Obstet. Gynecol 33*:759–779 (1990).
77. J. A. Mills. Dermatomyositis, *Dermatology in General Medicine*, 4th ed. (T. B. Fitzpatrick, A. Z. Eisen, K. Wolff, I. M. Freedberg, and K. F. Austen, eds.). McGraw-Hill, New York, 1993, pp. 2118–2155.
78. G. Rocha Costelar Pinheiro, J. Goldenberg, E. Atra, R. Borges Pereiva, L. Cameno, and B. Schmidt. Juvenile dermatomyositits and pregnancy: Report and literature review, *J. Rheumatol. 19*:1798–1801 (1992).

79. T. Ohno, A. Imai, and T. Tamaya. Successful outcomes of pregnancies complicated with dermatomyositis, *Gynecol. Obstet. Invest.* *33*:187–189 (1992).
80. G. J. Morgan and W. S. Chow. Clinical features, diagnosis, and prognosis in rheumatoid arthritis, *Curr. Opin. Rheumatol.* *5*:184–190 (1993).
81. N. R. Rowell. Skin manifestations of rheumatoid diseases, *Dermatology in General Medicine*, 4th ed. (T. B. Fitzpatrick, A. Z. Eisen, K. Wolff, I. M. Freedberg, and K. F. Austen, eds.), McGraw-Hill, New York, 1993, pp. 2190–2195.
82. T. D. Spectar and J. A. P. Silva. Pregnancy and rheumatoid arthritis: An overview, *Am. J. Reprod. Immunol.* *28*:222–225 (1992).
83. J. W. J. Bijlsma and H. R. van den Brink. Estrogens and rheumatoid arthritis, *Am. J. Reprod. Immunol.* *28*:231–234 (1992).
84. J. L. Nelson, K. A. Hughes, A. G. Smith, B. B. Nisperos, A. M. Branchaud, and J. A. Hansen. Remission of rheumatoid arthritis during pregnancy and maternal-fetal class III alloantigens disparity, *Am. J. Reprod. Immunol.* *28*:226–227 (1992).
85. W. H. James. Rheumatoid arthritis, the contraceptive pill, and androgens, *Ann. Rheum. Dis.* *52*:470–474 (1993).
86. C. M. Black. Systemic sclerosis and pregnancy, *Bailliere's Clin. Rheumatol.* *7*:105–124 (1990).
87. J. R. Karlen and W. A. Cook. Renal scleroderma and pregnancy. *Obstet. Gynecol.* *44*:349–354 (1974).
88. T. R. Johnson, E. A. Banner, and R. K. Winkelmann. Scleroderma and pregnancy, *Obstet. Gynecol.* *23*:467–469 (1964).
89. V. D. Steen, C. Conte, N. Day, R. Ramsey-Goldmann, and T. A. Medsger. Pregnancy in women with systemic sclerosis, *Arthritis Rheum.* *32*:151–157 (1989).
90. A. J. Silman. Pregnancy and scleroderma, *Am. J. Reprod. Immunol.* *28*:238–240 (1992).
91. N. S. Goldberg, C. DeFeo, and N. Kirshenbaum. Pemphigus vulgaris and pregnancy: risk factors and recommendations, *J. Am. Acad. Dermatol.* *28*:877–879 (1993).
92. D. Green and J. C. Maize. Maternal pemphigus vulgaris with in vivo bound antibodies in the stillborn fetus, *J. Am. Acad. Dermatol.* *7*:388–392 (1982).
93. N. Wasserstrum and R. K. Laros. Transplacental transmission of pemphigus, *JAMA* *249*:1480–1482 (1983).
94. R. W. Eyre and J. R. Stanley. Maternal pemphigus foliaceus with cell surface antibody bound in neonatal epidermis, *Arch. Dermatol.* *124*:25–27 (1988).
95. R. Rocha-Alvarez, H. Friedman, I. T. Campbell, L. Souza-Aguiar, R. Martins-Castro, and L. A. Diaz. Pregnant women with endemic pemphigus foliaceus (fogo selvagem) give birth to disease-free babies, *J. Invest. Dermatol.* *99*:78–82 (1992).
96. D. R. Bickers, M. A. Pathak, and H. W. Lim. The porphyrias, *Dermatology in General Medicine*, 4th ed. (T. B. Fitzpatrick, A. Z. Eisen, K. Wolff, I. M. Freedberg, and K. F. Austen, eds.). McGraw-Hill, New York, 1993, pp. 1855–1893.
97. J. Günther. Die Hämatoporphyrie, *Dtsch. Arch. Klin. Med.* *105*:89–106 (1991).
98. J. Waldenström. Studien über Porphyrie, *Acta Med. Scand.* *82*(Suppl.):1 (1937).
99. J. Waldenström. The porphyrias as inborn errors of metabolism, *Am. J. Med.* *22*:758 (1957).
100. C. J. Watson. The manifestations of the different forms of porphyria in relation to chemical findings, *Trans. Assoc. Am. Physicians* *64*:345 (1951).

101. M. Doss. Porphyrie and hormonale Kontrazeptiva, *Dtsch. Med. Wochenschr. 109*:1701–1702 (1984).
102. H. Ippen, D. Aust, and G. Goerz. Klinisch-experimentelle Untersuchungen zur Entstehung der Porphyrien. III. Wirkung einiger Steroidhormone auf die "latente" Hexachlorbenzol-Porphyrie der Ratte, *Arch. Dermatol. Forsch. 245*:305–307 (1972).
103. A. G. Smith and J. E. Francis. Increased inhibition of hepatic uroporphyrinogen decarboxylase in male rats given the oestrogenic drugs diethylstilbestrol and chlorotrianisene, *Chem. Pharmacol. 30*:1849–1853 (1981).
104. B. Wintzen. Porphyrin-Ausscheidung bei östrogenbehandelten Prostata-Carcinom-Trägern. M. D. Thesis, University of Düsseldorf, 1973.
105. G. Linss and C. Schmechel. Porphyria cutanea tarda nach Behandlung mit Depot-Östrogenen bei Patienten mit Prostatakarzinom, *Z. Urol. Nephrol. 83*:229–231 (1990).
106. M. J. Lamon and C. B. Frykholm. Pregnancy and porphyria cutanea tarda, *Johns Hopkins Med. J. 145*:235–237 (1979).
107. R. Marks. Porphyria cutanea tarda, *Arch. Dermatol. 118*:452 (1982).
108. G. Goerz and G. Hammer. Porphyria cutanea tarda and pregnancy, *Dermatologica 166*:316–318 (1983).
109. G. Rajka. Pregnancy and porphyria cutanea tarda, *Acta Derm. Venereol. (Stockh.) 64*:444–445 (1984).
110. L. V. Baxi, T. J. Rubeo, and B. Katz. Porphyria cutanea tarda and pregnancy, *Am. J. Obstet. Gynecol. 146*:333–334 (1983).
111. L. Malina and C. K. Lim. Manifestation of familial porphyria cutanea tarda and childbirth, *Br. J. Dermatol. 118*:243–245 (1988).
112. W. M. Lee. Pregnancy in patients with chronic liver disease, *Gastroenterol. Clin. North Am. 21*:889–903 (1992).
113. U. F. Kroh, M. Frank, C. Schwerk, and M. O. Doss. Anästhesie mit Propofol bei einem exacerbierten Verlauf der akuten intermittierenden Porphyrie, *Anästhesiol. Intensivmed. Notfallmed. Schmerzther. 28*:531–533 (1993).
114. R. Milo, M. Neumann, C. Klein, E. Caspi, and S. A. Alazoroft. Acute intermittent porphyria in pregnancy, *Obstet. Gynecol. 73*:450–452 (1989).
115. A. Olund. Acute intermittent porphyria complicated by pregnancy, *Clin. Exp. Obstet. Gynecol. 15*:168–189 (1988).
116. M. Isenschmid, Ch. König, C. Fässli, A. Haend, W. Hänggi, and H. Schneider. Akute intermittierende Porphyrie in der Schwangerschaft: Therapie mit Glukose oder Hämatin?, *Schweiz. Med. Wochenschr. 122*:1741–1745 (1992).
117. M. K. Polano. Xanthomas and dyslipoproteinemias, *Dermatology in General Medicine*, 4th ed. (T. B. Fitzpatrick, A. Z. Eisen, K. Wolff, I. M. Freedberg, and K. F. Austen, eds.). McGraw-Hill, New York, 1993, pp. 1901–1916.
118. D. S. Frederickson, R. I. Levy, and R. S. Lees. Fat transport in lipoproteins—An integrated approach to mechanisms and disorders, *N. Engl. J. Med. 276*:34, 94, 148, 215, 273 (1967).
119. F. Davidoff, S. Tishler, and C. Rosoff. Marked hyperlipidemia and pancreatitis associated with oral contraceptive therapy, *N. Engl. J. Med. 289*:552–555 (1973).
120. C. J. Glueck, D. Scheel, and J. Fishback. Estrogen-induced pancreatitis in patients with previously covert familial type V hyperlipoproteinemia, *Metabolism 21*:657–666 (1972).

121. T. M. B. DeChalain, W. L. Michell, and G. M. B. Berger. Hyperlipidemia, pregnancy and pancreatitis, *Surg. Gynecol. Obstet. 167*:469–473 (1988).
122. C. J. Glueck, C. Christopher, and M. A. Mishkel. Pancreatitis, familial hypertriglyceridemia and pregnancy, *Am. J. Obstet. Gynecol 136*:755–761 (1980).
123. P. W. Jaber, B. B. Wilson, D. W. Johns, P. H. Cooper, and J. E. Ferguson. Eruptive xanthomas during pregnancy, *J. Am. Acad. Dermatol. 27*:300–302 (1992).
124. K. H. Neldner. Acrodermatitis enteropathica and other zinc-deficiency disorders, *Dermatology in General Medicine*, 4th ed. (T. B. Fitzpatrick, A. Z. Eisen, K. Wolff, I. M. Freedberg, and K. F. Austen, eds.). McGraw-Hill, New York, 1993, pp. 1826–1832.
125. E. J. Moynahan and P. M. Barnes. Zinc-deficiency and a synthetic diet for lactose intolerance, *Lancet 1*:676 (1973).
126. D. M. Bronson, R. Barsky, and S. Barsky. Acrodermatitis enteropathica: Recognition at long last during a recurrence in a pregnancy, *J. Am. Acad. Dermatol. 9*:140–144 (1983).
127. K. M. Hambidge, K. H. Neldner, and P. A. Walravens. Zinc, acrodermatitis enteropathica and congenital malformations, *Lancet 1*:577–578 (1975).
128. J. S. Vedder and S. Griem. Acrodermatitis enteropathica (Danboldt-Closs) in five siblings, *J. Pediatr. 48*:212–219 (1956).
129. D. P. Brenton, M. J. Jackson, and A. Young. Two pregnancies in a patient with acrodermatitis enteropathica treated with zinc sulphate, *Lancet 2*:500–502 (1981).
130. R. J. Wenstrup and S. R. Pinnell. Heritable disorders of connective tissue with skin changes, *Dermatology in General Medicine*, 4th ed. (T. B. Fitzpatrick, A. Z. Eisen, K. Wolff, I. M. Freedberg, and K. F. Austen, eds.), McGraw-Hill, New York, 1993, pp. 1961–1974.
131. D. E. Hammerschmidt, M. A. Arneson, and S. L. Larson. Maternal Ehlers-Danlos syndrome type X: Successful management of pregnancy and parturition, *JAMA 248*:2487–2488 (1982).
132. P. Kiilholma, M. Grouros, and V. Nanto. Pregnancy and delivery in Ehlers-Danlos syndrome: Role of copper and zinc, *Acta Obstet. Gynecol. Scand. 63*:437–439 (1984).
133. L. Leduc and N. Wasserstrum. Successful treatment with the Smith-Hodge pessary of cervical incompetence due to defective connective tissue in Ehlers-Danlos syndrome, *Am. J. Perinatol. 9*:25–27 (1992).
134. S. R. Ainsworth and P. L. Aulicino. A survey of patients with Ehlers-Danlos syndrome, *Clin. Orthop. Rel. Res. 286:* 250–256 (1993).
135. P. Beighton. *The Ehlers-Danlos Syndrome*, Heinemann, London, 1970.
136. J. D. Schulman and J. L. Simpson. *Genetic Disease in Pregnancy*, Academic Press, New York, 1981, pp. 2–83.
137. M. E. Rivera-Alsina, P. Kwan, and F. G. Zavisca. Complications of the Ehlers-Danlos syndrome in pregnancy: A case report, *J. Reprod. Med. 29*:757–759 (1984).
138. N. L. Rudd, C. Nimrod, and K. A. Holbrook. Pregnancy complications in type IV Ehlers-Danlos syndrome, *Lancet 1*:50–53 (1983).
139. M. Lebwohl, K. Neldner, F. M. Pope, A. De-Paepe, A. M. Christiano, C. D. Boyd, J. Uitto, and V. A. McKusick. Classification of pseudoxanthoma elasticum: Report of a consensus conference, *J. Am. Acad. Dermatol. 30*:103–107 (1994).
140. I. Baratte, J. P. Schaal, and R. Laurent. Association of pseudoxanthoma and pregnancy, *Rev. Fr. Gynecol. Obstet. 86*:243–245 (1991).

141. T. T. Lao, B. N. J. Walters, and M. De Swiet. Pseudoxanthoma elasticum and pregnancy: Two case reports, *Br. J. Obstet. Gynaecol. 91*:1049–1050 (1984).
142. C. Berde, D. C. Willis, and E. C. Sandberg. Pregnancy in women with pseudoxanthoma elasticum, *Obstet. Gynecol. Surv. 38*:339–344 (1983).
143. D. L. Viljoen, S. Beatty, and P. Beighton. The obstetric and gynecological implications of pseudoxanthoma elasticum, *Br. J. Obstet. Gynaecol. 94*:884–888 (1987).
144. F. F. Broekhuizen and P. R. Hamilton. Pseudoxanthoma elasticum and intrauterine growth retardation, *Am. J. Obstet. Gynecol. 148*:112–114 (1984).
145. B. R. Elejalde, M. M. de Elejalde, and T. Samter. Manifestations of pseudoxanthoma elasticum during pregnancy: A case report and review of the literature, *Am. J. Med. Genet. 18*:755–762 (1984).
146. E. F. Cava and R. L. Drier. The Marfan syndrome in pregnancy: A case report, *Trans. Pac. Coast. Obstet. Gynecol. Soc. 38*:129–133 (1970).
147. S. Elias and R. L. Berkowitz. The Marfan syndrome and pregnancy, *Obstet. Gynecol. 47*:338–361 (1976).
148. W. Mandel, E. W. Evans, and R. L. Walford. Dissecting aortic aneurysm during pregnancy. *N. Engl. J. Med. 251*:1059–1061 (1954).
149. S. Sutiner and O. Piiroinen. Marfan's syndrome, pregnancy and fatal dissection of aorta, *Acta Obstet. Gynecol. Scand. 50*:295–300 (1971).
150. R. Hanno, E. R. Saleeby, and E. A. Krull. Disorders of pregnancy, *Clinical Dermatology* (D. I. Demis, ed.). Lippincott, Philadelphia, 1991, pp. 1–15.
151. S. N. Bhaskar and J. R. Jacoawy. Pyogenic granuloma—Clinical features, incidence, histology, and result of treatment: Report of 242 cases, *J. Oral Surg. 24*:391–398 (1966).
152. E. Lance, C. Schatz, R. Nach, and P. Thomas. Pyogenic granuloma gravidarum of the nasal fossa: CT features, *J. Computer Ass. Tomogr. 16*:663–664 (1992).
153. J. L. Powell, C. L. Bailey, A. T. Coopland, C. N. Otis, J. L. Frank, and I. Meyer. Nd:YAG laser excision of giant gingival pyogenic granuloma of pregnancy, *Lasers Surg. Med. 14*:178–183 (1994).
154. J. MacVicar and M. F. Dunn. Pregnancy tumor of the gums. A report of two cases, *J. Obstet. Gynaecol. Br. Commonw. 76*:260–263 (1969).
155. P. D. Hellreich. The skin changes of pregnancy, *Cutis 13*:82–86 (1974).
156. D. Satge, J. Grande-Goburdhun, and E. Grosshans. Microcapillary hemangioma, *Ann. Dermatol. Venereol. 120*:297–298 (1993).
157. E. Graham, A. W. Cohen, M. Soulen, and R. Faye. Symptomatic liver hemangioma with intra-tumor hemorrhage treated by angiography and embolization during pregnancy, *Obstet. Gynecol. 81*:813–816 (1993).
158. A. Weissmann, R. Talmon, and P. Jakobi. Cavernous hemangioma of the uterus in a pregnant woman, *Obstet. Gynecol. 81*:825–827 (1993).
159. I. H. Tekkok, B. Acikgoz, S. Saglam, and B. Onol. Vertebral hemangioma symptomatic during pregnancy—Report of a case and review of the literature, *Neurosurgery 32*:302–306 (1993).
160. Y. K. Kim, H. J. Kim, and K. G. Lee. Acquired tufted angioma associated with pregnancy, *Clin. Exp. Dermatol. 17*:458–459 (1992).
161. S. R. Uhlin and K. S. McCarty. Unilateral nevoid telangiectatic syndrome, *Arch. Dermatol. 119*:226–228 (1983).

162. G. M. Swapp and R. A. Main. Neurofibromatosis in pregnancy, *Br. J. Dermatol. 80*:431–435 (1973).
163. C. T. Jarvis and A. C. Crompton. Neurofibromatosis and pregnancy, *Br. J. Obstet. Gynaecol. 85*:844–846 (1978).
164. A. Weissmann, P. Jakobi, I. Zaidisc, and A. Drugan. Neurofibromatosis and pregnancy. An update, *J. Reprod. Med. 38*:890–896 (1993).
165. A. H. Ansari and N. Nagamani. Pregnancy and neurofibromatosis, *Obstet. Gynecol. 47*(Suppl.):255–295 (1976).
166. S. J. Sherman and D. B. Schwartz. Eclampsia complicating a pregnancy with neurofibromatosis. A case report. *J. Reprod. Med. 37*:469–472 (1992).
167. S. Strauss, M. Pansky, and G. Lewinsohn. Hemorrhagic pheochromocytoma in a pregnant patient with neurofibromatosis: Sonographic appearance, *J. Ultrasound Med. 9*:165–167 (1990).
168. J. G. Schenker and M. Granat. Pheochromocytoma and pregnancy: An updated appraisal, *Aust. NZ J. Obstet. Gynaecol. 22*:1–4 (1982).
169. I. Blickstein and M. Lancet. Fetal growth retardation as a complication of pregnancy in patients with neurofibromatosis, *Am. J. Obstet. Gynecol. 157*:343–346 (1987).
170. S. R. Belton, J. E. Ferguson, and V. A. Catanzarite. Neurofibromatosis and pregnancy: Report of a case complicated by intrauterine growth retardation and oligohydramnios, *Am. J. Obstet. Gynecol. 149*:468–470 (1984).
171. D. L. Ellis. Pregnancy and sex steroid hormone effects on nevi of patients with the dysplastic nevus syndrome, *J. Am. Acad. Dermatol. 25*:467–482 (1991).
172. V. Beral, S. Ramcharan, and R. Faris. Malignant melanoma and oral contraceptive use among women in California, *Br. J. Cancer 36*:804–809 (1977).
173. S. Franceschi, A. E. Baron, and C. LaVecchia. The influence of female hormones on malignant melanoma, *Tumors 76*:439–449 (1990).
174. E. A. Holly, N. S. Weiss, and J. M. Liff. Cutaneous melanoma in relation to exogenous hormones and reproductive factors, *J. Natl. Cancer Inst. 70*:827–831 (1983).
175. I. Jatoi and M. E. Gore. Sex, pregnancy, hormones and melanoma. Exogenous oestrogens do not seem to have a role in causation, *Br. Med. J. 307*:2–3 (1993).
176. H. M. Shaw, G. W. Milton, G. Farago, and W. H. McCarthy. Endocrine influences on survival from malignant melanoma, *Cancer 42*:689–677 (1978).
177. D. Raderman, S. Giler, A. Rothem, and M. Ben-Bassat. Late metastases (beyond ten years) of cutaneous malignant melanoma, *J. Am. Acad. Dermatol. 15*:374–378 (1986).
178. J. S. Lederman, R. A. Lew, H. K. Koh, and A. J. Sober. Influence of estrogen administration on tumour characteristics and survival with cutaneous melanoma, *J. Natl. Cancer Inst. 74*:981–985 (1985).
179. L. M. Duncan, R. L. Travers, F. C. Koerner, M. C. Mihm, and A. J. Sober. Estrogen and progesterone receptor analysis in pregnancy associated melanoma: Absence of immunohistochemically detectable hormone receptors, *Hum. Pathol. 25*:36–41 (1994).
180. G. T. Pack and I. M. Scharnagel. The prognosis for malignant melanoma in the pregnant woman, *Cancer 4*:324–334 (1951).
181. B. F. Byrd and W. J. McGanity. The effect of pregnancy on the clinical course of malignant melanoma, *South. Med. J. 47*:196–200 (1954).
182. P. A. George and I. G. Fortner. Melanoma with pregnancy: a report of 115 cases, *Cancer 13*:854–859 (1960).

183. L. P. White, G. Linden, and L. Breslow. Studies on melanoma: The effect of pregnancy on survival in human melanoma, *JAMA 177*:235–238 (1961).
184. M. H. Shiu, D. Schottenfeld, and B. Maclean. Adverse effect of pregnancy on melanoma: A reappraisal, *Cancer 37*:181–187 (1976).
185. C. L. Slinguff and H. F. Seigler. Malignant melanoma and pregnancy, *Ann. Plast. Surg. 28*:95–99 (1992).
186. A. N. Houghton, J. Flannery, and M. V. Viola. Malignant melanoma occurring during pregnancy, *Cancer 48*:407–410 (1981).
187. D. S. Colbourn, L. Nathanson, and E. Belilos. Pregnancy and malignant melanoma, *Semin. Oncol. 16*:377–387 (1989).
188. D. S. Reintgen, K. S. McCarty, and R. Vollmer. Malignant melanoma and pregnancy, *Cancer 55*:1340–1344 (1985).
189. D. S. McManamny, A. L. H. Moss, and P. V. Pocock. Melanoma and pregnancy: A long-term follow-up, *Br. J. Obstet. Gynaecol. 96*:1419–1423 (1989).
190. J. H. Wong, E. E. Sterns, and K. H. Kopald. Prognostic significance of pregnancy in stage I melanoma, *Arch. Surg. 124*:1227–1231 (1989).
191. C. L. Slinguff, Jr., D. S. Reintgen, and R. T. Vollmer. Malignant melanoma arising during pregnancy: a study of 100 patients, *Ann. Surg. 211*:552–559 (1990).
192. R. M. MacKie, R. Bufalino, and A. Morabito. Lack of effect of pregnancy on outcome of melanoma, *Lancet 337*:653–655 (1991).
193. M. S. Driscoll, C. M. Grin-Jorgensen, and J. M. Grant-Kels. Does pregnancy influence the prognosis of malignant melanoma?, *J. Am. Acad. Dermatol. 29*:619–630 (1993).
194. E. Kjems and C. Krag. Melanoma and pregnancy, *Acta Oncol. 32*:371–378 (1993).
195. H. J. Hurley. Apocrine glands, *Dermatology in General Medicine*, 4th ed. (T. B. Fitzpatrick, A. Z. Eisen, K. Wolff, I. M. Freedberg, and K. F. Austen, eds.). McGraw-Hill, New York, 1993, pp. 753–766.
196. T. W. Turner. Hormonal levels in Fox-Fordyce disease, *Br. J. Dermatol. 94*:317–320 (1976).
197. *Dermatology* (O.Braun-Falco, G. Plewig, H. H. Wolff, and R. K. Winkelmann, eds.). Springer-Verlag, Berlin, 1991, pp. 744–746.
198. J. S. Strauss. Sebaceous glands, *Dermatology in General Medicine*, 4th ed. (T. B. Fitzpatrick, A. Z. Eisen, K. Wolff, I. M. Freedberg, and K. F. Austen, eds.). McGraw-Hill, New York, 1993, pp. 709–726.
199. O. Fyrand, H. J. Fiskaadal, and E. Trygstad. Acne in pubertal boys undergoing treatment with androgens, *Acta Derm. Venereol.* (*Stockh.*) *72*:148–149 (1992).
200. G. Plewig and A. M. Kligman. *Acne—Morphogenesis and Treatment*. Springer-Verlag, Berlin, 1975, p. 33.
201. J. S. Fitzsimmons, P. R. Guilbert, and E. M. Fitzsimmons. Evidence of genetic factors in hidradenitis suppurativa, *Br. J. Dermatol. 113*:1–8 (1985).
202. P. S. Mortimer, R. P. R. Dawber, M. A. Gales, and R. A. Moore. Medication of hidradenitis suppurativa by androgens, *Br. Med. J. 292*:245–248 (1986).
203. F. Lewis, A. G. Messenger, and J. K. H. Wales. Hidradenitis suppurativa as a presenting feature of premature adrenarche, *Br. J. Dermatol. 129*:447–448 (1993).
204. F. Gruneberg. Psoriasis and pregnancy, *Hautarzt 3*:155–159 (1982).
205. R. Church. The prospect of psoriasis, *Br. J. Dermatol. 70*:139–143 (1958).

206. M. Ostensen. The effect of pregnancy on ankylosing spondylitis, psoriatic arthritis, and juvenile rheumatoid arthritis. *Am. J. Reprod. Immunol. 28*:235–237 (1992).
207. F. Ott, A. Krakowski, and E. Tur. Impetigo herpetiformis with lowered serum level of vitamin D and its diminished intestinal absorption, *Dermatologica 164*:360–365 (1982).
208. M. Gligora and Z. Kolacio. Hormonal treatment of impetigo herpetiformis, *Br. J. Dermatol. 107*:253–256 (1982).
209. E. M. Farber and L. Nall. Pustular psoriasis, *Cutis 51*:29–32 (1993).
210. O. Y. Oumeish, S. E. Farraj, and A. S. Bataineh. Some aspects of impetigo herpetiformis, *Arch. Dermatol. 118*:103–105 (1982).
211. H. Gordon. Erythema nodosum. A review of cases, *Br. J. Dermatol. 73*:393–409 (1961).
212. F. Holcomb. Erythema nodosum associated with the use of oral contraception, *Obstet. Gynecol. 25*:136–157 (1965).
213. M. A. Salvatore and P. J. Lynch. Erythema nodosum, estrogens and pregnancy, *Arch. Dermatol. 116*:557–558 (1980).
214. J. A. Bartelsmeyer and R. H. Petric. Erythema nodosum, estrogens and pregnancy, *Clin. Obstet. Gynecol. 33*:777–781 (1990).
215. P. O. Fritsch and P. M. Elias. Erythema multiforme and toxic epidermal necrolysis, *Dermatology in General Medicine*, 4th ed. (T. B. Fitzpatrick, A. Z. Eisen, K. Wolff, I. M. Freedberg, and K. F. Austen, eds.). McGraw-Hill, New York, 1993, pp. 585–600.
216. M. Beckmann, D. Mühlenstedt, and R. Happle. Schwangerschaft und Entbindung beim hereditären angioneurotischen Ödem, *Geburtsh. Frauenheilk. 39*:338–340 (1979).
217. M. M. Frank, J. A. Gelfand, and G. P. Atkinson. Hereditary angioedema, the clinical syndrome and its management, *Ann. Intern. Med. 84*:580–593 (1976).
218. R. J. Stiller, B. M. Kaplan, and J. W. Andreoli. Hereditary angioedema and pregnancy, *Obstet. Gynecol. 64*:133–137 (1984).
219. M. Böckers and K. Bork. Kontrazeption und Schwangerschaft beim hereditären Angioödem, *Dtsch. Med. Wochenstr. 112*:507–509 (1987).

5

Skin Diseases Seriously Affecting Fetal Outcome and Maternal Health

Betty Bellman and Brian Berman
University of Miami School of Medicine, Miami, Florida

I. INTRODUCTION

Some cutaneous diseases during pregnancy run a benign course, whereas others are associated with significant maternal and/or fetal morbidity and mortality. Pregnant women are susceptible to the exacerbation of various skin diseases because of endocrine, hormonal, vascular, and immunological changes. This chapter initially focuses on diseases specifically associated with pregnancy: pruritus gravidarum, pruritic urticarial papules and plaques of pregnancy, herpes gestationis, impetigo herpetiformis, and papular dermatitis of pregnancy. We have also included cutaneous changes resulting from altered physiology and cutaneous tumors influenced by pregnancy such as malignant melanoma and cutaneous T-cell lymphoma. Finally, we discuss infectious skin diseases in pregnancy and the puerperium and other uncommon skin conditions affecting maternal and fetal outcome.

II. SKIN DISEASES SPECIFICALLY ASSOCIATED WITH PREGNANCY

Pregnant patients are no more affected by skin diseases than persons in the general population (1,2); however, a small group of dermatoses occur predominantly, if not exclusively, during pregnancy and the puerperium. These four conditions have a firm clinical, histological, or laboratory basis and stand out as distinct entities.

A. Pruritus Gravidarum

One of the most frequent cutaneous symptoms of pregnancy is pruritus. Itching occurs to some extent in approximately 17% of pregnant patients (2). This subjective symptom may seem out of proportion to the visible changes on the skin. Pruritus in the absence of a skin eruption may be generalized or localized to the abdominal, vulvar, or perianal areas. Pruritus may also be an associated symptom of many of the dermatoses of pregnancy or may be the result of any of the numerous causes of pruritus that occur in the nonpregnant state. Prurigo gestationis was first reported by Besnier and colleagues (3) in 1904, and it was clinically described by Nurse (4) in 1962 as "early onset prurigo of pregnancy." No maternal or fetal complications have been reported with prurigo gestationis (5).

Pruritus gravidarum is a condition in which there is intense generalized pruritus in the absence of any skin eruption. It is considered to be the result of a mild anicteric cholestasis resulting from disturbances of bilirubin excretion likely due to the effects of estrogens and progestins (6).

1. Incidence

The incidence of pruritus gravidarum is reported to be 0.02–3.0% worldwide; however, there have been higher rates reported in Chile (14%) (7).

2. Clinical Presentation

Pruritus gravidarum usually begins in the third trimester, with initial intermittent pruritus that is limited to the trunk, abdomen, and extremities. There are usually no other symptoms such as nausea, vomiting, or abdominal pain. Pruritus eventually becomes constant and generalized, leading to excoriations, particularly on the abdomen. Symptoms remit within a few days after delivery but tend to recur in subsequent pregnancies (8) or following oral contraceptive use. If the disorder progresses to cholestatic jaundice, icterus eventually may become detectable within 2–4 weeks after the onset of pruritus. The liver may become enlarged and tender, the urine darkens, and stools become clay colored.

3. Laboratory Diagnosis

The serum level of direct bilirubin may be normal or slightly increased and rarely exceeds 8 mg/dl. Mild to moderate transaminase elevations may be found. The most marked laboratory abnormality found in patients with significant obstetrical cholestasis is the serum concentration of bile acids. The most abnormally elevated acid is cholic acid. In fact, the measurement of cholic acid conjugates provides the most sensitive test for the diagnosis of obstetrical cholestasis (9). In rare instances, a liver biopsy may be required to substantiate the diagnosis of cholestasis and is reported to be as safe in pregnant women as in nonpregnant women (10). Systemic disorders such as thyroid dysfunction, diabetes, parasites, malignancy, and liver disease must be excluded as possible causes of pruritus.

4. Histology

Because there are no primary skin lesions in pruritus gravidarum, cutaneous histology has not been reported in pertinent reviews. Liver biopsy reveals nonspecific cholestasis with widely dilated, enlarged bile canaliculi, staining of parenchyma with bile pigments, and little to no inflammatory response (11). The abnormalities are completely reversible and do not lead to any permanent functional or structural hepatic damage.

5. Pathophysiology

The pruritus in pruritus gravidarum is caused by the elevated concentration of bile acids in the skin. The intensity of the pruritus does not always correlate with the serum bile acid levels. The increase in serum bile acids during pregnancy is related to a decreased capacity for hepatic excretion of organic anions such as bilirubin, bile acids, and bromsulfophthalein. In the genetically susceptible person, physiological concentrations of estrogens and progestins are believed to interfere with hepatic excretion of bile acids. Synthetic agents in oral contraceptives have also been shown to induce decreased hepatic function in women who developed cholestasis in earlier pregnancies (12).

6. Prognosis

Pruritus gravidarum subsides rapidly postpartum but may recur with variable severity in subsequent pregnancies or with the use of estrogen-containing medications. Restoration of normal liver function and structure may lag behind improved symptomatology by several weeks. Maternal morbidity is limited to the inconvenience caused by pruritus. The question of fetal prognosis is more controversial. The fetus usually suffers no ill effects. There is, however, a significantly higher incidence of premature labor, low birth weight babies, and postpartum hemorrhage in pregnancies complicated by severe frank obstetrical cholestasis (12,13). Pregnancy complicated only by pruritus may be associated with a tendency toward earlier delivery and meconium staining of amniotic fluid, which are features that can be considered less serious variations of those encountered with maternal jaundice (12,14). Fisk et al. reviewed 83 pregnancies complicated by cholestasis. Intrapartum distress occurred in 22% of their patients, and there was a 45% incidence of meconium-stained amniotic fluid and two stillbirths. Therefore, fetal monitoring may be necessary, and if it is warranted, amniocentesis to detect meconium fluid starting as early as 30 weeks' gestation. (15,16)

7. *Treatment*

Mild forms of pruritus gravidarum may be treated with bland antipruritic preparations. More severe cases may require ion-exchange resins, such as cholestyramine, which bind bile acids in the intestine. Cholestyramine is a nonresorbable resin and is considered to be harmless to the fetus (17). Cholestyramine will usually relieve pruritus within 2 weeks. Dosages of 12–16 g daily cause infrequent side effects. One of the adverse side effects of cholestyramine is malabsorption of fat-soluble vitamins. Profuse bleeding at delivery and an increased prothrombin time because of vitamin K deficiency have been reported in patients treated with cholestyramine (18,19). Prothrombin time should be measured periodically to evaluate vitamin K requirements.

B. Pruritic Urticarial Papules and Plaques of Pregnancy

Pruritic urticarial papules and plaques of pregnancy (PUPPP) was first described by Lawley and colleagues (20) in 1979. An intensive review of the literature suggests that a considerable overlap exists between PUPPP and several other eruptions that have been described to occur during pregnancy. These include toxemic rash of pregnancy (21), late-onset prurigo of pregnancy (4), and toxic erythema of pregnancy (22). Holmes and Black (23) introduced the term *polymorphic eruption of pregnancy* as a more accurate and descriptive name that would include these entities as well as PUPPP. Therefore, the dermatological and obstetrical literature has contained several reports that attach two names to what is now considered to be the same disease.

1. *Incidence*

Many cases of PUPPP have been reported (24–28) since its description. Apart from pruritus gravidarum, which has no clinical lesions, it is the most common dermatosis of pregnancy (20,29). Estimates of the incidence of PUPPP range between 1 in 120 pregnancies to 1 in 240 pregnancies (23).

2. *Clinical Presentation*

The skin eruption of PUPPP usually begins in the third trimester after the thirty-fourth week. The most frequent week of onset is the thirty-ninth week (28). Occasionally, PUPPP will develop in the immediate postpartum period. Generally, PUPPP is a disease of the first pregnancy (24,28), and most patients do not experience a recurrence in subsequent pregnancies. The lesions consist of pruritic erythematous papules that coalesce to form urticarial plaques. Papules may be surrounded by a pale halo and may blanch easily on pressure. Although pruritus is a major symptom of PUPPP, excoriations are rare. The eruption almost always begins on the abdomen, particularly in the abdominal striae (30,28). Lesions then spread over the next several days to involve the buttocks, waistline, thighs, lower thorax, lower back, and upper inner arms. The face usually is spared as well as the hands and feet and mucous membranes. The eruption generally clears within several weeks after delivery. No laboratory abnormalities have been detected in PUPPP, and the pathophysiology of the condition is unknown. Urticarial vasculitis during pregnancy can present within striae distensae, especially on the lower extremities, and therefore should be considered in the differential diagnosis of PUPPP (31).

3. *Histology*

Two histological patterns have been described in PUPPP (20): a superficial type that consists of perivascular lymphohistiocytic infiltration associated with some edema of the papillary dermis with local spongiosis, parakeratosis, and crusts in the epidermis; and a deeper pattern marked by an uninvolved epidermis and perivascular and interstitial infiltrates in the mid and deep dermis. The papillary dermis may be edematous and some eosinophils may be present in the infiltrate. Immunofluorescent studies are consistently negative (23).

4. *Prognosis*

The importance of recognizing PUPPP is to distinguish it from the more uncommon herpes gestationis which may be associated with fetal morbidity and mortality. In cases of early nonbullous urticarial herpes gestationis, the clinical appearance of both diseases can be similar. Histological and immunofluorescence examinations can be helpful in distinguishing between the two disorders.

5. *Treatment*

Pruritus is the major complaint of patients who have PUPPP, and almost all describe it to be severe enough to interfere with sleep. Most patients respond to mid- to high-potency topical steroid creams. Severe cases of PUPPP may require a brief course of systemic corticosteroids.

6. *Pathophysiology*

Immunological studies done on patients with PUPPP have not been helpful. The possibility of an autoimmune mechanism was postulated by Alcalay et al. (32); however, most of the serum autoantibodies and immunofluorescent results were negative. Cohen et al. studied 30 patients during a 5-year period and found a significantly increased maternal weight gain of 18.1 ± 0.9 kg in women with PUPPP versus 14.6 ± 1.0 kg for parity-matched controls (excluding twin gestation) (33). They also noted a significant increase in the mean newborn birth weight of 3.60 ± 0.09 kg for the PUPPP group versus 3.30 ± 0.08 kg in the control group. Thus, excessive maternal weight gain coupled with increased newborn birth weight may play a role in the etiology of PUPPP, because it increases abdominal girth. Cohen et al. suggest that the rapid distension of the abdomen, which is always involved, and trauma to abdominal skin may trigger the inflammatory response of PUPP. Unlike herpes gestationis, there appears to be no HLA association among patients with PUPP.

C. Herpes Gestationis

Herpes gestationis is a rare, pruritic recurrent urticarial and vesiculobullous skin disease of pregnancy and the puerperium. Diagnosis rests on a distinctive clinical presentation and specific histopathological and immunopathological findings. Herpes gestationis bears a close clinical and immunopathological similarity to bullous pemphigoid. On this basis, it has been proposed by various researchers that herpes gestationis be renamed *pemphigoid* gestationis (23).

Incidence. The incidence of herpes gestationis has been estimated as 1 in 3,000–60,000 pregnancies (15,17,34,35).

1. Clinical Presentation

The onset of the disease is anywhere from the first trimester of pregnancy to the first 5 days of the postpartum period. It is most common during the second trimester (36), with an average time of onset of 21 weeks (37). The disease may begin with a prodrome of malaise, fever, nausea, headache, and alternate hot and cold sensations. Burning and severe pruritus may precede the eruption by several days. The earliest skin lesions are erythematous edematous papules and plaques with an urticarial quality. These plaques may assume circinate configurations and have a predilection for the trunk, especially the abdomen, and in particular the umbilical area. Within days, papules, vesicles, and tense bullae develop. Target lesions like those of erythema multiforme sometimes appear. The eruption may also involve the buttocks, back, forearms, palms, and soles. The mucous membranes are uncommon sites for lesions. Bilateral symmetry is not a constant feature and lesions may spread centrifugally. With rupture of the bullae or vesicles, denuded areas become covered with a brownish yellow or hemorrhagic crust. Bacterial infection and excoriations may be present. Resolution of lesions leaves little or transient hyperpigmentation, but deep excoriations may leave scars. Transverse pitting and grooving of fingernails and toenails may be observed corresponding to the time of onset of the eruption.

The clinical course of herpes gestationis is one of recurring crops of blisters, which, if untreated, usually resolve within a few days to 3 months postpartum. The dermatosis may wane in late pregnancy and exacerbation occurs with delivery in approximately 75% of the cases (38). Cases that have spontaneously resolved during pregnancy or that have lasted as long as 2 years after delivery have been reported (39).

2. *Histology*

Histologically, the urticarial lesions of herpes gestationis are characterized by a moderately dense, perivascular, mixed, inflammatory cell infiltrate of lymphocytes, histiocytes, and eosinophils around the vessels of the superficial and deep dermal plexuses. There is papillary dermal edema, spongiosis, and focal necrosis of basal cells over the tips of the dermal papillae (36). Eosinophils may be found in spongiotic foci within the epidermis. Neutrophils may be present in the dermal infiltrate in small numbers. Bullous lesions are the result of subepidermal separation with the basal lamina forming the floor of the blister (40). Eosinophils are usually found within blister fluid. The presence of eosinophils is the most constant histological feature of herpes gestationis, being seen in nearly every case (23).

Direct immunofluorescence of lesions of herpes gestationis reveals the third component of complement to be deposited at the dermal-epidermal junction in a linear pattern, with or without immunoglobulin G (IgG). Less commonly IgA, IgM, C1, C2, C4, C5, and properdin are present. Ten percent of patients have IgG deposits at the dermal-epidermal junction visible on direct immunofluorescence.

Immunoelectron microscopy has demonstrated a fairly uniform deposition of reaction products throughout the lamina lucida that contrasts only slightly with findings in bullous pemphigoid. The events leading to these findings may occur by the generation of IgG antibody reacting against the basement membrane zone of the skin. The antigen apparently is a component of the lamina lucida and may be identical to the antigen of bullous pemphigoid. Because there is so much more C3 than IgG present at the basement membrane zone, C3 is detectable by direct immunofluorescence, whereas IgG usually is not.

Fewer than 20% of patients have circulating skin-reactive IgG antibodies, as detected by routine indirect immunofluorescence (41). Herpes gestationis factor is present in the sera of most patients and can induce exogenous complement (C3) to be deposited at the basement membrane zone of normal skin or mucous membranes, as detected by a technique called complement indirect immunofluorescence. Recent studies have shown that herpes gestationis factor is most likely an IgG, but it is usually not demonstrable on routine direct immunofluorescence and is not demonstrable in the sera of all patients. (42) In fact, herpes gestationis factor titers, although playing a role in causing the disease, correlate poorly with disease activity.

3. *Pathophysiology*

Herpes gestationis may be induced by placental antigens that cross react with the skin. Experimental support exists for the hypothesis that Ortonne et al. (43), using complement-fixing immunofluorescence and immune electron microscopy, showed herpes gestationis factor could bind to the basement membrane zone of the amnion and chorion laeve of the placenta. Kelly et al. (44) have also shown that antibody binds to the amnion layers and to the umbilical cord. Women with herpes gestationis have evidence of abnormal immune reactions within their placental villi, which may lead to placental insufficiency causing the increased incidence of prematurity and low birth weights (38).

Eosinophils may play an important role in herpes gestationis, because there often is striking tissue eosinophilia and frequent peripheral blood eosinophilia in patients who have herpes gestationis. The presence of products of eosinophil degranulation in lesional skin suggests their role in the tissue damage in herpes gestationis.

4. *Differential Diagnosis*

Herpes gestationis can be differentiated from the other specific dermatoses of pregnancy, because it is the only such condition that produces bullae. Early urticarial lesions of herpes gestationis may resemble PUPPP, leading some clinicians to suggest performing direct immunofluorescence in all cases of presumed PUPPP to rule out the possibility of herpes gestationis (35). They point to the occurrence of urticarial herpes gestationis without blisters during one pregnancy followed by typical bullous disease during subsequent pregnancies. Herpes gestationis must be differentiated from other bullous diseases that may coincidentally occur during pregnancy: bullous pemphigoid, pemphigus, dermatitis herpetiformis, bullous drug eruption, and erythema multiforme.

5. *Treatment*

Therapeutic goals in herpes gestationis include controlling maternal blister formation and pruritus and lessening the risks for fetal complications. Treatment of mild cases may require only antihistamines and topical steroids, but most patients will require the use of systemic corticosteroids. The preferred treatment for more severe disease is prednisone 40–60 mg/day in divided doses, which may be tapered and modified to an alternate-day schedule once clearing is achieved. Cases unresponsive to oral corticosteroids require immunosuppressive agents such as azathioprine. Azathioprine should not be given during pregnancy without weighing risk versus benefit. Plasmapheresis has been used successfully in herpes gestationis as well. Postpartum flare-ups, which are not uncommon, often require aggressive therapy.

6. *Course and Prognosis*

Herpes gestationis is a disease of exacerbations and remissions. Clearing generally occurs within 3 months of delivery. Exacerbations have occurred prior to normal menses and following the use of progesterone-containing oral contraceptives (45). The disease usually occurs in subsequent pregnancies, with a tendency for earlier onset and more severe manifestations. Maternal prognosis is usually excellent in the absence of secondary infection or steroid therapy side effects.

The question of whether herpes gestationis is associated with significant fetal morbidity and mortality has been debated. Holmes et al. did not find an increased tendency for stillbirths or neonatal death in 24 patient cases (22). Similar findings were noted by Shornick et al. (38), who determined the rate of spontaneous abortion to be 13% of 28 cases of herpes gestationis (10–15% is cited as the rate in the normal population). Herpes gestationis is associated with an increase in prematurity and small-for-gestational-age infants (38), and recent studies using immunological criteria suggest an increased risk of stillbirths and prematurity (46–48).

In the majority of cases, transmission of the herpes gestationis factor antibody from mother to fetus occurs asymptomatically for the infant. However, cutaneous involvement of the newborn of an affected mother occurs in only 10% of cases (38). The lesions may be present at birth or appear within hours or by the third day of life. They vary from fleeting erythematous papules to frank bullae and spontaneously regress by 3 weeks of age. No correlations have been made between the occurrence of skin lesions in the newborn and the maternal serum antibody titer (49). Interestingly, positive immunofluorescence results from newborn skin biopsy specimens in the absence of clinically apparent disease have been demonstrated repeatedly (35).

D. Impetigo Herpetiformis

Impetigo herpetiformis is a rare but serious generalized pustular eruption resembling pustular psoriasis. Although originally described by von Hebra in 1872 as a disease specific for pregnancy, impetigo herpetiformis may occur in nonpregnant women and male patients. Hypoparathyroidism and hypocalcemia are frequently associated with impetigo herpetiformis whether the patient is pregnant or not. Interestingly, some patients with impetigo herpetiformis have a family history of psoriasis (15), but the clinical significance of such an association is unknown; however, impetigo herpetiformis has been considered to be a variant of psoriasis.

1. *Incidence*

Impetigo herpetiformis is a rare entity with just under 200 reported cases in the world literature (50).

2. *Clinical Presentation*

The onset of impetigo herpetiformis in pregnant women is from late in the first trimester to the end of the third trimester. Peak incidence occurs in the last 3 months of gestation. Impetigo herpetiformis affects pregnant women who usually have no personal or family history of psoriasis. The disease usually recurs with every successive pregnancy and recurs earlier and with increased morbidity.

Cutaneous lesions of impetigo herpetiformis begin as irregular patches or slightly raised plaques of erythema with peripherally studded superficial white to greenish yellow sterile pustules which may become secondarily infected. These areas of involvement gradually enlarge by peripheral extension of the annular margin, whereas the more central areas are broken down, becoming denuded or crusted. The eruption may become confluent, so that in severe cases, the entire skin surface (save the hands, feet, and face) may be covered with active pustules or older crusted lesions.

Usually, cutaneous lesions of impetigo herpetiformis first involve the intertriginous regions such as the groin, axillae, inframammary folds, gluteal crease, and umbilicus. Lesions also occur commonly on the medial thighs and lower abdomen. In flexural areas, moist vegetating plaques may resemble pemphigus vegetans. Lesions generally heal without scarring, although postinflammatory hyperpigmentation is regularly seen. Subungual pustules may cause onycholysis. Mucous membrane lesions have been reported to involve the oral and esophageal mucosa. These pustules leave painful erosions arranged in a circinate pattern.

Pruritus is not usually a problem in impetigo herpetiformis. Severe constitutional symptoms are present in a majority of cases and include fever, chills, nausea, vomiting, prostration, and diarrhea. Delirium, tetany, and convulsions may occur and are frequent in cases associated with hypocalcemia.

3. *Histology*

The histology of impetigo herpetiformis is in many respects identical to that of pustular psoriasis. The characteristic lesion is the spongiform pustule of Kogoj, a spongelike cavity containing a collection of neutrophils in the epidermis. Pierard et al. (51) found histological differences from pustular psoriasis. The pustules did not show any tendency to confluence and they contained both neutrophils and mononuclear cells that had abundant cytoplasm and large, irregularly shaped nuclei. Parakeratosis, with regular elongation of rete ridges, and migration of mononuclear cells from dermal capillaries into the epidermis may also be seen.

4. *Laboratory Diagnosis*

Leukocytosis with a left shift and an elevated erythrocyte sedimentation rate are seen during severe exacerbations of impetigo herpetiformis. Bacterial culture of pus from the lesions or peripheral blood are negative providing no infection is present. Hypocalcemia secondary to hypoparathyroidism is found in some patients, and one may find albuminuria, pyuria, and hematuria. (15)

5. *Pathophysiology*

Whether or not impetigo herpetiformis is a variant of pustular psoriasis triggered by the metabolic state of pregnancy or a disease sui generis is unclear. Those who consider impetigo herpetiformis as a true dermatosis of pregnancy point out that between pregnancies affected patients are free from the skin disorder and often have no prior manifestations or history of psoriasis, whereas the majority of patients with pustular psoriasis, both pregnant and nonpregnant, have had preexisting typical or atypical psoriasis.

6. *Differential Diagnosis*

Impetigo herpetiformis must be differentiated from other pustular conditions such as pustular psoriasis, candidiasis, subcorneal pustular dermatosis, impetigo, dermatitis herpetiformis, and herpes gestationis. Another dermatosis of pregnancy having a pustule as a primary lesion is pruritic folliculitis of pregnancy, which has no serious sequelae for mother or child.

7. *Treatment*

Corticosteroids are the treatment of choice for impetigo herpetiformis but most clinicians report only moderate responses to these agents (52). Lotem et al. (52) reported a case in which improvement after delivery failed to occur until complete removal of all pregnancy products was established. In classic pustular psoriasis, systemic corticosteroids have an immediate therapeutic effect. Fluid and electrolyte balance should be maintained and hypocalcemia corrected if present.

8. *Course and Prognosis*

Prior to the use of corticosteroids and antibiotics, a gloomy maternal prognosis for impetigo herpetiformis was common. Maternal mortality is now rare, but stillbirth and placental insufficiency may still occur even when the disease appears to be controlled with corticosteroids. The more severe and long-standing the impetigo herpetiformis, the greater the risks of placental insufficiency leading to stillbirth, neonatal death, or fetal abnormalities (53). The disease remits promptly postpartum, usually without residual psoriatic plaques, but may recur in successive pregnancies.

E. Papular Dermatitis of Pregnancy

Papular dermatitis of pregnancy (PDP) was described by Spangler et al. (54) in 1962. It has since received attention because of the investigators' contention of increased fetal risk. Subsequent analysis of this report has revealed that the fetal mortality data were overestimated and were presented in a way that has precluded valid reassessment (23).

Spangler and associates (54) may have represented severe cases of prurigo gestationis or PUPPP. Incidentally, a large number of patients in Spangler's series were Rh negative, and the high incidence of fetal loss may have been related to that condition (15). We include it in this chapter but question whether it truly represents a specific dermatosis of pregnancy.

1. *Incidence*

PDP is rare and is estimated by Spangler to have an incidence of 1 per 2500 pregnancies (55).

2. *Clinical Presentation*

The onset of PDP has been reported from the first to the last month of pregnancy. It is characterized by generalized, intensely pruritic papules involving all areas of the body and may involve the face and scalp. Individual lesions are 3- to 5-mm soft erythematous edematous papules topped by slightly firmer acuminate papules. These are often scratched off, leaving a hemorrhagic crust. Lesions appear gradually rather than in crops, so that three to eight lesions may appear daily, whereas older lesions may heal in 7–10 days with slight hyperpigmentation and no true scarring. Delivery abruptly terminates the eruption with clearing of lesions within days. The dermatitis tends to recur in subsequent pregnancies.

3. *Laboratory Diagnosis*

In 12 patients with PDP studied by Spangler and Emerson (55), urinary chorionic gonadotropin levels were greatly increased in the last trimester. Low urinary estriol, low plasma by hydrocortisone, and reduced plasma hydrocortisone halflife were also reported. Histopathology has not been reported.

4. *Pathophysiology*

The eruption of PDP improves abruptly after delivery. The one exception to this pattern occurred when the dermatitis persisted for 6 weeks' postpartum, after which time a placental fragment retained in the uterus was discovered. The rash subsequently disappeared after curettage.

5. *Course and Prognosis*

No maternal complications have occurred in PDP, yet controversy surrounds the disease because of the 27% incidence of fetal stillbirths and spontaneous abortions reported by Spangler and associates (54) in their initial study. The prognosis has made dermatologists reluctant to diagnose prurigo eruptions as PDP. Review of Spangler's data by Winton (30) reveals that the 27% incidence of fetal death included all pregnancies of the initial study group regardless of the presence of PDP. When only those pregnancies associated with the rash are considered, the incidence of fetal death was considerably lower (12.5%).

6. *Treatment*

Spangler and Emerson (55) found that diethylstilbestrol (DES) in doses of 1000–2500 mg per day controlled PDP. The subsequent discovery of genital adenocarcinoma in the offspring of mothers given DES during pregnancy has led to the avoidance of this therapy. Systemic corticosteroids are usually effective; however, doses up to 100 mg per day may be required to control the disease and reduce fetal loss to 12% or less (2,55). Topical corticosteroids may control the eruption and should be the first line of treatment.

III. SKIN DISEASES NOT RESTRICTED TO PREGNANCY

A. Varicosities

Vascular changes during pregnancy lead to vessel proliferation, resulting in vascular spiders (spider nevi, spider angiomas), and to vasomotor instability and congestion which may cause gingival hyperemia and vestibular congestion (Jacquemier-Chadwick sign). Palmar erythema is seen in approximately 66% of pregnant patients. These skin and mucous membrane changes are generally cosmetic in nature and of limited duration.

Varicosities, most frequently of the saphenous, vulvar, and hemorrhoidal veins, appear in 40% of pregnant women (2). They are a result of increased venous pressure in the femoral and pelvic vessels caused by the gravid uterus. A familial tendency for varicose veins may also be important. Varicosities tend to regress after delivery but often not completely. Hemorrhoidal varicosities are also common and may cause pain and bleeding. Deep venous thrombosis (DVT) has been reported to occur in 0.018–0.29% of all deliveries. The period of greatest risk for thrombosis and embolism appears to be the immediate puerperium, especially after cesarean delivery. Postpartum DVT occurs 3–5 times more than antepartum DVT and is 3–16 times more common after cesarean section (56). Signs of DVT include pain, swelling, a palpable cord, and a positive Homan sign of the involved limb. There is usually a 2-cm measured difference in circumference between the affected versus the normal limbs. Thrombi in larger veins with fewer valves may be clinically silent and have a greater chance of embolization. Symptomatic or occult pulmonary embolism may occur.

Pregnancy is a hypercoagulable state with an increased potential for thrombosis. Risk factors include a previous history of thromboembolism (5–15% recurrence risk), operative delivery, immobilization, protein C or S deficiency, obesity, older age, and pelvic trauma. Autoimmune disorders may be linked to thrombosis, fetal death, and pregnancy loss (56). Diagnosis can be made by noninvasive duplex Doppler.

B. Cutaneous Tumors Influenced by Pregnancy

1. *Cutaneous Hemangiomas*

Cutaneous hemangiomas may develop and enlarge during pregnancy (57). In view of the effects of gestational hormones on vascular structures, the association of pregnancy with the spontaneous development of hemangioma, hemangioendothelioma, and glomus tumor is not surprising (30). Vascular tumors generally arise in the second or third trimesters, increase in size, and regress after delivery (57). Large hemangiomas resulting in arteriovenous shunting have been reported with subsequent high-output cardiac failure (30). These lesions regress postpartum only partially, tending to enlarge again in subsequent pregnancies (57). Small lesions need not be treated if cosmetically acceptable but may be treated by electrodesiccation or laser therapy after delivery.

2. *Eruptive Xanthomas*

Eruptive xanthomas may occur during pregnancy in association with hypertriglyceridemia. The added stimulus of increased estrogens during pregnancy may play a role in the elevation of triglycerides. Complications include severe pancreatitis which can result in adult respiratory distress syndrome and fetal loss (58). Acute pancreatitis during pregnancy may carry a mortality rate of 21%. Treatment consists of dietary restriction, cholestyramine, and nicotinic acid.

3. *Neurofibromatosis*

Von Recklinghausen neurofibromatosis (NF) is an autosomal dominantly inherited disorder with a markedly variable expression. This disease may be inherited from a patient who has NF or may be the result of new, spontaneous mutation in the developing fetus. Each child of an affected parent has a 50% chance of inheriting the disease and of developing some stigmata of NF (59). Neurofibromatosis is relatively common, with a frequency of about 1 in 3000 births (60). Café au lait spots are present in well over 99% of patients who have neurofibromatosis. Crowe et al. (60) designated the presence of six or more café au lait spots larger than 1.5 cm in diameter in adults as a criterion in their study.

Neurofibromas always involve the skin; however, they may occur in deeper peripheral nerves and nerve roots in or on viscera and blood vessels innervated by the autonomic system. Neurofibromas of the skin and elsewhere increase in size and number in both sexes at puberty and in women during pregnancy (61,62). Although lacking a specific rationalization for this feature, the accumulation of intercellular glycosaminoglycans has been suggested as the cause (63), as has the stimulation of neurofibroma growth by sex steroids, directly by or through mediation of nerve-growth factor (64). Lesions may show a complete or partial regression following delivery (62).

Strange (65) and Ansari and Nagamani (62) have reported cases that typify the serious effects that pregnancy can have on patients who have NF as a result of enlargement of neurofibromas. They described a patient who had large neurofibromatous lesions that enlarged greatly during the latter part of pregnancy as the result of massive hemorrhage within the tumors. In addition, the patient developed partial paralysis of the lower extremities either because of the enlargement of a preexisting intraspinal lesion or because of the development of new intraspinal neurofibromas.

Although rare, vascular changes with subsequent hypertension in NF may occur (66). The association of NF and hypertension during pregnancy has been reported by Swapp and Main (67), who reported 24 pregnancies. Eleven of these patients had neurofibromatosis; 10 of these patients developed hypertension. In five patients, lesions of neurofibromatosis appeared for the first time during pregnancy. In the others, café au lait macules and neurofibromas increased in size and number, and the nodules regressed considerably after delivery. The investigators postulated that patients who have NF could not expand their intravascular space adequately because of diseased arterioles (atrophy of the media and elastic layer) and, therefore, could not accommodate the increased plasma volume, red cell mass, and cardiac output of pregnancy, thus inducing hypertension. Jarvis and Crompton (13), in a study of 27 pregnancies of 10 patients who had NF, could not confirm a higher incidence of hypertension. Ansari and Nagamani (62) suggested that there is an increased incidence of abortion and stillbirth in NF; however, this has not been confirmed in other studies (30).

Based on the well-documented severe deformity and disability which may be precipitated by pregnancy, and the autosomal dominant mode of inheritance by the fetus, genetic counseling is mandatory for the family. Elective interruption of pregnancy at an early stage or elective tubal ligation to prevent future pregnancies may considered on a case by case basis.

4. *Melanocytic Nevi and Melanoma*

During pregnancy, there may be increased growth and darkening of existing melanocytic nevi, with occasional production of new, small, flat, brown nevi.

Fortunately, most of these lesions are benign and do not require treatment. Those of sufficient cosmetic and diagnostic concern should be excised completely and examined histologically. The influence of pregnancy on melanoma is controversial. Malignant melanoma not infrequently presents during the active reproductive years of women, and the effects of pregnancy on the course of the disease can be of considerable concern and controversy. The estimated incidence of malignant melanoma ranges from 0.14 to 2.8 cases per 1000 deliveries (68), making it one of the most frequent cancers occurring during pregnancy.

Although melanoma is not generally regarded as a hormone-dependent neoplasm (such as mammary carcinoma), circumstantial evidence suggests that endocrine factors may have a bearing on the tumor's biological behavior. Case reports of rapidly growing tumors, the appearance of multiple primary tumors, and malignant transformation of congenital and dysplastic nevi during pregnancy point toward an unfavorable impact of estrogens on melanoma, especially with the regression of metastases after delivery (69,70). It has recently been demonstrated that estrogen can bind to melanoma cells in a nonspecific manner. Feucht et al. identified a specific estrogen-binding protein in three human melanoma lines. Chronic exposure to estradiol resulted in slowed tumor growth, suggesting that estradiol may have indirect effects on melanoma cells in addition to receptor-mediated effects (71). Shaw et al. (72), in a retrospective study of 938 women who had melanoma, found that endocrine influences in patients who have melanoma may be complicated by tumor formation and metastases as well as in the distribution of the anatomical site of the primary lesion. They found no adverse effect on the survival rate among 17 patients who were pregnant at the time of diagnosis of their melanoma. They also noted that patients not exposed to high circulating levels of endogenous or exogenous estrogens (e.g., nulliparous women and postmenopausal women) had more widespread disease initially and a lower 5-year survival rate than women who were exposed to high levels of endogenous or exogenous estrogens. These findings led the investigators to suggest that estrogens may play a protective role in the development and progression of melanoma. Multiparity seems to confer a protective effect. The demonstration of an increased amount of melanocyte-stimulating hormone (MSH) in the blood and urine of pregnant women heightened the clinical suspicion of an adverse hormonal influence, although a direct association between MSH and melanoma was not found (73,74). George et al. (75), in a study of 115 cases of pregnancy coinciding with melanoma, failed to substantiate this impression and found no statistically significant difference in prognosis compared with a control group of 330 nonpregnant women who had melanoma. Other studies have substantiated these findings (76,77).

In 1975, Shiu et al. (78) retrospectively reviewed 251 surgically treated cases of cutaneous melanoma in women of childbearing age. Their study revealed a statistically significant difference in prognosis of melanoma in some patients with associated pregnancy, depending on the clinical stage of the disease. No statistical difference in survival at 5 years, free of disease, could be demonstrated in melanoma between nulliparous, parous, nonpregnant, and pregnant women. For stage II melanoma, however, a significantly lower survival rate was observed for pregnant patients (29%) and parous women who had experienced activation (ulceration, bleeding, itching, scaling, elevation) of the lesion in a previous pregnancy (22%) compared with nulliparous patients (55%) and other patients in the parous group (51%). The investigators suggested that a lack of deleterious effects of pregnancy on stage I melanoma could be explained by the probable total surgical eradication compared with stage II melanoma in which occult foci could carry a potential for recrudescence stimulated by pregnancy. Melanomas occurring on the trunk were also found to occur in greater frequency among the pregnant patients (78).

Slingluff et al. studied 100 patients diagnosed with melanoma during pregnancy, who were followed for a mean of 6.8 years. When compared with a nonpregnant female population with melanoma, there was a significantly shorter disease-free interval for the pregnant group, with nodal metastases developing in 48% of the pregnant patients and only 26% of the nonpregnant patients at a 10-year follow-up. Thus, pregnancy at the time of diagnosis of malignant melanoma was significantly associated with the development of metastatic disease (79).

Despite all evidence, no conclusive data exist to support the belief that pregnancy has inevitable adverse effects on malignant melanomas. Until such data are available, it is wise to deal with each case individually with the knowledge that there have been cases in which, directly or indirectly, pregnancy did or did not affect the course of the neoplasm adversely. Therapeutic abortion, oophorectomy, adrenalectomy, or hypophysectomy is not advocated, because no evidence exists to show that these measures improve the outcome of melanoma. The disease should be treated alike in nonpregnant and pregnant patients (80).

Observations made in the study by Shiu et al. (78) suggest that, for stage II melanoma, pregnancy, even after treatment for melanoma, may be hazardous. It has been suggested that a waiting period of 2–3 years after melanoma diagnosis before attempting pregnancy, because the majority of recurrences develop thicker tumors within 3 years of diagnosis. For those patients who have had activation of a lesion in a previous gestation, it would seem wise to counsel against subsequent pregnancies. The use of oral contraceptives in those patients likewise would be unwise until the cellular effects of estrogen and progesterone on melanoma are better understood (78). Two of four studies (81,82) comparing oral contraceptive use in women who had melanoma and in those who did not found use to be significantly greater statistically in the melanoma group.

The best treatment of melanoma is prevention. Prenatal examination of the mother should include a survey of all pigmented nevi at the first antenatal examination. Careful observation should be made of changes in size, alteration in uniformity or intensity of pigmentation, ulceration, pain, or bleeding at the site of any nevus. Attention should be given to irregular borders, elevations, shading of red, white, or blue, and especially changes in a preexisting pigmented lesion. Special evaluation should be given to lesions on the trunk, palms, soles, and vulvar area. The development of a new mole adjacent to one already present may be another indication of possible malignancy. All suspicious lesions should be examined by an experienced dermatologist, biopsied, and sent for histopathological analysis.

The treatment of primary melanoma is surgical excision with wide margins. Elective lymph node dissection has been controversial. Metastatic disease has been very resistant to many forms of therapy. Dacarbazine is the agent of choice for the initial treatment of metastatic disease; however, maternal salvage must be balanced against fetal risks. In some instances, early delivery of the infant may be necessary so that chemotherapy can be used as palliative therapy (68). Metastatic lesions to the fetus and placenta are very rare occurrences. Gross and microscopic examination of the placenta should be performed on all pregnant patients diagnosed with malignant melanoma.

5. *Carcinoid Tumors*

Carcinoid tumors are rare; however, 22 cases associated with pregnancy have been reported. Most cases were appendiceal in origin and did not cause problems for either mother or fetus. However, the presence of metastatic disease with resulting carcinoid syndrome may cause serious maternal and fetal complications and fetal death (83). Cutaneous manifestations of carcinoid syndrome include flushing affecting the face and upper extremities which is transient in nature and a persistent erythema with or without telangiectases. Less common manifestations include sclerodermalike change, pigment anomalies, and a pellagralike dermatitis (84).

6. *Cutaneous T-Cell Lymphoma*

Cutaneous T-cell lymphoma (CTCL) may flare during pregnancy with the development of secondarily infected eczematous lesions and the appearance of new infiltrated plaques (85). Treatment of CTCL during pregnancy with cytotoxic agents is contraindicated, especially during the first trimester. Mechlorethamine is also contraindicated, because it may cause fetal malformations.

C. Infectious Skin Diseases in Pregnancy and the Puerperium

1. *Condylomata Acuminata*

Condylomata acuminata (genital warts) are fleshy verrucae that occur at mucocutaneous junctions and intertriginous areas as soft, flesh-colored, pedunculated or polypoid nodules. In some patients, particularly young women, these lesions multiply and coalesce into large cauliflowerlike masses. Condylomata acuminata are caused by a human papilloma virus (HPV) antigenically related to the agents for common skin warts (verruca vulgaris) and may be transmitted by sexual contact (venereal warts) or may be associated with other forms of verrucae. Condylomata acuminata must be differentiated from the moist, wide-based 1- to 3-cm plaquelike papular or nodular lesions of secondary syphilis (condylomata lata) that occur in similar anatomical sites.

Pregnancy appears to act as a stimulus to the growth or enlargement, sometimes to massive size, of condylomata acuminata (86–90). There is no widely accepted explanation for the propensity of these leions to enlarge during pregnancy. Suggested explanations include increased vascularity, increased perineal moisture, and stimulation by elevated estrogen levels, because spontaneous resolution of warts may occur after pregnancy (87). Any consideration during pregnancy must be taken with two aspects in mind: the management of pregnancy itself and the treatment of the disease. Severe hemorrhage, an extended febrile course, sepsis, and even death have been reported as results of massive condylomata acuminata of the vulva complicating labor (86). Condylomata may grow to such an extent as to cause mechanical obstruction of the birth canal, resulting in swelling, bleeding, pain, dysuria, and trauma during vaginal delivery. There is an increased risk of infection, most commonly with fusospirochetal, streptococcal, and staphylococcal organisms. Perinatal infection may ensue, with premature rupture of the fetal membranes and chorioamnionitis (91). If a cesarean section is not to be performed, surgical removal of the condylomata may be required to avoid a vaginal delivery through large, partially necrotic and infected lesions. Surgical treatment of large vascular condylomata should not be attempted when the risks of removal are greater than the risk of an elective cesarean section.

The inadequacies and danger of conservative therapy of larger growths through the long practice of applying 25% podophyllin are well described (92,93). Podophyllin therapy during pregnancy is contraindicated, because this agent has been associated with maternal toxicity, premature labor, and fetal death following absorption of the antimitotic resin into the maternal circulation. Podophyllin can produce bizarre histological forms of epithelial cells that can be indistinguishable from those of squamous cell carcinoma; thus biopsies of the cervix and vulva should be done before treatment(s) are instituted. Fluorouracil creams and treatment with interferon alpha are contraindicated in pregnancy.

Massive lesions are best treated by electrodesiccation and curettage or by laser therapy under general or spinal anesthesia (94). Surgical removal of large warts in pregnant women is difficult, because the lesions are highly vascular and hemostasis often is difficult to achieve. Postoperative vulvar edema is the most common complication, but this responds rapidly to supportive therapy. Associated vaginitis should be treated vigorously, and systemic antibiotics should be used to treat infected lesions before undertaking therapy. Although sometimes effective for small lesions

(95), cryosurgery generally is not effective in lesions massive enough to require therapy during pregnancy (94). Carbon dioxide laser photocoagulation and vaporization resulted in 80% of patients cured after a single treatment, and there was a 91% cure rate with multiple treatments (96). Trichloroacetic acid is one of the treatments of choice, because it is not absorbed systemically and denatures on contact with tissue. Electrocautery can also be used safely during pregnancy; however, care must be exercised to avoid excess tissue destruction which may result in scarring (91).

The strongest evidence implicating HPV infections in the pathogenesis of genital tract malignancies comes from investigations of human tissues with molecular hybridization techniques. Beckmann et al. (97) tested 32 women with a history of multicentric squamous cell carcinoma of the anogenital region for the presence of HPV with polymerase chain reaction (PCR) or DNA hybridization technique. In 28 of 32 women, HPV was detected at all sites (most frequently types 6, 16, and 33). Two hundred and forty-five women with vulvar condylomata were studied over a 4-year period. Eighteen patients were diagnosed with vulvar intraepithelial neoplasia, grade 3, and four patients were diagnosed with invasive carcinoma (91). Therefore, it is important to biopsy genital condylomata, because it is not possible to differentiate clinically between benign and malignant lesions.

2. *Recurrent Respiratory Papillomatosis*

Recurrent respiratory papillomatosis (RRP) can develop as a result of perinatal vertical transmission of human papilloma virus (HPV) transmitted via neonatal aspiration of vaginal secretions during vaginal delivery (98). Neonates appear to be at greater risk of HPV infection in the oropharyngeal tract than in the genital region. HPV types 6 and 11 appear to be the primary types that have been detected in RRP. A report by Cook et al. (99) associated maternal genital warts with the development of infant laryngeal papillomas in nine patients, and they suggest that the virus of genital warts (papilloma virus types 6 and 11) may be acquired at birth by neonates who subsequently develop papillomas of the larynx. Seventy-two women were tested during the third trimester and again during labor prior to delivery for the presence of HPV-DNA in exfoliated cevical cells. These results were compared with swabs from the oropharyngeal cavity and genitalia of neonates 24–72 hr after delivery. Eighteen percent (13 of 72) of the mothers were found to be HPV positive, and 2.8% (2/72) of the neonates tested positive for HPV from the oropharyngeal secretions, supporting the hypothesis that RRP may develop as a result of perinatal vertical transmission of HPV. Prepartum treatment of HPV lesions may not protect against the neonatal acquisition of HPV.

Complications of RRP can be severe or fatal, and they include hoarseness, airway obstruction, and recurrent disease (100). There is a prolonged latency period between infection and clinically obvious lesions, making the true incidence of RRP difficult to estimate. However, the incidence in the pediatric population is thought to be seven new cases of RRP annually per million persons. Adult-onset disease comprises up to 40% of all RRP cases (91).

3. *Candidiasis*

a. Monilial Vaginitis and Vulvitis. Monilial vaginitis and vulvitis occurs 10–20 times more frequently during pregnancy, and the neonates of affected women are susceptible to developing candidiasis (57,101). Pregnancy seems to predispose to monilial vaginitis, perhaps because of the effect of glycosuria on vaginal acidity (102) and the altered hormonal milieu in which elevated estrogen levels favor the growth of *Candida albicans* (103). It has been estimated that 25% of pregnant women suffer from candidal vulvovaginitis and that up to 50% of their offspring show clinical signs of mucocutaneous candidiasis (104). Possibly for the same reason, monilial vaginitis appears more frequently in women who take progestins for contraceptive purposes or for the treatment of endometriosis (102). Broad-spectrum antibiotics that radically alter the bacterial flora of the vagina also predispose to monilial infection.

Acute vulvitis due to infection by *C. albicans* sometimes accompanies primary monilial vaginal infections but may also occur after secondary monilial colonization of macerated lesions of intertrigo and pruritus ani et vulvae. Candidal vulvitis presents with itching, burning, soreness, and painful micturition and is associated with a thick, creamy white vaginal discharge. Typically, a beefy red, moist erythema of the vaginal mucous membranes exists with the vulval skin being flecked with a curdy white discharge. There may be spread onto the perineum, perianal region, gluteal folds, and upper inner aspects of the thighs. In extensive involvement, subcorneal pustules may be seen at the periphery of the fringed irregular margin of the moist areas.

The diagnosis of monilial vaginitis is established by the clinical signs and symptoms and by demonstration of the pseudohyphae of the yeast by potassium hydroxide (KOH) microscopic examination and yeast culture.

Treatment consists of the use of vaginal suppositories that contain nystatin (100,000 units), deposited high in the vagina by means of an applicator (twice daily for 2 weeks and then nightly for an additional 2 weeks) or clotrimazole vaginal tablets inserted at bedtime for 1 week (105). Clotrimazole has not been studied during the first trimester, however, its use during the second and third trimesters of pregnancy has not been associated with ill effects.

Inflammatory vulvar and perineal lesions can be compressed three to five times daily with water or Burow solution (1:30 dilution) or oilated oatmeal baths to cool and soothe as well as to remove irritant endotoxin produced by *C. albicans*. After compressing and thorough drying, a nystatin cream or powder or a steroid-nystatin cream is applied to the affected areas. Clotrimazole and miconazole creams also are effective topically (106); however, only when they are considered essential to the welfare of the patient should they be used in the first trimester of pregnancy. The safety of oral ketoconazole during pregnancy has not been studied and lowered testosterone levels have been associated with its use in high doses. In severe cases, gentian violet (0.25%) may be applied; however, it tends to be messy and will stain clothing, linen, and skin. For further control of vulvar pruritus, an antipruritic cream or lotion may be necessary (see Section I.A). Conditions leading to moisture and maceration must be eliminated. Air conditioning, drying of the groin with a fan or blow dryer, and wearing loose clothing may be necessary. After lesions resolve, application of a starch-free drying powder or nystatin powder should be continued.

b. Neonatal Candidosis. Neonatal candidosis is acquired by an infected birth canal. Skin lesions appear as a diaper dermatitis and/or oral thrush sometime after the first week of life. Presumably, the organisms are acquired during passage through an infected birth canal or by contact with the mother during the early postpartum period (107).

c. Congenital Cutaneous Candidiasis. Congenital cutaneous candidiasis (CCC) is due to ascending infection of fetal skin by candidal organisms via the birth canal. Infection can occur through intact membranes, yet it is facilitated by subclinical rupture of the membranes (108). Whyte et al. reported a high percentage (94%) of prematurity in infected infants with candida (109). Prematurity may enhance the possibility of systemic spread of candida before or after birth (104).

The eruption of CCC is noted at birth or within 12 hr after delivery, yet it may appear at 2 and 7 days of age (110). The eruption is diffuse and may involve the trunk, neck, face, and extremities. Different evolutionary stages may coexist in the same area of the body, even at birth, and pass through macular, papular, vesicular, and pustular phases. Bullae formation may also occur, and the palms and soles are frequently involved. Desquamation is a prominent feature of CCC in the recuperative period (110). The lesions of CCC last 5–20 days, and the condition is usually characterized by an absence of constitutional signs and normal white blood cell and platelet counts; however, asymptomatic systemic dissemination may occur (110,104). A fatal outcome of CCC has been reported in infected neonates with low birth weight and signs of respiratory distress (111). Some infants with CCC may present with respiratory distress, hepatosplenomegaly, or clinical signs of sepsis during the first 2 days of life (104).

CCC is diagnosed by a careful history of maternal infection, fungal culture, and direct KOH examination from the pustules. This condition does not appear to be related to maternal age, parity, type of delivery, or duration of labor.

4. Chlamydia Trachomatis Infection

Chlamydia trachomatis infection is the most prevalent sexually transmitted disease. *C. trachomatis* comprises several serotypes, some of which cause blinding trachomas and others cause lymphogranuloma venereum (LGV) and a mucopurulent cervicitis/salpingitis. Chlamydial infections have been associated with preterm delivery, intrauterine growth retardation, premature rupture of the membranes, and increased perinatal mortality (112,113). Conjunctivitis and pneumonia are the most frequent complications of infants infected with chlamydiae during birth. Conjunctivitis occurs in 18–50% of neonates born to infected mothers (113) and pneumonia occurs in 11–18% of such neonates (112). LGV infection can present with painful inguinal adenopathy, which is unilateral in 60% of the cases. Patients may present with periproctitis with fever, constipation, tenesmus, thin stools, and perianal pruritus. Later complications include esthiomene, with genital scarring and vulvar lymphedema, chronic fistulae, and draining abscesses. Pharmacological treatment of choice for chlamydial infection during pregnancy is oral erythromycin 500 mg q.i.d for 7 days.

5. *Leprosy*

Leprosy will exacerbate in more than one-third of infected patients during pregnancy or during the initial 6 months of lactation. There is a concomitant increase in the number and viability of the lepra bacilli in slit-skin smears, a rise in the proportion of viable bacilli in smears, the appearance of new lesions, the extension of old lesions, or the development of erythema in tuberculoid lesions of leprosy (114,115). Patients may relapse despite being formerly under good control with chemotherapy, and subclinical disease may clinically become apparent during pregnancy. The reactional states of leprosy are greatly influenced by pregnancy. The type 1 reaction occurs with greater frequency during the first trimester, subsides until delivery, and increases once again. This reaction is associated with the reversal phenomenon. The type 2 lepra reaction increases in frequency during the second and third trimesters and during the first 9 months of lactation. Hypersensitivity reactions (i.e., erythema nodosum leprosum) may develop (116) from the third trimester through the first 15 months postpartum (114), and the clinical state may deteriorate (2). Cutaneous involvement during gestation is common, whereas one usually sees nerve involvement postpartum (114).

Leprosy may have severe effects on the fetus, causing low birth weight and small placenta, which may account for the high incidence of infant mortality (117). Patients of childbearing age who have leprosy should be warned against pregnancy during the years when their disease is active. If leprosy is diagnosed during pregnancy or if pregnancy occurs during treatment, the patient can be assured that transplacental infection does not occur. The baby will be free of leprosy at birth, and there will be no need to separate baby from mother unless the mother has bacilli in skin smears when the birth takes place. This is possible in lepromatous leprosy, and the baby should be removed at birth and returned to maternal care only after living bacilli have disappeared from skin slit smears.

Dapsone is the treatment of choice for uncomplicated cases of leprosy (118). However, the decline in the immune status of the mother may cause an increased incidence of drug resistance. Thalidomide suppresses reactional states, yet is contraindicated in pregnancy because of its teratogenic effects. Clofazimine may be effective in dapsone-resistant cases and may suppress reactional states (116, 118). Its use is limited by its side effects, and clofazimine has been associated with unexplained neonatal deaths (114); therefore, current recommendation is that clofazimine not be used before the second trimester.

6. *Measles (Rubeola)*

Measles is a highly infectious viral infection caused by a paramyxovirus which mostly affects children, and it has an incubation period of 9–11 days. Prodromal signs such as fever, cough, coryza, and conjunctival infection occur. Pathognomonic Koplik spots appear on day 2 or 3, which are described as blue-gray specks which occur on the lateral buccal mucosa. The morbilliform rash appears on day 4, and patients remain contagious from the onset of symptoms to about 4 days after the rash fades. The eruption usually begins on the neck, spreads to the face and trunk, and then to the extremities over a 3-day period and then becomes confluent.

Measles may occur during pregnancy and can be associated with serious complications. Rubeola virus, although not a teratogen, has been associated with increased perinatal mortality and spontaneous abortions (119). Measles has been associated with the following complications: pneumonia, encephalitis, hepatitis, elevated liver enzymes, and otitis media. Pregnant women with measles should be evaluated for volume depletion, preterm labor, hypoxemia, and secondary bacterial pneumonia (120). All susceptible women should receive postpartum vaccination along with the rubella vaccine to women who are rubella nonimmune. A pregnant woman exposed to measles should receive immune globulin at a dose of 0.25 ml/kg (not to exceed 15 ml) within 6 days of exposure to measles. The live vaccine is not recommended during pregnancy. Rare cases of life-threatening pneumonia and encephalitis have been treated with Ribavirin, a nucleoside analogue of guanosine.

7. *Herpes Simplex Infection*

Genital herpes simplex virus (HSV) infections may cause congenital (intrauterine) or neonatal infection. Congenital HSV is transplacentally transmitted and frequently leads to spontaneous abortion, cardiac abnormalities, and limb hypoplasia in early infection (first 8 weeks of gestation). Late infection (9 weeks' gestation to term) may involve the fetal skin with the presence of cutaneous vesicles, bullae, erosions, and scarring. Neonatal HSV is caused by ascending maternal infection after premature rupture of the membranes or by direct contact through an infected birth canal (49). Postnatal horizontal contact associated with kissing or breast-feeding and horizontal transmission from other siblings, nurses, or caretakers may cause

HSV infection. Infants are at increased risk owing to their porous integument and exposure to invasive procedures such as the placement of scalp monitors. Neonatal infection with HSV in variable, yet all cases need immediate diagnosis and management. The most frequent presentation of neonatal HSV is localized disease of the skin, eyes, or oral mucosa. Recurrent disease occurs in 60–80% of infants with primary neonatal HSV-2 limited to skin and mucous membranes. Disseminated disease, if left untreated, has a mortality rate of 85%, and with treatment, it has a 60% morbidity rate and a 55% mortality rate (122). The presentation of fever, poor feeding, and decreased alertness may be the only initial symptoms of infection. Babies born with HSV infection have an astounding mortality rate of 60%, with serious neurological and ophthalmological complications. Fifty percent of infants who develop HSV infection are premature (91). Manifestations of dissemination include encephalitis, hepatitis, pancreatitis, myocarditis, and coagulopathies, with mortality approaching 50% for mother and fetus (114).

Women infected with genital herpes infection may be asymptomatic in 78–97% of the time or unaware of a previous exposure to HSV infection. Asymptomatic viral shedding of HSV can be detected in only 15% of pregnant women with recurrent herpes infection, yet it may have occurred at the time of delivery in as many as 70% of neonatal herpes cases (122,123). Results of cervical cultures taken before labor may not reflect the status of viral shedding intrapartum. Shedding from the cervix is more likely to result in neonatal infection then shedding from the vulva (91). Only 25% of mothers of infants with neonatal herpes infection give a history of a previous HSV infection. There are different risks to the neonate depending on the status of maternal exposure to HSV before pregnancy. Women with a history of genital herpes before pregnancy are less likely to deliver infants who will develop neonatal herpes than woman who develop an initial infection of herpes during pregnancy (124). Babies born to mothers with primary herpes at the time of vaginal delivery have a 50% risk of neonatal infection, yet less than 5% of babies born to mothers with recurrent disease develop symptomatic neonatal infection (91). This is thought to be due to maternal antibodies that may neutralize the smaller viral inoculum associated with recurrent disease. Frenkel et al. studied 1355 pregnant women with no history of genital herpes (122). Antibody to HSV-2 was detected in 32% (439 of 1355) of the women. Asymptomatic viral shedding was detected in 0.43% (5 of 1160) viral cultures obtained in late pregnancy and during delivery, which is similar to the rate of that seen in women with symptomatc genital herpes infection. Sixteen percent (43 of 262) of HSV-2 seropositive women recognized a first episode of clinical genital herpes infection during their pregnancy.

The mode of delivery for women with recurrent HSV infections should be based on the presence or absence of genital lesions at the time of labor. Cesarean section is recommended for herpetic disease especially accompanied by prodromal symptoms. Serial genital cultures for HSV are not predictive of neonatal infection and do not predict viral shedding at the time of delivery. Topical analgesics and anesthetics are recommended for relief of pain.

Acyclovir may safely be prescribed to those patients with a primary genital HSV outbreak with tapering of the drug as symptoms improve. Patients should be educated to recognize the diverse symptoms of genital herpes. It is recommended that fetal scalp monitoring be avoided during active HSV infection at delivery (122).

8. *Varicella-Zoster Infection*

Varicella-zoster virus (VZV) is a highly contagious viral infection which is characterized by a vesicular eruption after an incubation period of 14–21 days. Successive crops of new vesicles appear as "dew drops" on an erythematous base on the face and trunk and may involve the mucous membranes. There may be constitutional symptoms such as a low-grade fever, malaise, backache, and headaches. Clinical diagnosis can be confirmed by a Tzanck smear taken from the floor of the vesicle base and by viral culture. Varicella-zoster immune globulin should be given to those infants whose mothers have had VZV during the last 7 days of pregnancy, because maternal varicella can result in neonatal infection if the eruption is noted 2–5 days before delivery (125).

VZV infection may produce significant morbidity and mortality in the mother. Although it rarely occurs in women during their reproductive years, VZV has been associated with congenital anomalies and pneumonia may occur in 14% of pregnant patients, 3% of whom may have a fetal outcome (114). First-trimester maternal infection has a risk of being transplacentally transferred in 0.02–9.1%. Second- and third-trimester maternal infection has not been associated with congenital abnormalities. The congenital varicella syndrome is characterized by limb hypoplasia, cutaneous scars, microcephaly, cortical atrophy, cataracts, and chorioretinitis (126). In a prospective study of 43 pregnancies complicated by varicella, 9 of 43 patients had associated morbidity: 4 women had pneumonia, 1 woman died, and 4 had premature labor (126). The congenital varicella syndrome occurred in 1 of 11 infants (9%) after first-trimester varicella. None of the infants whose mothers had varicella in the second or third trimester had birth defects; however, skin lesions were observed in two infants and one infant developed herpes zoster, which can be associated with asymptomatic intrauterine varicella infection. If a mother has varicella within 4 days before to 2 days after term, the neonate would have no maternal antibody and is at risk of severe varicella infection with a mortality rate of up to 30% in the absence of treatment. Balducci et al. studied 40 pregnant women with first-trimester varicella (127): Three patients had first-trimester spontaneous abortions; 2 of 36 had preterm deliveries, and 1 patient had premature rupture of the membranes at 31 weeks. One of 36 neonates was born with an abdominal omphalocele, yet all others had no clinical evidence of the congenital varicella syndrome. Two of 27 infants whose mothers had first-trimester varicella developed congenital defects; 1 developed microcephaly and the other a cataract (128).

9. *Parvovirus B19/Erythema Infectiosum*

Human parvovirus B19 is the etiological agent of fifth disease (erythema infectiosum), which occurs mainly in children as a "slapped cheek" facial rash that spreads to the trunk and extremities. Infection during pregnancy usually presents between weeks 15–29 of gestation. The rash is usually confluent, reticulated, and macular, and it is often preceded by malaise, fever, myalgias, and upper respiratory symptoms. Pruritus may be severe, and the eruption may involve the palms and soles. In adults, arthritis involving the hands, wrists, and knees may be present and constitutional symptoms may be pronounced, whereas the rash may be faint or absent (125). In one-third of the cases, maternal infection is asymptomatic; however, the majority of women present with a rash in 91% of the cases (129). Thus far, there have been 37 documented cases of parvovirus during pregnancy; 14 cases (38%) resulted in fetal demise (130).

The diagnosis of recent infection is confirmed by the presence of parvovirus B19–specific IgM and IgG antibodies in serum. Serial maternal serum alpha-fetoprotein and sonographic examinations should be obtained if there is a high index of suspicion of infection. The maternal serum alpha-fetoprotein becomes elevated when the fetus is affected before detection of fetal hydrops by ultrasonography, and it may be an indicator of a poor fetal prognosis. Fetal death has occurred up to 12 weeks after maternal exposure to the virus and may follow asymptomatic maternal infection. Parvovirus B19 may be associated with both transient fetal hydrops and fatal fetal hydrops (129). There have been reports of maternal infection associated with normal fetal outcome (131). High-titered parvovirus B19 DNA in fetal tissue has been associated with aplastic anemia in the fetus as well as hydrops fetalis (125). During school outbreaks of fifth disease, pregnant personnel should remain at home until 2–3 weeks after the last identified case (130).

10. *Human Immunodeficiency Virus*

Currently, there is no evidence of a deleterious effect of pregnancy and childbirth on early human immunodeficiency (HIV) infection (133). Infants born to infected mothers who carry HIV can clinically develop acquired immunodeficiency syndrome (AIDS) from 3 weeks to 21 months of age. Perinatal transmission may occur through breast milk or most commonly via passage through an infected birth canal. Thus, breast-feeding is not recommended for HIV-infected mothers in the United States. The prenatal transmission rate is reported to be between 13 and 39% (133). Transplacental transfer of the HIV may lead to a variety of cutaneous diseases in the infant, including persistent oral or diaper candidiasis, impetigo, herpes zoster, herpes simplex infection, ecthyma, and molluscum contagiosum (49). Congenitally infected infants present with recurrent infections by the age of 2 years, and intrauterine growth retardation and prematurity have been observed. Recently, a new dysmorphic syndrome has been described in 20 children with AIDS or AIDS-related complex who were born to mothers with AIDS. The clinical features of this syndrome have been attributed to the embryopathy caused by the immunodeficiency virus and include ocular hypertelorism, microcephaly, flat nasal bridge, boxlike forehead, short nose, obliquity of the eyes, triangular philtrum, blue sclerae, and patulous lips (114,133).

Maternal cutaneous manifestations of HIV infection are numerous, with most not seriously affecting the mother's health, but they serve as markers for possible HIV infection and/or AIDS. However, the following cutaneous manifestations of HIV infection are associated with significant maternal morbidity and life-threatening systemic disease: bacillary angiomatosis, disseminated protozoal and deep fungal infections, disseminated herpes zoster infection, and Kaposi sarcoma (134, 135). Treatment of an HIV-positive pregnant mother with azidothymidine (AZT) has been shown to decrease the rate of transmission from mother to fetus by 50–75%.

11. Human T-Cell Lymphotropic Virus Type 1

Human T-cell lymphotropic virus type 1 (HTLV-1) is a retrovirus that is endemic in Africa, Japan, and the Caribbean, as well as parts of Europe, yet its influence on pregnancy is not well known. In endemic areas, the prevalence of HTLV-1 infection can be as high as 10–20% and can rise to 30–40% in families of patients. Children in families where both parents are seropositive have the highest rates of seropositivity. The major route of transmission of HTLV-1 is from infected mother to child via breast milk, with a transmission rate of 20–25% (136). Maternal IgG antibodies can be identified in some infants, although they soon decline over the first 6–12 months of life, suggesting that transfer is passive. Seroconversion in babies usually occurs between the ages of 12 and 19 months, which suggests that transplacental and intrapartum infections account for a proportion of early infections (137). Cutaneous manifestations of HTLV-1 occur only when associated with HTLV-1 lymphoma and include erythematous indurated skin nodules, exfoliative dermatitis on the palms and soles, and a hyperpigmented eruption on the face that may spread to the trunk and extremities (137). The mortality rate of HTLV-1 lymphoma approaches 100% in all patients (138).

The effects of HTLV-1 on the course and outcome of pregnancy remain unknown. Ville et al. (139) studied 45 HTLV-1–seropositive pregnant women matched with 90 seronegative pregnant women and found that none of the infants seroconverted to HTLV-1 even up to 1 year of age.

12. Lyme Disease

Lyme disease is a multisystemic disease caused by the spirochete *Borrelia burgdorferi*, which is transmitted by a deer tick. The effects of Lyme disease on pregnancy are unknown. The hallmark sign is called erythema migrans, an expanding red annular lesion with central clearing that usually appears 4–21 days after the tick bite and can be accompanied by flulike symptoms. Complications include arthritis, cardiac disease, and neurological manifestations (140).

Most treated pregnant patients have a favorable outcome; however, both early and late infections may result in intrauterine growth retardation, fetal death, prematurity, and malformations. Transplacental transmission of *B. burgdorferi* is associated with increased fetal loss. Markowitz et al. evaluated 19 pregnant women with Lyme disease, 5 of whom had adverse outcomes including syndactyly, cortical blindness, intrauterine fetal death, prematurity, and rash in the newborn (141). It is thought that many patients are bacteremic early in Lyme disease and that later manifestations are due to tissue invasion and persistence of the organism. Conventional laboratory tests may be inadequate or give false-negative results; thus, it is important to rely on the clinical signs and physical examination as well as the history.

13. Syphilis

The eliotogical agent of syphilis, *Treponema pallidum*, may cross the placenta as early as the eighth week of gestation; however, it is usually transmitted during the second trimester. Primary syphilis usually presents as a solitary chancre, which is a painless round ulcer that is indurated. Bilateral regional lymphadenopathy is usually seen with firm, nonfluctuant, slightly tender nodes; however, systemic symptoms are not usually present.

Secondary syphilis most commonly presents as a generalized papulosquamous nonpruritic eruption, often involving the palms and soles. However, syphilis may simply present with patchy alopecia or mucous membrane patches. Condylomata lata, flat-topped genital or perianal excrescences that are highly infectious, may be mistaken for human papillomavirus-induced condylomata acuminata. Systemic manifestations include pharyngitis, fever, nuchal rigidity, generalized lymphadenopathy, hepatitis, and cranial nerve abnormalities.

Tertiary (late) syphilis, is very rare and most commonly presented as gummas, which are locally destructive lesions involving skin, bone, liver, and the ascending aorta and other viscera. Late neurosyphilis presents as tables dorsalis and general paresis.

Transplacental transfer may result in congenital syphilis, which ranges in severity from asymptomatic to fatal. Clinical disease presents before the age of 2 years. Neonates commonly have vesicobullous lesions on the palms and soles, rhinitis (snuffles), and perioral and perianal fissures. Infants less than 6 months of age have skin lesions in 52% of the cases presenting as a papulosquamous rash as early as 2–6 weeks of age (49). Hepatic dysfunction, consumption coagulopathy, and multiple organ failure may occur. Later complications include osteitis of the long bones, dental malformations, keratitis, and hearing loss.

Pregnant patients with syphilis may experience spontaneous abortions and premature labor (49,142). Rawstron studied 403 pregnancies associated with positive syphilis serologies (143). Seventy-three pregnancies (18%) resulted in congenital syphilis, with 35 liveborn and 40 stillborn neonates. A syphilitic stillborn is defined as a stillbirth born to a mother with untreated or inadequately treated syphilis. Syphilitic infection in utero may manifest as nonimmune hydrops fetalis (144). Adequate treatment for the mother before the fourth month of pregnancy prevents the disease in the newborn. Treatment instituted after 18 weeks of gestation may effect an intrauterine cure but will not prevent permanent bone, joint, neural, or ocular complications. Penicillin is the drug of choice, and desensitization should be implemented if the patient is penicillin allergic.

14. Coccidiodomycosis

In the United States, over 20,000 cases of mild coccidiodomycosis and over 200 cases of severe coccidiodomycosis occur each year, with nearly 60 deaths caused by the disease. In endemic areas in the United States, 1 in 1000 pregnant women has coccidiodomycosis and is at high risk for dissemination. The rate of dissemination of the disease during pregnancy is 40–100 times that of the general population. In endemic areas, disseminated coccidiodomycosis has become a significant cause of maternal mortality, with mortality rates of 20–60% (145).

There are three cutaneous signs which are helpful in making a diagnosis of coccidiodomycosis, toxic erythema, erythema nodosum, and erythema multiforme, when found in conjunction with pulmonary symptoms such as productive cough, pleuritic chest pain, abnormal roentgenogram, and blood-streaked sputum. Toxic erythema occurs in 10% of infected patients with coccidiodomycosis and presents as a diffuse, macular, erythematous rash in the first few days of illness. Erythema multiforme and erythema nodosum (described later in this chapter) are more commonly associated skin findings.

Primary coccidiodomycosis appears to have a more virulent course during pregnancy with an increased risk of dissemination. In the nonpregnant state, chronic pulmonary disease develops in 5% of patients and extrapulmonary dissemination in 0.2% of cases. The first-trimester rate of dissemination is 23%, the second-trimester rate is 59%, and the third-trimester rate is 68% (146). There have been approximately 109 reported cases in the literature, with 90 cases being described fully, and 55 cases that were complicated by disseminated disease. Those patients without disseminated disease experienced no maternal deaths, but there were five stillbirths and there was perinatal mortality rate of 14%. In patients with disseminated disease, overall 34 maternal deaths occurred among 55 patients (62%), and the perinatal mortality rate increased to 50%, with placental infection occurring in 37.5% of the cases. Pregnant patients who develop coccidiodomycosis should undergo regular physical examinations and serological studies to assess them for possible dissemination. Women with a history of antecedent infection are usually not at a risk for relapse or dissemination; however, reactivation can occur (146). The most common association with disease reactivation is related to immunosuppression induced by certain diseases such as HIV infection, and the use of corticosteroids. Infection is thought to occur via aspiration of infected decidua and/or placental infection. Cervicovaginal cultures before delivery are recommended; however, it is unclear if a positive culture warrants a cesarean section (145). An uncommon manifestation of maternal disseminated coccidiodomycosis is the development of osteomyelitis in neonates and infants (147).

D. Connective Tissue Skin Diseases in Pregnancy

1. Antiphospholipid Syndrome and Lupus Anticoagulant

Antiphospholipid syndrome (APS) is defined by the presence of antiphospholipid antibody or lupus anticoagulant, usually in high titer and associated with all or some of the following clinical events: recurrent fetal losses, recurrent thromboses, and thrombocytopenia. Primary antiphospholipid syndrome often occurs in patients with systemic lupus erythematosus who have antiphospholipid antibodies and may experience occlusive vascular disease, neurological disease, or false-positive results of a syphilis test. The presence of the antibody alone does not define APS, because there must be associated clinical events. The lupus anticoagulant (LA) is an immunoglobulin acquired by some patients with systemic lupus erythematosus. The LA prolongs phospholipid-dependent coagulation times and is paradoxically associated with an increased risk of thrombotic episodes (148).

Livido reticularis is often a cutaneous marker for APS (149). Less common cutaneous manifestations include distal acral ischemia and necrosis, blue toe syndrome, splinter hemorrhages, porcelain white scars, and superficial thrombophlebitis (150). Patients may develop neurological syndromes, renal hypertension, pulmonary thrombosis, endocrinopathies, cardiac manifestations, and hemolytic anemia.

The antiphospholipid antibody is identified by ELISA (enzyme-linked immunosorbent assay), which uses cardiolipin as the phospholipid antigen or by finding a lupus anticoagulant via clotting tests. It has been suggested that the LA is a better predictor of thrombotic complications than the antiphospholipid antibody. Identification of the LA is based on the observation of an increased activated partial thromboplastin time and abnormal results on a tissue thromboplastin-inhibition test. The presence of the LA is an important clinical marker for recurrent first-trimester spontaneous abortion as well as for second- and third-trimester fetal death (151).

Treatment includes high doses of prednisone, subcutaneous heparin therapy, and low-dose aspirin. Experimental therapies include intravenous gamma-globulin and plasmapheresis (149). The corticosteroid and low-dose aspirin regimen appears to improve perinatal outcome in cases in which the mother has the LA; however, careful fetal monitoring and appropriate preterm delivery are important to successful obstetrical management (148). There is very little information on the long-term outcome of children born to mothers with APS. Most of the complications of treated patients with APS include maternal autoimmune disorders, preeclampsia, fetal growth retardation, preterm delivery, and fetal distress (148). Twenty-three mothers with APS and their 29 newborn infants were compared with controls. All of the women with APS were receiving therapeutic regimens, including prednisone, low-dose aspirin, and heparin. Neonatal complications in this study included hyperbilirubinemia (14 patients), respiratory distress syndrome (3 patients), bronchopulmonary dysplasia (2 patients), necrotizing enterocolitis (2 patients), intraventricular hemorrhage (2 patients), sepsis (1 patient), coarctation of the aorta (1 patient), hypothyroidism (1 patient), hypoglycemia (1 patient), and death in one patient. They found no increase in the overall rate of neonatal complications (152).

There are various obstetrical complications that can occur in women with antiphospholipid antibodies, including (a) late intrauterine death, (b) second-trimester miscarriages, (c) intrauterine growth retardation, (d) preeclampsia, (e) HEELP (hemolysis, elevated liver enzymes, and thrombocytopenia) syndrome, and (f) spontaneous abortion (150). Women with APS who have very high titers and a history of prior fetal loss may have completely normal pregnancies in 20% of the cases (149). Abnormal pregnancies progress from early normality to slowed fetal growth rate in mid pregnancy, decreased amniotic fluid, abnormal fetal testing, and either fetal death or emergent delivery of a premature infant. Placentas are usually small, and these have been shown to have infarcts and unusual vasculopathy involving the decidual and placental blood vessels (150). It is estimated that 10% of women with a history of two or more unexplained fetal losses have the antiphospholipid antibody.

A retrospective review of the obstetrical histories of 43 women with the LA recorded 162 pregnancy losses and only 20 (12%) surviving infants (148,151). Pollard et al. found that 13 of 28 women with APS developed preeclampsia and subsequent preterm delivery (152). The investigators concluded that complications seen in neonates of women with APS resulted from prematurity rather than from maternal APS or its treatments. Three-quarters of the infants born to the women in this study were growing and developing normally at the time of childhood follow-up.

2. *Systemic Lupus Erythematosus*

Systemic lupus erythematosus (SLE) is a common disease with a female to male incidence ratio of 10:1. Its frequent occurrence in women of childbearing age makes the occurrence of SLE and pregnancy an important clinical problem. Little consensus exists as to whether pregnancy adversely affects the course of SLE or vice versa and whether the maternal or fetal outcome is compromised. Nevertheless, an increasing number of reports have determined that the outcome is more favorable than formerly believed (114,153). Pregnancy is tolerated best by mothers who have been in remission for 3 months before conception and who do not have significant nephropathy or cardiac disease (149).

Patients who develop SLE for the first time during pregnancy have a higher frequency of severe manifestations, including fever, heart failure, renal disease, lymphadenopathy, abdominal pain with jaundice, and pancreatitis. However, these patients may experience postpartum remission, and successful subsequent pregnancy may occur in approximately two-thirds of the cases (114,154). During acute and subacute SLE, approximately 50% of pregnant patients will worsen during gestation; however, this exacerbation rate is the same in nonpregnant women with similar disease severity (114). Although poor fetal outcome may occur in pregnant patients who are in remission and patients with mild disease, the effects of SLE on fetal outcome are generally proportional to the severity of maternal disease.

Pregnancy can incite exacerbation of SLE in as many as 38% of patients at any time from the first month of pregnancy to 8 weeks postpartum (30,155). Women with SLE have an increased incidence if abortion, two to four times normal, as well as premature births, which occur in 16–37% of pregnancies (114,156). A retrospective analysis by Barnett (153) of 52 pregnancies in 39 patients who had SLE showed that pregnancy did not seem to affect the course of uncomplicated (nonrenal) SLE nor did the onset of SLE significantly coincide with the onset of pregnancy. Patients who had moderate renal involvement rarely became pregnant, and fewer than 15% of those who had milder renal dysfunction experienced an exacerbation during pregnancy (153). These and other recent findings (157,158) contrast with previous studies that reported a high frequency of flares of SLE and lupus nephritis during gestation or the postpartum period, with subsequent postpartum maternal mortality ranging between 50 and 82% (159–161). Postpartum manifestations such as rash, arthritis, and fever were reported (153) in 31% of patients who received no glucocorticoids during pregnancy and the postpartum period and in 9.5% of those who did.

In Barnett's study of SLE, fetal complications tended to be much more common than maternal ones (153). Only 31% of the 52 pregnancies ended in full-term delivery, and patients who had apparent renal involvement accounted for the major proportion of poor fetal outcome. There were 5.1% spontaneous abortions, 22.4% therapeutic abortions, 17.2% stillbirths, and 24% premature deliveries. One review of the literature estimates an average pregnancy rate loss of 28% (156). The prevalence of fetal wastage (22.3%) was higher than the 10% average for the general population (153). Although previous reports have indicated that spontaneous and therapeutic abortions may affect maternal SLE adversely, this study showed no maternal deleterious effects in 15 first-trimester abortions. Neonates did not demonstrate any increased incidence of neonatal complications, although growth retardation and poor head growth, possibly secondary to maternal glucocorticoid therapy, were reported. In cases where maternal SS-A/Ro antibodies are present, neonates may develop the neonatal lupus syndrome, with congenital heart block, liver and hematological abnormalities, and skin lesions (162).

Neonatal lupus erythematosus (NLE) occurs in mothers with clinical or subclinical autoimmune connective tissue disease and is thought to occur via the transplacental passage of maternal autoantibodies, specifically, SS-A/Ro antibody. The SS-A antigen is present in fetal skin and heart tissue (164). Most infants do not have significant titers of antinuclear antibodies. Approximately 50% of mothers of infants with NLE have signs of SLE, subacute cutaneous lupus erythematosus, or the Sicca syndrome. The remaining 50% of women are at greater risk of the development of autoimmune disease in the future.

Skin lesions in NLE are transient in nature and are usually present at birth or appear shortly thereafter. They appear clinically as well-demarcated scaly annular plaques with a predilection for the periorbital/facial region. Late sequelae include telangiectases and atrophy, especially around the temples and scalp. Infants rarely have both skin and cardiac lesions. Infants with skin lesions and systemic features other than heart block show little evidence of disease after the age of 1 year. The risk of recurrence in further pregnancies is 25% (165). Treatment is usually not necessary, and sun protection is advisable.

There is less concern if women who have SLE become pregnant as long as they have maintained good renal function. The major risk to the pregnant patient with SLE is a permanent decline in renal function, which was observed in fewer than 10% of cases in Barnett's study (153). Women who have SLE and who become pregnant should be informed that, although they are at a somewhat greater risk, most pregnancies do not affect the mother adversely. In contrast, the fetus is at a relatively higher risk, with fetal wastage being high and prognosis adversely affected even if mild renal involvement is detected in the mother (153).

Management of the pregnant patient who has SLE is more difficult, because the usual monitors of disease activity, such as antinuclear antibody (including anti–double stranded DNA) titers and the erythrocyte sedimentation rate, do not reflect disease activity during pregnancy. Complement levels may not correlate with disease activity. Drugs such as chlorambucil and cyclophosphamide are highly teratogenic. Dapsone and azathioprine should be avoided during pregnancy (164). Hydroxychloroquine and chloroquine have been the mainstay of systemic therapy for SLE; however, these antimalarial drugs have been known to accumulate in the eyes of the fetus and potentially cause blindness, and they should be avoided during pregnancy (164). Modifications in the pharmacological management of the disease during labor and in the postpartum period include an increase in the dosage of glucocorticosteroids, which may reduce postpartum exacerbation. Judiciously administered, prednisone is a justified medication to be used during pregnancy in light of its degradation by the placenta (153,165). The use of hemodialysis during pregnancy offers a difficult but suitable means of managing those patients who have severe renal disease. In most cases, such pregnancies result in a viable but premature or small infant (153).

3. *Scleroderma*

Scleroderma affects women during their reproductive years, and if it is uncomplicated by renal disease, does not affect pregnancy adversely (30,166,167). In general, with the exception of renal disease, pregnancy does not alter the course of scleroderma, and fetal outcome is relatively unaffected (168). Steen et al. (170) compared 48 women with age- and race-matched controls and found no differences in the frequencies of miscarriage or perinatal death. However, preterm births occurred slightly more frequently and there were more small full-term infants. Ballou (171) reviewed the obstetrical histories of 19 women with systemic sclerosis and followed 2 women in whom 3 pregnancies occurred. Maternal complications included hypertension in two of these three pregnancies and congestive heart failure during one. There were two premature deliveries, and all three infants survived. Ballou suggested that women with systemic sclerosis may have decreased fertility, accounting for the few pregnancies observed in his patients, and that the more frequent complications of pregnancy necessitates close monitoring for premature birth and intrauterine growth retardation. Scleroderma may involve the genital areas and reproductive tract, which leads additional rationale for the possibility of decreased fertility (170,171).

The pregnancies of those patients with scleroderma who have preexisting renal involvement or of those in whom renal involvement develops during pregnancy, however, have been adversely affected (172,173). Unfortunately, kidney involvement may not be detectable by standard clinical means at the onset of pregnancy, so that it may be difficult to predict which patients will develop complications (30). In a review of renal scleroderma and pregnancy, Karlen and Karlen (174) noted that many pregnancies were uneventful until the early third trimester, at which time the symptoms and signs of preeclampsia suddenly developed, renal failure ensued, and a fulminant clinical course led to maternal death within days. Most maternal deaths occurred in patients who had renal involvement. The investigators concluded that pregnancy associated with scleroderma represents a high-risk situation for mother and fetus alike, and serious consideration should be given to permanent contraception in women who have widespread systemic involvement or kidney involvement. Black et al. (174) reviewed 29 pregnancies from 23 patients and found that over 50% of these women developed deterioration of their disease and 33% died from renal failure. Women with early rapidly progressive, diffuse skin thickening should avoid becoming pregnant, because they are at a higher risk of developing renal crisis (175).

Antiphospholipid antibodies have been implicated in the etiology of pregnancy loss in women with systemic sclerosis (156). The greatest concern in pregnant women with scleroderma apart from disease exacerbation is the risk of fetal death, which is estimated to be 15% (176). Steen et al. found that 20 of 133 pregnancies (15%) of women with scleroderma ended in miscarriage (168). If a woman with scleroderma decides to proceed with pregnancy, therapeutic interruption may be advisable at the first sign of preeclampsia associated with a decrease in renal function (173).

There is new hope for treatment of pregnant women with systemic sclerosis with nifedipine. Wilson and Kirby (177) reported successful conception and pregnancy in a woman with systemic sclerosis who received continuous treatment with nifedipine after having a poor obstetrical record and secondary infertility.

4. *Dermatomyositis/Polymyositis*

The peak incidence of dermatomyositis (DM) occurs during the reproductive years with twice as many cases reported in women than in men. Although there is a paucity of data concerning the outcome of pregnancy in this disease, DM appears harmful to both mother and fetus. The disease may manifest itself first in pregnancy (179), and high fetal mortality (46%) and neonatal prematurity death have been reported (181). A facial rash and/or proximal muscle weakness may occur in 50% of affected patients, and fetal loss can occur in over 50% of the cases due to abortion, stillbirth, or premature neonatal death. Eighteen women with dermatomyositis/polymyositis (DM/PM) had a total of 77 pregnancies before disease onset; of these, seven (9%) ended in abortion and two (2.5%) ended in perinatal death. Three premature infants survived. There were 10 pregnancies in seven women with active disease at the time of pregnancy; three (30%) ended in abortion, three of the remainder ended in perinatal death (25%), and half the infants were born prematurely. The total fetal loss was 11.5% before and 55% after the onset of DM/PM (179). King and Chow noted a more favorable outcome in three patients with five successful pregnancies complicated by DM (181). They concluded that women with disease in remission may have successful pregnancies, and that if exacerbation occurs, treatment with corticosteroids can minimize fetal loss. Pregnancy should be avoided during active DM but not necessarily during remission. Recently, it has been reported that pharmacological control of disease activity, usually through administration of prednisone, is associated with a more successful pregnancy. Surviving children of patients with DM/PM are not affected by the illness (114).

E. Erythema Nodosum

Reports of erythema nodosum occurring in pregnant (182,183) and lactating (184) women as well as in women taking oral contraceptives (183,185,186) lend support to a contributory role of estrogen in the pathogenesis of this disease.

Erythema nodosum is characterized by painful, nonsuppurative red cutaneous nodules that usually occur over the extensor surfaces of the extremities. Lesions are sometimes associated with fever, swelling of the legs, and arthralgias. Individual nodules last several weeks before disappearing spontaneously. New lesions appear while old ones are resolving, and the entire course of the disease may last weeks to months.

Drug reactions (e.g., sulfonamides, anovulatories, penicillin), infections (e.g., streptococcal, mycobacterial, fungal), sarcoidosis, and inflammatory bowel diseases are causative factors of erythema nodosum and should be excluded. The diagnosis of erythema nodosum usually can be made clinically and confirmed histologically. Lesions associated with pregnancy tend to resolve spontaneously and may recur with subsequent oral contraceptive therapy. Bed rest with elevation of the legs gradually will reduce pain and edema, and analgesics may relieve arthralgias. In chronic or recurrent cases unresponsive to supportive therapy, intralesional injection of a corticosteroid suspension may cause involution of treated lesions. A 1- to 2-week course of oral corticosteroids may also be effective. There is an association between pregnancy and erythema nodosum, because it may occur with consecutive pregnancies (187). It appears as though female hormones may influence the onset of erythema nodosum, because it occurs predominantly during the years after menarche and before the menopause.

F. Erythema Multiforme

Pregnancy is one of the many causes of erythema multiforme. Erythema multiforme is an acute, usually self-limiting, frequently recurrent, and distinctive morphological mucocutaneous reaction that is a hypersensitivity response involving immune complex formation to numerous factors. The exact mechanism of the development of erythema multiforms involved in pregnancy cannot be explained simply by considering the developing fetus as foreign tissue. Characteristically, there are symmetrical polymorphous skin lesions (macules, papules, urticaria, and bullae) that range in color from bright red to dusky purple. The development of iris or target lesions is seen most often on the hands and consists of a central vesicle or livid erythema surrounded by a pale ring and then by a concentric red ring. Iris lesions are characteristic of erythema multiforme but need not be present in order to make the diagnosis clinically.

Sites of predilection include the oral mucosa, palms and soles, distal extremities, extensor surfaces, and face. Burning and itching are the chief complaints. At times, only the mucous membranes of the lip, mouth, pharynx, or vagina may be involved.

These lesions may progress to denuded raw ulcerations that become crusted, tender, and painful and may interfere with nutrition if they involve the upper alimentary tract.

In severely affected persons, there is widespread cutaneous, mucosal, and ocular involvement with large bullae. This severe mucocutaneous bullous form of the disease is frequently designated erythema multiforme bullosum, or Stevens-Johnson syndrome. The mild form of erythema multiforme heals spontaneously within 2–3 weeks; the severe form, with widespread mucosal involvement, may last 6–8 weeks and is a life-threatening disease.

A pregnant patient who develops erythema multiforme requires a workup to rule out other causal agents. Antecedent infection (e.g., herpetic, streptococcal, mycoplasma, deep fungal, viral hepatitis), drug administration (e.g., penicillin, barbiturates, sulfonamides), or illness occurring up to 3 weeks before the rash appears should be investigated.

Specific therapy is possible when a specific cause is found. Local treatment consists of measures to minimize burning and pruritus. Bullae may be drained, but the blister roof should be left intact. Open wet compresses for erosive, denuded, or bullous lesions can be used to clean involved areas. Antihistamines may decrease pruritus. General supportive measures and systemic steroid therapy may be required in episodes of severe involvement. Prednisone given in a short-term, tapering course may be effective; however, its effectiveness and the appropriateness of its use is controversial.

G. Pemphigus Vulgaris

Pemphigus vulgaris (PV), pemphigus foliaceus, and pemphigus vegetans may occur during pregnancy for the first time or may be exacerbated by pregnancy. The onset of pemphigus vulgaris during pregnancy is very uncommon, with very few cases reported (57,188,189). Pemphigus vulgaris is characterized by bullae appearing on apparently normal skin and mucous membranes. At first, the bullae are tense but soon become flaccid and rupture to form erosions and raw surfaces that ooze and bleed easily. Lateral traction on normal skin may cause the epidermis to shear off, and this is called a positive Nikolsky sign. Pemphigus usually manifests itself with lesions first appearing in the mouth as well as on the groin, scalp, face, neck, axillae, and genitals. Healing occurs without scarring, and there may be postinflammatory hyperpigmentation. Involvement of the periumbilical area is a characteristic feature. Although the cause of pemphigus is unknown, an autoimmune mechanism is clearly the basic mechanism. Intercellular antibodies are demonstrable throughout the epidermis or the oral epithelium, and circulating intercellular antibodies are present in the serum in most cases.

The pemphigus IgG antibodies are thought to be transplacentally transferred, because it has been demonstrated in fetal plasma and is deposited intercellularly in fetal skin (191). Active maternal PV skin lesions during pregnancy are not obligatory for the transfer of pemphigus antibodies to the infant. Maternal indirect immunofluorescence antibodies do not appear to influence fetal outcome (192).

The course of the disease tends to be chronic and not affected by pregnancy, with the pregnancy terminating normally in most instances. Samitz et al. (189) reported a case of pemphigus vulgaris that began before conception. The disease was mild in the first and last trimesters but became aggravated in the mid trimester and immediately after parturition. This variation in severity was attributed to the effects of varying adrenocortical activity during the different trimesters. A stillborn infant with pemphiguslike skin lesions, direct immunofluorescence findings, and circulating pemphigus antibodies (indirect immunofluorescence findings) has been reported in a case in which the mother developed a recurrence of pemphigus in the third trimester of pregnancy (191,193). Pregnant women with PV may experience intrauterine death despite careful antepartum monitoring (191). Erosions may occur on the infant's skin, and gradual healing skin lesions correlate with a decrease in their circulating pemphigus antibodies. There is usually a complete diappearance of the skin lesions by 6 weeks of age (192).

The trauma of vaginal delivery may result in an exacerbation of vulvovaginal and perineal erosions which may result in secondary infection and significant morbidity for the patient. Poor wound healing may occur, and this can also be seen at the site of cesarean section. Nevertheless, vaginal delivery is recommended and increased fetal monitoring is recommended (194).

Clinically, pemphigus can resemble herpes gestationis (see Sec. II.C) and may be differentiated by skin biopsy and immunofluorescence studies. The causes for stillbirths in 4 of 29 pregnancies complicated by pemphigus are unknown (195); however, the high dose of prednisone required or the use of azathioprine may be contributory, as well as intercurrent infection or placental insufficiency. Blistering disease of the fetus is unlikely to be the sole cause of death.

High-dose steroids have been the treatment of choice for PV during pregnancy, and they are relatively safe, yet they have been implicated as possibly causing placental failure. Doses of steroids greater than 160 mg daily may be required for initial control with subsequent tapering (114). Choices of drug therapy are limited owing to the possible teratogenic effects of immunosuppressants such as cyclophosphamide, azathioprine, gold, and methotrexate. Pemphigus titers may be helpful in assessing and controlling disease activity (196). Plasmapheresis should be considered in severe cases or in patients with very high titers.

H. Psoriasis

Pregnancy and parturition have an influence on psoriasis that is neither constant nor predictable (57). Gruneberg (197) claims that, as a rule, this influence is a favorable one. Localized forms of psoriasis are most refractory, whereas generalized forms tend to improve. In another study, Church (198) reviewed the effect of pregnancy on psoriasis in 43 women. During pregnancy, 33% of the patients with psoriasis cleared, 21% displayed worsening, and 14% showed no change. In 44% of the patients, parturition was accompanied by exacerbation of the psoriasis (199). Farber et al. noted that 32% of 1018 patients surveyed reported improvement of their psoriasis during pregnancy, whereas 18% claimed their disease worsened and 50% reported no change. Fluxes in hormones, such as adrenocorticotropin (ACTH), may play an important role in those flares and improvements. It appears that there is a definite tendency toward remission and/or improvement of psoriasis during pregnancy.

I. Acrodermatitis Enteropathica

Acrodermatitis enteropathica may be exacerbated by pregnancy, with a measurable decline in serum zinc concentrations beginning early in gestation owing to increased fetal demand for zinc and the effects of estrogens (200). Some patients may be diagnosed for the first time with the disease during pregnancy. The skin manifestations may be mild during puberty, and diarrhea may be slight or absent. During the late first or second trimester, the disease progressively worsens until delivery, and then it rapidly clears postpartum.

Most pregnancies produce normal offspring (201); however, there have been isolated reports of achondroplastic dwarfism, anencephaly, and neonatal death associated with untreated maternal acrodermatitis enteropathica (118,202). These reports coupled with the known teratogenic effects of a zinc deficiency in mice make it essential to diagnose properly and treat acrodermatitis enteropathica during pregnancy (114). Treatment with zinc along with monitoring of serum zinc levels are effective in preventing adverse fetal outcome.

J. Androluteoma Syndrome of Pregnancy

A persistent corpus luteum can produce excess testosterone and may cause severe abnormalities to both the mother and fetus. The mother can become masculinized with hypertrichosis, seborrhea, papulopustular acne, and a deep voice. Female fetuses are more at risk, because they may be born with signs of masculinization. The diagnosis of androluteoma syndrome of pregnancy is based on ultrasonic identification of the tumor in the ovary and by blood levels of excess androgens. Approximately 15 cases have been reported. Surgical removal of the androgen-producing corpus luteum during pregnancy is curative (203).

K. Hereditary Angioedema

Hereditary angioedema (HAE) is an autosomal dominant disease marked by a deficiency or dysfunction of the serum protein inhibitor of the first complement component, the C1 esterase inhibitor (C1-1NH) (204). Clinically, the illness is characterized by intermittent episodes of edema that may affect the limbs, face, pharynx, and vulva and may cause abdominal pain. Often antecedent minor trauma or dental manipulation is identified as the precipitating factor. Endogenous hormones may play a role in the precipitation of attacks. Gelfand et al. (205) noted attacks were more prevalent during menstrual periods in 5 of 12 patients. Androgen administration has been associated with prompt and prolonged remission. Danazol, a synthetic androgenic steroid with minimal virilizing effects, has been used to prevent attacks with good success. Danazol suppresses ovulation in women and increases serum levels of C1 esterase inhibition in both men and women who have the disorder (205).

In view of the hormonal influence on the disease, it is not surprising that pregnancy would have a definite effect on the clinical severity of HAE. Gelfand et al. (205) noted that among the 25 pregnancies in 10 women, there were significantly fewer or no attacks during the last two trimesters. There were no episodes of angioedema at delivery despite the significant tissue trauma associated with childbirth. The fetal outcome of pregnancy in women who have HAE would be expected to be normal.

The possibility that female fetuses can become virilized as a result of maternal danazol therapy must be considered. The safe use of the drug in pregnancy has not been established because of its potential androgenic effects on the fetus, which, to this date, have been limited to clitoral hypertrophy and labial fusion of the external genitalia in the female fetus.

L. Ehlers-Danlos Syndrome

There are presently at least 10 variants of Ehlers-Danlos syndrome. Type I (classic or gravis) and type IV (ecchymotic or arterial) are the most likely types to cause complications during pregnancy (114,201). Type I is inherited in an autosomal dominant manner, so that an affected mother will have a 50% chance of having an affected child. Pregnancy in Ehlers-Danlos syndrome type I involves risks for both mother and fetus (206,207). During pregnancy, affected mothers may manifest increased bruisibility (208), develop abdominal wall, inguinal, umbilical, and femoral hernias, and develop varicosities of the leg and vulva (206). Pregnant women with either type of the syndrome are susceptible to poor wound healing, wound dehiscence, uterine lacerations, and bladder and uterine prolapse (207,209), as well as severe postpartum hemorrhage with bleeding from the episiotomy sites and formation of perineal hematomas. Patients commonly develop papyraceous scars, and owing to the fragility of the fetal membranes, prematurity is common (210). Ainsworth and Aulicino evaluated 151 patients and determined a miscarriage rate of 60% for type I Ehlers-Danlos syndrome (210). Premature rupture of the membranes, uterine prolapse, and cervical tears were common complications.

Type IV (ecchymotic or arterial) Ehlers-Danlos syndrome is similar to type I, but rupture of the aorta and the pulmonary and other major arteries as well as the uterus and bowel may be more common, leading to a maternal death rate of nearly 25% (211). Type II (mitis) Ehlers-Danlos syndrome may have a more favorable outcome of pregnancy with normal vaginal delivery. Episiotomy sites and cesarean section incision sites may heal slowly and may extend spontaneously. All sutures should remain at least twice the usual length of time to prevent wound dehiscence. Previous cesarean scars also may rupture during labor, and cesarean section should be avoided unless it is strictly indicated. Spontaneous rupture of the intact uterus has not been reported. Forceps should be used with caution during delivery (206). Interestingly, women who have Ehlers-Danlos syndrome apparently do not develop striae gravidarum. Striae gravidarum (striae distensae, albicantes, atrophicans) occur to some degree in approximately 90% of pregnant women (2), and there often is a familial tendency (212).

Managing the pregnant patient with ED is very difficult because complications are most likely to occur during labor, parturition, or postpartum (211). Pregnancies frequently terminate prematurely either because of premature rupture of the fetal membranes (if the child is affected) or because of lax cervical tissues (incompetent cervix). Rapid effacement and dilation of the cervix may lead not only to premature delivery but also to precipitous delivery. Cesarean section may not result in fewer complications than vaginal delivery (211). The clinician should consider early termination of pregnancy if ultrasonic examination of the aortic root reveals more than a 20% enlargement above baseline or a diameter greater than 4 cm (213).

M. Pseudoxanthoma Elasticum

Pseudoxanthoma elasticum (PXE), both autosomal dominant and recessive, is a syndrome which affects the gastrointestinal system, eyes, heart, vascular system, and skin. Cutaneous changes progressively develop in the second decade, around the neck, axillary folds, umbilicus, genitals, face, and antecubital fossae. The ocular hallmark of PXE is the finding of angioid streaks which often precedes the infiltrative yellow, lax, redundant plaques and patches on the skin. Complications in pregnant women include gastrointestinal hemorrhage with massive hematemesis that may require blood transfusions. Biopsy of the gastric mucosa shows degeneration of the elastic fibers in medium-sized arteries and the formation of microaneurysms. Other complications in pregnancy include epistaxis and congestive heart failure with ventricular arrhythmias (214). Hematuria, angina, mitral valve prolapse, hypertension, and intermittent claudication may occur in all patients with PXE. It is thought that pregnancy may aggravate the vascular effects of the disease; thus, careful monitoring of blood pressure to decrease the risk of hemorrhage is necessary.

There is no proven fetal risk in PXE, although intrauterine growth retardation associated with placental abnormalities has been reported (215).

N. Marfan Syndrome

Marfan syndrome is adversely affected by pregnancy (2). The life-threatening cardiovascular complication seen in the Marfan syndrome is cystic medial necrosis of the wall of the aorta, which predisposes to aneurysm formation. Aortic aneurysms (216) as well as dissection and rupture of aortic aneurysms (216–219,162) occur with increased frequency during pregnancy. The most stressful period on the aorta seems to be in the third trimester. Although no explanation for the increased susceptibility to vascular aneurysm is available, increased circulating estrogen levels and increased cardiac output may play a role. Women who have Marfan syndrome do not seem to be more prone to problems related to cesarean section and apparently have normal wound healing. Hernias and striae gravidarum occur more frequently during pregnancy in the Marfan syndrome. No specific complications either for the affected or unaffected newborn are expected.

O. Porphyrias

From reported clinical experience and the literature review concerning pregnancy in the acute porphyrias, the general consensus is that the disease worsens during pregnancy. Zimmerman et al. (221) noted a high incidence of prematurity and spontaneous abortion coinciding with acute exacerbations of porphyria; however, most premature infants survived the neonatal period. A study of Brodie et al. (222) revealed a 13% fetal loss rate in 95 pregnancies of mothers with acute intermittent porphyria. Infants born to mothers who experienced an acute attack during pregnancy had significantly lower birth weights compared with infants born to asymptomatic mothers with acute intermittent porphyria. It is unclear whether there is a permanent effect on the newborn.

1. Porphyria Cutanea Tarda

Cutaneous porphyrias (porhyria cutanea tarda [PCT], erythropoietic protoporphyria, and erythropoietic porphyria) during pregnancy are of far less concern than the attacks of acute porphyria. The use of oral contraceptives in recent years has exposed a group of predisposed young women to the risk of developing PCT. Estrogens, iron, and alcohol have been known to affect PCT adversely; however, there have been case reports of patients with successful pregnancies, leading to speculation that endogenous estrogens may not be harmful (223). In comparison, other reports demonstrate a clear worsening of disease during pregnancy with increased plasma and urine porphyrin levels. Lamon and Frykholm measured serum iron, iron-binding capacity, and urine porphyrin levels during gestation

(224). They noted a physiological rise in serum estrogen and a high rate of porphyrin excretion coinciding with clinical exacerbation of skin fragility during the first trimester. As fetal iron requirements rose later in pregnancy, the skin disease improved and a concomitant decrease in serum iron and urinary porphyrins occured, supporting the tendency of pregnancy to worsen PCT. The maternal loss of iron to the fetus could be therapeutic owing to increased blood volume and hemodilution. Fetal morbidity and erythrodontia were not seen in the two offspring of women who had PCT (225). The use of iron supplementation possibly could exacerbate underlying PCT, and chloroquine use should be avoided because of reported birth defects, including mental retardation, neurosensory hearing loss, and neonatal convulsions (226). Phlebotomy treatment during pregnancy has been used successfully to control PCT (227,228).

2. *Erythropoietic Protoporphyria*

Five women who had erythropoietic protoporphyria (EPP) followed by Schmidt et al. (229) showed a marked decrease or disappearance of their cutaneous symptoms during pregnancy. No information has been reported on the outcome of gestation or on fetal effects.

3. *Congenital Erythropoietic Porphyria*

The small number of reports of offspring from congenital erythropoietic (CEP) affected mothers reflects the rarity of this autosomal recessive disease. Affected patients have a shortened life span, and they may have difficulty finding mates because of the severe cutaneous disfigurement (230). Offspring of persons who have CEP invariably would be obligate heterozygotes. Townes (230) reported one woman with CEP who experienced a normal, uncomplicated pregnancy and delivery.

REFERENCES

1. G. M. Crawford and R. W. Leeper. Disease of the skin in pregnancy, *Arch. Dermatol. Syphilol. 61*:753 (1950).
2. R. B. Scoggins. Skin changes and diseases in pregnancy, *Dermatology in General Medicine* (T. B. Fitzpatrick et al., eds.). McGraw-Hill, New York, 1979, pp. 1363–1370.
3. E. Besnier, L. Brocq, and L. Jacquet, *La Pratique Dermatologigue.* Vol. IV. Masson, Paris, 1904, p. 74.
4. D. S. Nurse. Prurigo of pregnancy, *Aust. J. Dermatol. 9*:258–267 (1968).
5. M. J. Costello. Eruptions of pregnancy, *N.Y. State J. Med. 41*:849–855 (1941).
6. R. T. Hozbach. Jaundice in pregnancy, *Am. J. Med. 61*:367–376 (1976).
7. Itching in pregnancy (editorial), *Br. Med. J. 3*:608 (1975).
8. U. P. Haemmerli. Jaundice during pregnancy, *Acta Med. Scand. 179*(Suppl.):444 (1966).

9. M. Lunzer, P. Barnes, Byth, and M. O'Halloran, Serum bile acid concentrations during pregnancy and their relationship to obstetric cholestasis, *Gastroenterology 91*:825–829 (1986).
10. T. E. Bynum. Hepatic and gastrointestinal disorders in pregnancy, *Med. Clin. North Am. 61*:129 (1977).
11. M. B. Johnston and T. F. Baskett. Obstetric cholestasis: A 14 year review, *Am. J. Obstet. Gynecol. 133*:299–301 (1979).
12. H. Adlercruetz, A. Svanborg, and A. Anberg. Recurrent jaundice in pregnancy: A study of estrogens and their conjugates in late pregnancy, *Am. J. Med. 49*:630 (1970).
13. G. T. Jarvis and A. C. Crompton. Neurofibromatosis and pregnancy, *Br. J. Obstet. Gynecol. 85*:844–846 (1978).
14. A. Ferhoff. Itching in pregnancy, *Acta Med. Scand. 196*:402–410 (1974).
15. J. V. Dacus. Pruritus and pregnancy, *Clin. Obstet. Gynecol. 33*:737–746 (1990).
16. N. M. Fisk and G. N. Storey. Fetal outcome in obstetric cholestasis, *Br. J. Obstet. Gynecol. 95*:1137 (1988).
17. D. Sasseville, R. D. Wilkinson and J. Y. Schrader. Dermatoses of pregnancy, *Int. J. Dermatol. 20*:223–241 (1981).
18. E. E. Lutz and A. T. Margolis. Obstetric hepatosis: Treatment with cholestyramine and interim response to steroids, *Obstet. Gynecol. 33*:64 (1969).
19. X. Noguera, L. Puig, and J. M. de Moragas. Prurigo gravidarum, *Cutis 39*:437–440 (1987).
20. T. S. Lawly, K. C. Hertz, and T. R. Wade, et al. Pruritic urticarial papules and plaques of pregnancy, *JAMA 241*:1696–1699 (1979).
21. G. Bourne. Toxemic rash of pregnancy, *Proc. R. Soc. Med. 55*:462 (1962).
22. R. C. Holmes, M. M. Black, J. Dann, D. C. O. James, and B. Bhogal. A comparative study of toxic erythema of pregnancy and herpes gestationis, *Br. J. Dermatol. 106*:499–510 (1982).
23. R. C. Holmes and M. M. Black. The specific dermatoses of pregnancy. *J. Am. Acad. Dermatol. 8*:403–412 (1983).
24. A. R. Ahmed and R. Kaplan, PUPPP, *J. Am. Acad. Dermatol. 4*:679–681 (1981).
25. E. Hershel. Pruritic urticarial papules and plaques of pregnancy, *JAMA 243*:2156 (1980).
26. R. A. Schwartz, R. C. Hansen, and P. J. Lynch. PUPPP, *Cutis 27*:425–432 (1981).
27. S. R. Uhlin. PUPPP: Involvement of mother and infant, *Arch. Dermatol. 117*(3):238–239 (1981).
28. K. B. Yancey, R. P. Hall, and T. J. Lawley. Pruritic urticarial papules and plaques of pregnancy: Clinical experience in twenty-five patients, J. Am. Acad. Dermatol. *10*:473–480 (1984).
29. J. Alcalay and J. E. Wolf. Pruritic urticarial papules and plaques of pregnancy: The enigma and the confusion, (editorial), *J. Am. Acad. Dermatol. 19*:1115–1116 (1988).
30. W. B. Winton. Dermatoses of pregnancy, *J. Am. Acad. Dermatol. 6*:977–998 (1982).
31. W. L. Chang, T. K. Young, et al. Urticarial vasculitis developed on the striate distensae during pregnancy, *Int. J. Dermatol. 32*:751–752 (1993).
32. J. Alcalay, A. Ingber, B. Kafri, et al. Hormonal evaluation and autoimmune background in PUPPP, *Am. J. Obstet. Gynecol. 158*:417–20 (1988).
33. L. M. Cohen, E. L. Capeless, P. A. Krusinski, et al. PUPPP and its relationship to

maternal-fetal weight gain and twin pregnancy, *Arch. Dermatol. 125*:1534–1536 (1989).

34. B. Russell and N. A. Thorne. Herpes gestationis, *Br. J. Dermatol. 69*:339–357 (1957).
35. J. K. Shornick. Herpes gestationis, *J. Am. Acad. Dermatol. 17*:539–556 (1987).
36. H. W. Lim and J. C. Bystryn. Bullous disease, *Clin. Obstet. Gynecol. 21*:1007–1022 (1978).
37. R. C. Holmes and M. M. Black. Herpes gestationis, *Dermatol. Clin. 1*:195 (1983).
38. J. K. Shornick, J. L. Banget, et al. Herpes gestationis, Clinical and histological features of 28 cases, *J. Am. Acad. Dermatol. 8*:214 (1983).
39. K. C. Hertz, S. I. Katz, J. Maize, et al. Herpes gestationis: A clinicopathologic study, *Arch. Dermatol. 112*:1543–1548 (1976).
40. H. Yaoita, M. Gullino, and S. I. Katz. Herpes gestationis: Ultra-structure and ultra-structural localization of in vivo-bound complement, *J. Invest. Dermatol. 66*:383–388 (1976).
41. M. V. Dahl. *Clinical Immunodermatology*, Year Book, Chicago, 1981, pp. 153–155.
42. S. I. Katz, K. C. Hertz, and H. Yaoita. Herpes gestationis. Immunopathology and characterization of the HG factor, *J. Clin. Invest. 57*:1434–1441 (1976).
43. J. P. Ortonne, B. L. Hsi, P. Verrando, et al. Herpes gestationis factor reacts with the amniotic epithelial basement membrane, *Br. J. Dermatol. 117*:147–154 (1987).
44. S. E. Kelly, B. S. Bhogal, F. Wojnarowska, and M. M. Black. Expression of a pemphigoid gestationis-related antigen by human placenta. *Br. J. Dermatol. 118*:605–611 (1988).
45. J. K. Morgan. Herpes gestationis influenced by an oral contraceptive, *Br. J. Dermatol. 80*:456–458 (1968).
46. T. P. Chorzelski, S. Jabonski, E. H. Beutner, et al. Herpes gestationis with identical lesions in the newborn, *Arch. Dermatol. 112*:1129–1131 (1976).
47. K. D. Kolodny. Herpes gestationis, a new assessment of incidence, diagnosis, and fetal prognosis, *Am. J. Obstet. Gynecol. 104*:39–45 (1969).
48. T.J. Lawley, G. Stingle, and S. I. Katz. Fetal and maternal risk factors in herpes gestationis, *Arch. Dermatol. 114*:552–555 (1978).
49. P. A. Krusinski and J. H. Saurat. Transplacentally transferred dermatoses, *Pediatr. Dermatol. 6*:166–77 (1989).
50. R. H. Hayashi, F. Ott, A. Krakowski, et al. Impetigo herpetiformis with lowered serum levels of vitamin D and its diminished in intestinal absorption, *Dermatologica 164*:360 (1982).
51. G. E. Pierard, C. P. Pierard-Franchimont, and M. dela Brassine, Impetigo herpetiformis and pustular psoriasis during pregnancy, *Am. J. Dermatopathol. 3*: 215–220 (1983).
52. M. Lotem, V. Katzenelson, A. Rotem, et al. Impetigo herpetiformis: A variant of pustular psoriasis or a separate entity, *J. Am. Acad. Dermatol. 20*:338–341 (1989).
53. O. Y.Oumeish, S. E. Farraj, et al. Some aspects of impetigo herpetiformis, *Arch. Dermatol. 118*:103 (1982).
54. A. S. Spangler, W. Reddy, W. A. Bardawil, et al. Papular dermatitis of pregnancy, *JAMA 181*:577–581 (1962).
55. A. S. Spangler and K. Emerson, Jr. Estrogen levels and estrogen therapy in papular dermatitis of pregnancy, *Am. J. Obstet. Gynecol. 110*:534–537 (1971).

56. S. E. Rutherford and J. P. Phelan. Deep venous thrombosis and pulmonary embolism in pregnancy, *Obstet. Gynecol. Clin. North Am. 18*:345–370 (1991).
57. S. M. Peck, I. K. Rovinsky, and Guttmacher, *The Medical, Surgical, and Gynecologic Complications of Pregnancy,* 2nd ed. Williams & Wilkins, Baltimore, 1964, pp. 619–646.
58. P. W. Jaber, B. B. Wilson, et al. Eruptive xanthomas during pregnancy, *J. Am. Acad. Dermatol. 27*:300–302 (1992).
59. V. M. Ricardi. Medical process: Von Recklinghausen neurofibromatosis, *N. Engl. J. Med. 305*:1617–2166 (1981).
60. F. W. Crowe, W. J. Schull, and J. V. Neel. *A Clinical, Pathological, and Genetic Study of Multiple Neurofibromatosis*, Charles C Thomas, Springfield, IL, 1956.
61. L. Rosenbaum and S. S. Paley. Neurofibromatosis, *N.Y. J. Med. 35*:1350 (1955).
62. A. H. Ansari and M Nagamani. Pregnancy and neurofibromatosis, *Obstet. Gynecol.* 47(Suppl.):255–295 (1976).
63. R. P. Bolande. Neurofibromatosis—The quintessential neurocristopathy: Pathogenic concepts and relationships, *Adv. Neurol. 29*:67–75 (1981).
64. J. R. Perez-polo, K. Hall, K. Livingston, et al. Steroid induction of nerve growth factor synthesis in cell culture, *Life Sci. 21*:1535–1544 (1977).
65. H. H. Strange. Recklinghausen's disease and pregnancy, *Zentralbl. Gynakol. 73*:1787 (1951).
66. S. H. Cornell and W. B. Kirkendall. Neurofibromatosis of the renal artery, an unusual case of hypertension, *Radiology 88*:24 (1967).
67. G. H. Swapp and R. A. Main. Neurofibromatosis in pregnancy, *Br. J. Dermatol. 88*:431–435 (1973).
68. D. J. Wong and H. T. Strassner. Melanoma in pregnancy, *Clin. Obstet. Gynecol. 33*:782–789 (1990).
69. C. Riberti, G. Marola, and A. Bertoni. Malignant melanoma: The adverse effect of pregnancy, *Br. J. Plast. Surg. 34*:338–339 (1981).
70. B. K. Schwartz, S. J. Zashin, S. K. Spencer, et al. Pregnancy and hormonal influences on malignant melanoma, *J. Dermatol. Surg. Oncol. 13*:276–181 (1987).
71. K. A. Feucht, M. J. Walker, T. K. Dasgupta, et al. Effects of 17 beta-estradiol on the growth of estrogen receptor positive human melanoma in vitro and in athymic mice, *Cancer Res. 48*:7093 (1988).
72. H. M. Shaw, G. W. Milton, G. Farago, et al. Endocrine influence on survival from malignant melanoma, *Cancer 42*:669 (1978).
73. I. G. Ances and S. H. Pomerantz, Serum concentrations of beta-melanocyte stimulating hormone in human pregnancy, *Am. J. Obstet. Gynecol. 119*:1062 (1974).
74. B. Dahlberg. Melanocyte stimulating substances in the urine of pregnant women, *Acta Endocrinol.* (Suppl.) 60 (1961).
75. P. A. George, J. G. Fortner, and G. T. Pack Melanoma with pregnancy, *Cancer 13*:854–859 (1960).
76. R. S. Smith and P. Randall. Melanoma during pregnancy, *Surg. Gynecol. Obstet. 34*:825–829 (1969).
77. L. P. White, G. Lindon, L. Breslow, et al. Studies on melanoma: The effect of pregnancy on survival in human melanoma, *JAMA 177*:235 (1961).

78. M. H. Shiu, D. Schottenfield, M. B. Maclean, et al. Adverse effect of pregnancy on melanoma: A reappraisal, *Cancer 37*:181–187 (1976).
79. C. L. Slingluff and H. F. Seigler. Malignant melanoma and pregnancy, *Ann. Plast. Surg. 28*:95–99 (1992).
80. A. J. Sober, T. B. Fitzpatrick, and M. C. Mihm. Primary melanoma of the skin: Recognition and management, *J. Am. Acad. Dermatol. 2*:179–197 (1980).
81. S. A. Adam, J. K. Scheaves, N. H. Wright, et al. A case-control study of the possible association between oral contraceptives and malignant melanoma, *Br. J. Cancer 44*:45–50 (1981).
82. E. A. Holly, N. S. Weiss, and J. M. Liff. Cutaneous melanoma in relation to exogenous hormones and reproductive factors, *J.N.V.I. 70*:827–831 (1983).
83. I. R. Gough and R. W. Stitz. Metastatic carcinoid tumour: Stability throughout pregnancy, *Aust. N.Z. J. Surg. 61*:960–962 (1991).
84. V. C. Andreev. Skin manifestations of visceral cancer, *Curr. Probl. Dermatol.* Karger, Basel, 1978.
85. E. C. Vonderheid, D. L. Dellatorre, and E. J. Van Scott. Prolonged remission of tumor-stage mycosis fungoides by topical immunotherapy, *Arch. Dermatol. 117*: 586–589 (1981).
86. F. W. Benschine. Massive condylomata acuminata of vulva complicating labor, *Am. J. Obstet. Gynceol. 42*:338 (1941).
87. W. Footer. Spontaneous postpartum disappearance of massive condylomata of the vulva, *Am. J. Obstet. Gynecol. 48*:266 (1944).
88. H. L. Garoner and R. H. Kaufman. Condyloma acuminata, *Clin. Obstet. Gynecol. 8*:938–945 (1965).
89. R. L. Gortlay and M. A. Krembs. Vulvar condylomata complicating labor, *Obstet. Gynecol. 4*:67 (1954).
90. L. C. Powell. Condyloma acuminatum, *Clin. Obstet. Gynecol. 15*:448 (1972).
91. N. G. Osborne and M. D. Adelson. Herpes simplex and human papillomavirus genital infections: controversy over obstetric management, *Clin. Obstet. Gynecol. 33*:801–811 (1990).
92. E. A. Graber, H. R. K. Barber, and J. J. O'Rouke. Simple surgical treatment for condyloma acuminata of the vulva, *Obstet. Gynecol. 29*:247–250 (1967).
93. D. R. Ostergard and D. E. Townsend. The treatment of vulva condyloma acuminata by cryosurgery—A preliminary report, *Cryobiology 5*:340–342 (1969).
94. R. L. Young, A. A. Acosta, and R. H. Kaufman. The treatment of large condylomata acuminata complicating pregnancy, *Obstet. Gynecol. 41*:65–73 (1973).
95. J. Matsunaga, A. Berman, and N. N. Bhatia. Genital condylomata acuminata in pregnancy: Effectiveness, safety and pregnancy outcome following cryotherapy, *Br. J. Obstet. Gynaecol. 94*:168–172 (1987).
96. J. W. Calkins, B. T. Masterson, and J. F. Magrina. Management of condylomata acuminata with the carbon dioxide laser, *Obstet. Gynecol. 59*:105–108 (1982).
97. Beckmann et al. HPV Infection in women with multicentric squamous cell neoplasia, *Am. J. Obstet. Gynecol. 165*:1431–1437 (1991).
98. E. M. Smith, S. R. Johnson, et al. Perinatal Vertical Transmission of human papillomavirus and subsequent development of respiratory tract papillomatosus, *Ann. Otol. Rhinol. Laryngol. 100*:479–483 (1991).

99. T. A. Cook, A. M. Cohn, J. P. Brunschwig, et al. Wart viruses and laryngeal papillomas, *Lancet 1*:782 (1973).
100. T. V. Sedlacek, S. Lindheim, C. Eder, et al. Mechanism for human papillomavirus transmission at birth, *Am. J. Obstet. Gynecol. 161*:55 (1989).
101. A. Rook, D. S. Wilkinson, and F. J. G. Ebling. *Textbook of Dermatology,* 3rd ed. Blackwell, Oxford, UK, 1979, pp. 220–224.
102. D. N. Danforth. *Obstetrics and Gynecology*, 3rd ed. Harper & Row, New York, 1977, p. 873.
103. P. S. Porter and J. S. Lyle. Yeast vulvovaginitis due to oral contraceptives, *Arch. Dermatol. 93*:402–403 (1966).
104. L. A. Santos, J. Beceiro, R. Hernandez, et al. Congenital cutaneous candidiasis: Report of 4 cases and review of the literature, *Eur. J. Pediatr. 150*:336–338 (1991).
105. K. A. Arndt. *Manual of Dermatologic Therapeutics*, 2nd ed. Little, Brown, Boston, 1978, pp. 118–126.
106. H. C. S. Wallenburg and J. W. Wladimiroff. Recurrences of vulvovaginal candidiasis during pregnancy, *Obstet. Gynecol. 48*:491–494 (1976).
107. W. M. McCormick. Management of sexually transmissible infections during pregnancy, *Clin. Obstet. Gynecol. 18*:57–71 (1975).
108. A. Broberg and K. Thiringer. Congenital cutaneous candidiasis, *Int. J. Dermatol. 18*:464–465 (1989).
109. R. K. Whyte, Z. Hussain, et al. Antenatal infections with candida species, *Arch. Dis. Child. 57*:528–535 (1982).
110. N. Rudolph, A. A. Tariq, M. R. Reale, et al. Congenital cutaneous candidiasis, *Arch. Dermatol. 113*:1101–1103 (1977).
111. T. A. Chapel, C. Gagliard, and W. Nichols. Congenital cutaneous candidiasis, *J. Am. Acad. Dermatol. 6*:926–928 (1982).
112. L. S. Blackburn. Effective treatment of chlamydia trachomatis infection during pregnancy to prevent perinatal and infant complications, *Nurse Practitioner 17*:56–60 (1992).
113. R. L. Sweet, et al. Chlamydia trachomatis infection and pregnancy outcome, *Am. J. Obstet. Gynecol. 156*:824–831 (1987).
114. G. B. Winton. Skin diseases aggravated by pregnancy, *J. Am. Acad. Dermatol. 20*:1–13 (1989).
115. M. E. Duncan, J. M. H. Pearson, D. S. Ridley, et al. Pregnancy and leprosy: The consequences of alterations of cell-mediated and humoral immunity during pregnancy and lactation, *Int. J. Lepr. 50*:425–435 (1982).
116. M. E. Duncan and J. M. H. Pearson. The association of pregnancy and leprosy III, Erythema nodosum leprosum in pregnancy and lactation, *Lepr. Rev. 55*:129–142 (1984).
117. M. E. Duncan. Babies of mothers with leprosy have small placentas, low birth weights and grow slowly, *Br. J. Obstet. Gynaecol. 87*:471–479 (1980).
118. G. Kahn. Dapsone is safe during pregnancy (letter). *J. Am. Acad. Dermatol. 13*:838–839 (1985).
119. R. L. Atmar, J. A. Englund, and H. Hammill. Complications of measles during pregnancy, *Clin. Infect. Dis. 14*:217–26 (1992).
120. S. J. Stein and J. S. Greenspoon. Rubeola during pregnancy, *Obstet. Gynecol. 78*:925–929 (1991).

121. J. G. Wheeler and R. F. Jacobs. A practical approach to the use of acyclovir in herpes simplex and varicella-zoster infections, *Resident Staff Physician 40*:36–46 (1994).
122. L. M. Frenkel, E. M. Garratty, J. P. Shen, et al. Clinical reactivation of herpes simplex virus type-2 infection in seropositive pregnant women with no history of genital herpes, *Ann. of Int. Med. 118*:414–418 (1993).
123. R. J. Whitley, L. Corey, A. Arvin, et al. Changing presentation of herpes simplex infection in neonates. *J. Infect. Dis. 158*:109–116 (1988).
124. C. G. Prober, P. A. Hensleigh, F. D. Boucher et al. Use of routine viral cultures at delivery to identify neonates exposed to herpes simplex virus, *N. Engl. J. Med. 318*:887 (1988).
125. L. G. Smith and S. Faro. Cutaneous manifestations of bacterial and viral disorders in pregnancy, *Clin. Obstet. Gynecol. 33*:792–799 (1990).
126. S. G. Paryani and A. M. Arvin. Intrauterine infection with varicella-zoster virus after maternal varicella, *N. Engl. J. Med. 314*:1542–1546 (1986).
127. J. Balducci and J. F. Rodis, Rosengrens, et al. Pregnancy outcome following first trimester varicella infection, *Obstet. Gynecol. 79*:5–6 (1992).
128. M. Siegal. Congenital malformations following chickenpox, measles, mumps, and hepatitis: Results of a cohort study, *JAMA 226*:1521–1524 (1973).
129. A. L. Morey, J. W. Keeling, and H. J. Porter. Clinical and histopathological features of parvovirus B19 infection in the human fetus, *Br. J. Obstet. Gynaecol. 99*:566–574 (1992).
130. H. M. Feder, I. Anderson, et al. Fifth disease. A brief review of infections in childhood, in adulthood, and in pregnancy, *Arch. Int. Med. 149*:2176–2178 (1989).
131. J. S. Kinney, L. J. Anderson, J. Farrar, et al. Risk of adverse outcomes of pregnancy after human parvovirus B19 infection, *J. Infect. Dis. 157*:663–667 (1988).
132. W. El-Sadr, J. M. Oleske, et al. Evaluation and management of early HIV infection, *Clinical Practice Guideline*, U.S. Dept. of Health and Human Services *7*:6–70 (1994).
133. R.W. Marion, A. A. Wiznia, R. G. Hutcheon, et al. Human T-cell lymphotrophic virus type III (HTLV-III) embryopathy, *Am. J. Dis. Child. 140*:638–640 (1986).
134. N. S. Penneys. *Skin Manifestations of AIDS* (R. Marks, ed.), Lippincott, 1990.
135. L. E. Riley and R. E. Tuomala. Bacillary angiomatosis in a pregnant patient with acquired immunodeficiency syndrome, *Obstet. Gynecol. 79*:818–819 (1992).
136. A. Manns and W. A. Blattner. The epidemiology of the human T-cell lymphotrophic virus type 1 and 2: Etiologic role in human disease, *Transfusion 31*:67–74 (1991).
137. C. B. Bunker, S. Whittaker, L. Luzzatto, et al. Indolent cutaneous prodrome of fatal HTLV-1 infection, *Lancet 11*:426 (1990).
138. J. D. Temple. Personal communication, January, 1994.
139. Y. Ville, E. Delaporte, M. Peeters, et al. Human T-cell lymphotropic virus type I infection and pregnancy: A case control study and 12 month follow-up of 135 women and their infants, *Am. J. Obstet. Gynecol. 165*:1438–1443 (1991).
140. S. E. Schutzer, C. K. Janniger, R. A. Schwartz, et al. Lyme disease during pregnancy, *Cutis 47*:267–277 (1991).
141. L. E. Markowitz, A. C. Steere, J. L. Benach, et al. Lyme disease during pregnancy, *JAMA 255*:3394–3396 (1986).
142. P. A. J. Heaton and P. Lucas. Congenital syphilis despite pregnancy screening, *N.Z. Med. J. 103*:401 (1990).

143. S. A. Rawstron, S. Jenkins, S. Blanchard, et al. Maternal and congenital syphilis in Brooklyn, N.Y. Epidemiology, transmission, and diagnosis, *A.J.D.C. 147*:727–731 (1993).
144. M. Hallak, J. F. Peipert, A. Ludomirsky, et al. Nonimmune hydrops fetalis and fetal congenital syphilis, *J. Reprod. Med. 37*:173–176 (1992).
145. C. M. Peterson, K. Schuppert, P. C. Kelly, et al. Coccidiomycosis and pregnancy, *Obstet. Gynecol. Surv. 48*:149–156 (1993).
146. M. P. R. Walker, C. Z. Brody, et al, Reactivation of coccidiomycosis in pregnancy, *Obstet. Gynecol. 79*:815–817 (1992).
147. K. D. Bickel and B. H. Press, Successful treatment of coccidiomycosis osteomyelitis in an infant, *Ann. Plast. Surg. 30*:462–465 (1993).
148. D. W. Branch, J. R. Scott, N. K. Kochenour, et al. Obstetrical complications with the lupus anticoagulant, *N. Engl. J. Med. 313*:1322–1326 (1985).
149. M. D. Lockshin. Antiphospholipid antibody syndrome, *JAMA 268*:1451–1453 (1992).
150. M. Petri. Antiphospholipid antibodies: Lupus anticoagulant and anticardiolipin antibody, *Curr. Probl. Dermatol. 4*(5): (1992).
151. W. F. Lubbe, W. S. Butler, et al. Lupus anticoagulant and pregnancy, *Br. J. Obstet. Gynecol. 92*:357–363 (1984).
152. J. K. Pollard, J. R. Scott, and D. W. Branch. Outcome of children born to women treated during pregnancy for the antiphospholipid syndrome, *Obstet. Gynecol. 80*: 365–368 (1992).
153. E. V. Barnett. The influence of pregnancy, on the systemic manifestations of systemic lupus erythematosus. *Ann. Intern. Med. 94*:667–677 (1981).
154. J. P. Hyslett and E. A. Reece. Systemic lupus in pregnancy, *Clin. Perinatol. 12*:539–550 (1985).
155. C. D. McGee and E. L. Makowski. Systemic lupus erythematosus in pregnancy, *Obstet. Gynecol. 107*:1008–1012 (1970).
156. N. J. Mchugh, P. A. Reilly, L. A. Mchugh, et al. Pregnancy outcome and autoantibodies in connective tissue disease, *J. Rheumatol. 16*:42–46 (1989).
157. A. J. G. Swaak. Pregnancy in systemic lupus erythematosus, *Neth. J. Med. 27*:84–89 (1984).
158. C. H. Syrop and M. W. Varner. Systemic lupus erythematosus, *Clin. Obstet. Gynecol. 26*:547–557 (1983).
159. R. Bear. Pregnancy and lupus nephritis, *Obstet. Gynecol. 47*:715 (1976).
160. M. Garsenstein, V. E. Pollak, and R. M. Kark. Systemic lupus erythematosus and pregnancy, *N. Engl. J. Med. 267*:165 (1962).
161. J. I. Zulman, N. Talal, G. S. Hoffman, et al. Problems associated with the management of pregnancies in patients with systemic lupus erythematosus, *J. Rheumatol. 7*:37–49 (1980).
162. L. A. Lee, C. E. Harmon, J. C. Huff, et al. The demonstration of SSA/Ro antigen in human tissues and in neonatal and adult skin, *J. Invest. Dermatol. 85*:143–146 (1985).
163. L. A. Lee, P. J. Lillis, K. A. Fritz, et al. Neonatal lupus syndrome in successive pregnancies, *J. Am. Acad. Dermatol. 9*:401–406 (1983).
164. G. M. Horowitz and G. D. V. Hankins. Cutaneous manifestations of collagen vascular disease in pregnancy, *Clin. Obstet. Gynecol. 33*:759–766 (1990).

165. E. Sharon, J. Jones, H. Diamond, et al. Pregnancy and azathioprine in systemic lupus erythematosus, *Am. J. Obstet. Gynecol. 118*:25 (1974).
166. E. L. Dubois. Questions and answers: Raynaud phenomenon in pregnancy, *JAMA 233*:283 (1975).
167. R. K. Winkelman. Scleroderma and pregnancy, *Clin. Obstet. Gynecol. 8*:280 (1965).
168. T. R. Johnson, E. A. Banner, and R. K. Winkelmann. Scleroderma and pregnancy, *Obstet. Gynecol. 23*:467–469 (1964).
169. V. D. Steen, C. Conte, N. Day, et al. Pregnancy in women with systemic sclerosis, *Arthritis Rheum. 32*:151–157 (1989).
170. S. P. Ballou, J. J. Morley, and I. Kushner. Pregnancy and systemic sclerosis, *Arthritis Rheum. 27*:295–298 (1984)
171. M. A. Stenever, A. B. P. Ng. Scleroderma of the uterus and cervix, *Am. J. Obstet. Gynecol. 107*:965–966 (1970).
172. W. A. Cook. Letter and reply: Raynaud's phenomenon in pregnancy, *JAMA 235*:145–146 (1976).
173. J. R. Karlen and W. A. Cook. Renal scleroderma and pregnancy, *Obstet. Gynecol. 44*:349–354 (1974).
174. C. M. Black. Systemic sclerosis and pregnancy, *Baillieres Clin. Rheum. 7*:105–124 (1990).
175. V. D. Steen, T. A. Medsger, et al. Factors predicting the development of renal involvement in progressive systemic sclerosis, *Am. J. Med. 76*:779–786 (1984).
176. S. Mor-Yosef, D. Navot, R. Rabinowitz, et al. Collagen diseases in pregnancy, *Obstet. Gynecol. Surv. 30*:67–84 (1984).
177. A. G. Wilson and J. D. Kirby. Successful pregnancy in a woman with systemic sclerosis while taking nifedipine, *Ann. Rheum. Dis. 49*:51–52 (1990).
178. G. Gutierrez, R. Dagnino, and G. Mintz. Polymyositis/dermatomyositis and pregnancy, *Arthritis Rheum. 27*:291–294 (1984).
179. W. N. Spellacy. Scleroderma and pregnancy: Report of a case, *Obstet. Gynecol. 23*:297–300 (1964).
180. A. Tsai, M. D. Lindheimer, and S. I. Lamberg. Dermatomyositis complicating pregnancy, *Obstet. Gynecol. 41*:570–573 (1973).
181. C. R. King and S. Chow. Dermatomyositis and pregnancy, *Obstet. Gynecol. 66*:589–592 (1985).
182. S. Bombardieri, O. DiMunno, C. DiPunzio, et al. Erythema nodosum associated with pregnancy and oral contraceptives, *Br. Med. J. 1*:1509–1510 (1977).
183. M. A. Salvatore and P. J. Lyn. Erythema nodosum, estrogens and pregnancy, *Arch. Dermatol. 116*:557–558 (1980).
184. H. Gordon. Erythema nodosum: A review of 115 cases, *Br. J. Dermatol. 73*:393–409 (1961).
185. F. Holcomb. Erythema nodosum associated with the use of oral contraception, *Obstet. Gynecol. 25*:156–157 (1965).
186. M. H. Matz. Erythema nodosum and contraceptive medication, *N. Engl. J. Med. 276*:351–352 (1967).
187. J. A, Bartelsmeyer and R. H. Petrie. Erythema nodosum, estrogens and pregnancy, *Clin. Obstet. Gynecol. 33*:777–781 (1990).

188. M. G. Ross, B. Kant, R. Frieder, et al. Pemphigus in pregnancy: a reevaluation of fetal risk, *Am. J. Obstet. Gynecol. 155*:30–33 (1986).
189. M. H. Samitz, M. S. Greenberg and J. M. Coletti. Pemphigus in association with pregnancy: Observations of the effect of corticotrophin and cortisone on pemphigus, pregnancy and infant, *A.M.A. Arch. Dermatol. Syphilol. 67*:10 (1953).
190. H. Terpstra, M. C. J. M. DeJong, and A. M. Klakke. In vivo bound pemphigus antibodies in a stillborn infant, *Arch. Dermatol. 115*:316–319 (1979).
191. N. Wasserstrum and R. K. Laros. Transplacental transmission of pemphigus, *JAMA 249*:1480–1482 (1983).
192. P. Merlob, A. Metzger, B. Hazaz, et al. Neonatal pemphigus vulgaris, *Pediatrics 78*:1102–1105 (1986).
193. D. Green and J. C. Maize. Maternal pemphigus vulgaris with in vivo bound antibodies in the stillborn fetus, *J. Am. Acad. Dermatol. 7*:388–392 (1982).
194. N. S. Goldberg, C. DeFeo, and N. Kirshenbaum. Pemphigus vulgaris and pregnancy: Risk factors and recommendations. *J. Am. Acad. Dermatol. 28*:877–879 (1993).
195. M. G. Ross, B. Kant, R. Frieder, et al. Pemphigus in pregnancy: a reevaluation of fetal risk, *Am. J. Obstet. Gynecol. 155*:30–33 (1986).
196. R. H. Hayashi. Bullous dermatoses and prurigo of pregnancy, *Clin. Obstet. Gynecol. 33*:746–753 (1990).
197. T. Gruneberg. Psoriasis and pregnancy, *Hautartzt 3*:155 (1952).
198. R. Church. The prospect of psoriasis, *Br. J. Dermatol. 70*:139 (1958).
199. E. M. Farber and M. L. Nall. The natural history of psoriasis in 5,600 patients, *Dermatologia 148*:1–18 (1974).
200. D. M. Bronson, R. Barsky, and S. Barsky. Acrodermatitis enteropathica. Recognition at long last during recurrence in a pregnancy, *J. Am. Acad. Dermatol. 9*:140–144 (1983).
201. J. S. Schulman and J. L. Simpson. *Genetic Disease in Pregnancy*, Academic Press, New York, 1981, pp. 2–83.
202. K. M. Hambidge, K. H. Neldner, and P. A. Walravens. Zinc, acrodermatitis enteropathica and congenital malformations, *Lancet 1*:577–578 (1975).
203. J. Zander, H. Mickan, K. Holzmann, et al. Androluteoma syndrome in pregnancy, *Am. J. Obstet. Gynecol. 130*:170–177 (1978).
204. M. M. Frank, J. A. Gelfand, and J. P. Atkinson. Hereditary angioedema, *Ann. Intern. Med. 89*:580–593 (1976).
205. J. A. Gelfand and J. P. Atkinson. Hereditary Angioedema: The clinical syndrome and its management, *Ann. Intern. Med. 84*:580–593 (1976).
206. P. Beighton. *The Ehlers-Danlos Syndrome*, Heinemann, London, 1970.
207. V. A. McKusick. *Heritable Disorders of Connective Tissue*, 4th ed. Mosby, St. Louis, 1972.
208. M.A. Samuel, M. L. Schwartz, and M. M. Meister. The Ehlers Danlos syndrome, *U.S. Armed Forces Med. J. 4*:737 (1953).
209. M. E. Rivera-Alsina, P. Kwan, F. G. Zavisca et al. Complications of the Ehlers-Danlos syndrome in pregnancy, a case report, *J. Reprod. Med. 29*:757–759 (1984).
210. S. R. Ainsworth and P. L. Aulicino. A survey of patients with Ehlers-Danlos syndrome, *Clin. Orthop. Related Res. 286*:250–255 (1993).

211. N. L. Rudd, C. Nimrod, K. A. Holbrook et al. Pregnancy complications in type IV Ehlers-Danlos syndrome, *Lancet 1*:50–53 (1983).
212. T. R. Wade, S. L. Wade, and H. E. Jones. Skin changes and diseases associated with pregnancy, *Obstet. Gynecol. 52*:233–242 (1978).
213. D. E. Hammerschmidt, M. A. Arneson, S. L. Larson, et al. Maternal Ehlers-Danlos syndrome type X: Successful management of pregnancy and parturition, *JAMA 248*:2487–8 (1982).
214. C. Berde, D. C. Willis, and E. C. Sandberg. Pregnancy in women with pseudoxanthoma elasticuum, *Obstet. Gynecol. Surv. 38*:339–344 (1983).
215. F. F. Broekhuizen and P. R. Hamilton. PXE and intrauterine growth retardation, *Am. J. Obstet. Gynecol. 148*:112–114 (1984).
216. W. Mandel, E. W. Evans, and R. L. Walford. Dissecting aortic aneurysm during pregnancy, *N. Engl. J. Med. 251*:1059–1061 (1954).
217. E. F. Cava and R. L. Drier. The Marfan syndrome in pregnancy: A case report, *Trans. Pac. Coast Obstet. Gynecol. Soc. 38*:129–133 (1970).
218. S. Elias and R. L. Berkowitz. The Marfan syndrome and pregnancy, *Obstet. Gynecol. 47*:338–361 (1976).
219. A.E. Hirst, V. J. Johns, and S. W. Kime. Dissecting aneurysm of the aorta: A review of 505 cases, *Medicine 37*:270–279 (1958).
220. S. Sutiner and O. Piiroinen. Marfan's syndrome, pregnancy and fatal dissection of aorta, *Acta Obstet. Gynecol. Scand. 50*:295–300 (1971).
221. T. S. Zimmerman, J. M. McMillin, and C. J. Watson. Onset of manifestations of hepatic porphyria in relation to the influence of female sex hormones, *Arch. Intern. Med. 118*:229–240 (1966).
222. M. J. Brodie and M. R. Moore, G. G. Thompson et al. Acute intermittent porphyria, *J. Obstet. Gynecol. Br. Common. 84*:726–731 (1977).
223. R. Marks. Porphyria cutanea tarda, *Arch. Dermatol. 118*:452 (1982).
224. J. M. Lamon and B. C. Frykholm. Pregnancy and PCT, *Genet. Clin. Johns Hopkins Hosp. 145*:235–237 (1979).
225. J. M. Lamon, B. C. Frykholm, R. A. Hess, et al. Hematin therapy for acute porphyria, *Medicine 58*:252–269 (1979).
226. L. Tanenbaum and D. L. Tuffanelli. Antimalarial agents: chloroquine, hydroxychloroquine, and quinacrine, *Arch. Dermatol. 116*:587–591 (1980).
227. L. V. Baxi, T. J. Rubeo, B. Katz, et al. Porphyria cutanea tarda and pregnancy, *Am. J. Obstet. Gynecol. 146*:333–334 (1983).
228. G. Rajka. Pregnancy and porphyria cutanea tarda, *Acta Derm. Venerol (Stockh.) 64*:444–445 (1984).
229. H. Schmidt, G. Smitker, K. Thomsen, et al. Erythropoietic protoporphyria, *Arch. Dermatol. 110*:58–64 (1974).
230. P. L. Townes. Transplacentally acquired erythrodontia, *J. Pediatr. 67*:600–602 (1965).

6

Changes in the Mouth During Pregnancy

Sook-Bin Woo and Stephen T. Sonis
Brigham and Women's Hospital and Harvard School of Dental Medicine, Boston, Massachusetts

I. INTRODUCTION

The gingiva is the major target tissue for changes in the oral cavity during pregnancy. Pregnancy gingivitis and the formation of pyogenic granulomata are well-recognized entities. In addition, facial nerve paralysis, increased salivary flow, glossitis, and angular cheilitis have been reported.

II. PREGNANCY GINGIVITIS

As association between an increased gingival inflammatory state and pregnancy was first reported by Coles (1) in 1874. Since then, numerous reports have confirmed a relationship between pregnancy and an exuberant gingivitis characterized by edema, erythema, and especially bleeding. The frequency of pregnancy gingivitis has been reported at 55% (2), 76% (3), 86% (4), and 100% (5); the wide variation is probably due to differences in the criteria used for diagnosis.

Gingivitis appears to become more severe as pregnancy progresses (5–7) and may be the most severe in the second trimester. In a study of 120 pregnant patients and 40 nonpregnant, age-matched controls, Samant et al. (8) reported a significant and marked difference in gingivitis index between the two groups with patients in the second trimester demonstrating both a higher frequency of, and more severe gingivitis, than patients in other trimesters (Table 1). This finding was supported by other investigators (9).

Concomitant systemic disease may also affect the frequency of pregnancy gingivitis. Diabetes mellitus is a common systemic condition that can lead to severe gingivitis, periodontal disease, and bone loss at an early age. Whereas the prevalence of gingivitis was only 7% in 132 diabetic women before pregnancy, it rose to 96.2% during pregnancy (10). The intensity of the pregnancy gingivitis was unrelated to the severity of the patient's diabetes.

A. Etiology

Pregnancy gingivitis is probably influenced by three main factors: a shift in the gingival sulcular bacterial flora, the direct effect of hormones on the gingiva, and local immunomodulation.

Although there is clearly a relationship between increases in bacterial plaque and the severity of conventional gingivitis, the correlation is less clear in pregnancy gingivitis. Some studies report a direct correlation between gingivitis indices and plaque scores in pregnant patients (8,11). In contrast, others have noted increases in pregnancy gingivitis indices despite a relatively stable plaque mass (7,9) or even in the presence of reduced plaque mass (6,12). Silness and Löe (13) thought that the degree of gingivitis during pregnancy did not correspond with the amount of plaque present and that some other factor must play a role in the accentuated inflammatory changes.

Although plaque mass may not vary during pregnancy, its composition has been shown to change significantly. Kornman and Loesche (9) examined the subgingival microbial flora of 20 pregnant patients at monthly intervals. They found a fivefold

Table 1 Change in Severity of Gingivitis by Trimester[a]

	No gingivitis	Mild	Moderate	Severe
Pregnant controls (n = 40)	17.5	75.0	7.5	0.0
1st trimester (n = 40)	12.5	60.0	25.0	2.5
2nd trimester (n = 40)	7.5	40.0	45.0	7.5
3rd trimester (n = 40)	12.5	50.0	27.5	10.0
Overall pregnant patients (n = 120)	10.9	50.0	32.5	6.6

[a]The numbers represent the percentage of patients with gingivitis.
Source: From Ref. 8.

increase in the number of anaerobes, especially *Provetella intermedia*, which resulted in a significant increase in the ratio of anaerobes to aerobes. This finding peaked in the second trimester and was associated with high systemic levels of estradiol and progesterone. Increased uptake of these hormones by plaque was also noted. Jensen et al. (14) found a 55-fold increase in the same bacteria in pregnant women compared with controls. Kornman and Loesche (15) speculated that increased levels of estradiol and progesterone may substitute for vitamin K, an essential growth factor for *P. intermedia*, so that high gingival sulcular levels of these hormones provided a stimulus for growth for the bacterium.

A role for estrogens and progesterones in the development of pregnancy gingivitis was suggested by the clinical observation of an abrupt cessation of gingivitis following parturition (5,7,11). The finding of both progesterone- and estrogen-specific receptors in the gingiva gives teleological support for a potential role for these hormones (16,17).

Ojanotko-Harri et al. (18) found that the gingival metabolism of progesterone was reduced in pregnancy, resulting in increased gingival concentrations of the hormone. Increased gingival progesterone levels may be significant in pregnancy gingivitis at four levels. First, progesterone causes vascular proliferation (19) and increases the permeability of gingival blood vessels (20), resulting in increased exudation and localization of mediators of inflammation. Second, progesterone may affect the connective tissue matrix and collagen synthesis. When cultures of human gingival fibroblasts were exposed to progesterone at levels comparable to those seen during the third trimester, a significant reduction in glycosaminoglycan synthesis was osbserved (21). In addition, Lundgren et al. (22) reported that progesterone altered both the rate and pattern of gingival collagen production. These findings intimate that repair and maintenance of gingival tissues may be adversely affected by these hormones. Third, in vitro studies suggest that the presence of estradiol and progesterone results in an increase in the synthesis of prostaglandin E2, a potent mediator of inflammation (23), with the concentration of the hormones playing a regulatory role in prostaglandin synthesis (24). Finally, an alteration of folate metabolism is noted in response to both estrogen and progesterone. Whitehead et al. (25) noticed a relative deficiency of folate, as characterized by megaloblastic changes in the vaginal epithelium of women taking oral contraceptives; this could be reversed by the administration of systemic folate. This arose in the setting of normal serum folate levels and was termed "end-organ deficiency" by the investigators, ostensibly in response to estrogen and progesterone. Folate is essential for normal functioning and differentiation of many tissues, including epithelial cells. Patients treated with oral folate and folate rinses have shown significant reduction of pregnancy gingivitis (26), which led the investigators to conclude that pregnancy gingivitis may be in part secondary to hormonally induced end-organ deficiency.

A transient immunosuppression has been reported to occur during pregnancy

(27,28). Based on this finding, a number of studies have evaluated the possibility that changes in immune function may play a role in pregnancy gingivitis. Stashenko et al. (29) noted a reduction in the ratio of CD4 to CD8 cells in patients with periodontal disease. Since a similar change has been reported to occur in pregnant patients, Raber-Dulacher et al. (30) evaluated T-cell subsets and their response to mitogens, in particular *P. intermedia*. Of the seven patients they studied, reductions were noted in the numbers of CD3, CD4, and CD19 cells during the second trimester as compared to postpartum; there was no reduction in the proliferative response of peripheral blood lymphocytes to either mitogens or *P. intermedia*. The functional significance of these findings has yet to be elucidated. Another study also showed no detectable enhancement of lymphocyte blastogenic response to oral bacteria in pregnant subjects, possibly because of immunosuppression masking such enhancement which normally occurs in nonpregnant subjects (31).

B. Clinical Appearance

In its mildest form, pregnancy gingivitis presents as localized areas of edema and erythema, with a loss of the sharp, well-defined gingival contours normally seen in healthy tissues. In more advanced cases, diffuse gingival involvement may be noted which affects both the maxillary and mandibular arches (Fig. 1). The papillary gingiva tends to be affected more severely and frequently than the marginal gingiva. Edematous and boggy gingiva may extend over the tooth surfaces causing an increased depth of the gingival sulcus which may mimic

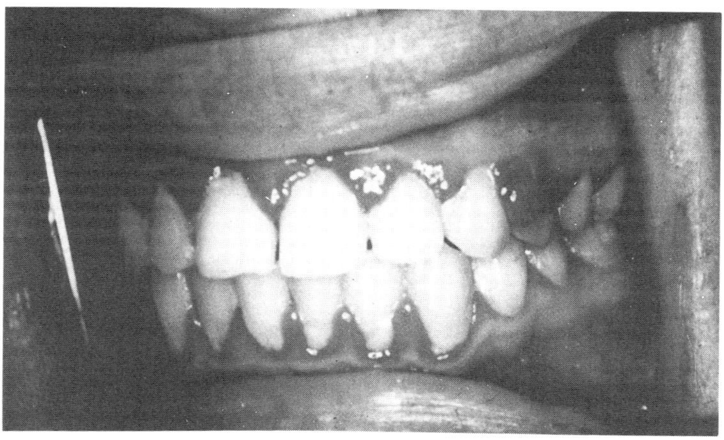

Figure 1 Generalized pregnancy gingivitis and early pyogenic granuloma in the maxillary left posterior area.

conventional periodontal disease. Consequently, plaque and food debris may be trapped and difficult to remove. In the most severe cases, the gingiva bleed readily on light pressure and during toothbrushing. Pain may not be significant.

C. Management

Treatment of pregnancy gingivitis entails removal of plaque and calculus and institution of a rigorous home oral care regimen. The former can be accomplished by a visit to the dentist or dental hygienist, at which time the deposits are removed by mechanical debridement. Patient education should be instituted early in pregnancy, and the patients should be motivated to maintain a high level of oral hygiene, adhering to a simple home care protocol of brushing and flossing. Antimicrobial rinses such as Peridex (32) (0.12% chlorhexidine digluconate, Proctor and Gamble, Cincinnati) and Listerine (33) used twice a day may be efficacious in killing plaque bacteria and reducing gingivitis.

If the gingival health is good at the onset of pregnancy and oral hygiene is maintained at a high level throughout pregnancy, gingivitis will only occur to a mild degree.

III. PYOGENIC GRANULOMA

Pyogenic granulomata are benign, localized, tumorlike proliferations of granulation tissue. They occur in approximately 0.5% (2) to 1.0% (34) of pregnant patients. In the oral cavity, the gingiva is the most common site of occurrence of these lesions and accounts for 45% (34) to 77% (35,36) of cases. Lesions may also occur on the lips, tongue, and buccal mucosa. The term *pyogenic* (pus producing) is a misnomer. The appearance of lesions is due to the fibrinous exudate on the surface, secondary to ulceration, from episodes of trauma.

Terms such as *epulis gravidarum*, *pregnancy epulides*, *angiogranuloma of pregnancy*, and *pregnancy tumor* have been applied to lesions in pregnant patients. Histologically and clinically, they are indistinguishable from simple pyogenic granulomata.

A. Etiology

Histologically, the oral pyogenic granuloma presents as an exuberant proliferation of fibrous and granulation tissue, with many proliferating endothelial cells, vascular spaces of varying sizes, and a mixed inflammatory infiltrate (Fig. 2). Older lesions tend to be less vascular and more fibrotic (34). Pyogenic granulomata result from an exaggerated reparative and healing response, often disproportionate to the severity of mechanical injury, or the presence of local irritants (such as bacterial plaque) (34,37).

In pregnancy, the pyogenic granuloma probably represents an extreme manifes-

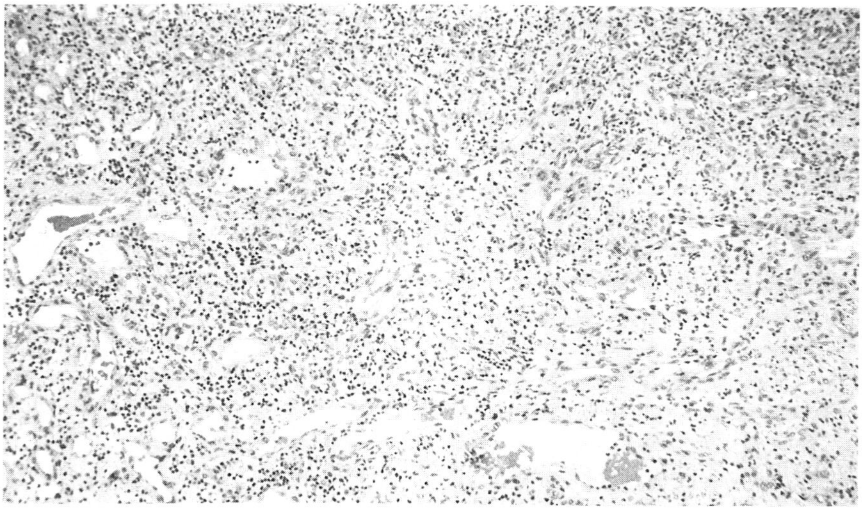

Figure 2 Photomicrograph of pyogenic granuloma showing characteristic proliferation of endothelial cells and vascular spaces.

tation of pregnancy gingivitis, in which inflammation, coupled with exuberant and ineffective repair and healing due to hormonal influences, causes a localized nodule of granulation tissue to persist and grow.

More recently, the term *lobular capillary hemangioma* has been suggested instead of pyogenic granuloma, because of the lobular arrangement of capillaries at the base of the lesions (38). This finding had been observed by previous investigators (34,37). It seems likely too that the "mucosal hemangiomas" mentioned by Rook (39) actually represent cases of pyogenic granulomata.

B. Clinical Appearance

The pyogenic granuloma consists of a polypoid or nodular mass, sessile or pedunculated, often erythematous, and focally covered by a yellowish fibrinous exudate if ulcerated. The size of the lesion may vary from a few millimeters in diameter to a few centimeters. It may be painful or asymptomatic, and it may occur in association with a supervening pregnancy gingivitis (see Fig. 1). Early lesions tend to be soft and spongy, whereas more mature lesions may be pink, firm, and fibrotic. Lesions may bleed with light pressure. The most common location for pyogenic granulomata is the gingiva anterior to the canines (35). Although unusual, large, long-standing lesions may cause resorption of the underlying bone (35,40).

C. Management

Some pyogenic granulomata spontaneously involute postpartum, although it is more likely that the larger ones will not regress completely (34,37), especially if the lesion has become predominantly fibrotic. Removal of local irritants may also lead to regression (37). Otherwise the treatment of choice is surgical excision. One report describes a case which regressed completely postpartum only to reappear again at the same site with a subsequent pregnancy (40).

As with pregnancy gingivitis, compliance with a rigorous oral hygiene regimen will probably reduce the risk of occurrence.

IV. FACIAL PALSY

A disproportionate number of pregnant or postpartum women present with idiopathic facial palsy or Bell palsy. Hilsinger et al. (41) reported that idiopathic facial palsy occurred with an incidence of 45.1 per 100,000 per year in pregnant women as compared with 16.9 per 100,000 per year in nonpregnant women. In the third trimester, however, the incidence rose to 118.2 per 100,000 per year. Another study found the incidence to be 41 per 100,000 pregnancies; two-thirds of the patients suffering from Bell palsy were in their third trimester, and the other one-third was in the first 2 weeks postpartum (42).

A. Etiology

Gestational Bell palsy is likely multifactorial, with patients having a predisposition to compression or inflammation of the seventh nerve (42). Two theories prevail. The "edema hypothesis" is based on the marked increase in interstitial fluid during the third trimester and immediate postpartum periods, which coincides with the highest incidence of Bell palsy in this population. This may result in direct nerve compression and subsequent facial palsy (41–43). Alternatively, the "viral hypothesis" is supported by a report that 100% of these patients had antibodies to the herpes simplex virus (41). Reactivation of the latent virus in a host that is compromised by high levels of cortisols may lead to transient neural damage.

B. Management

Earlier reports suggested improvement of gestational Bell palsy with prednisone treatment (41). However, current management is directed toward a thorough examination to exclude the presence of specific, recognized conditions that are potentially treatable (44). Otherwise, only supportive care is recommended, since in general, the majority of symptoms in most patients resolve within 6 months of onset regardless of treatment (42).

V. GLOSSITIS AND ANGULAR CHEILITIS

Pregnancy increases the demand for essential nutrients and vitamins, such as riboflavin and pyridoxine. A deficiency of these elements may result in an atrophic glossitis and angular cheilitis, the latter of which may become superinfected with *Candida albicans* (45).

A. Clinical Appearance

The tongue appears bald, shiny, and smooth with few papillae, and it may be sore. The commissures of the mouth become cracked, fissured, and macerated, often with erythema and crusting. These areas are often painful.

B. Management

Following serological documentation of the vitamin deficiency, treatment consists of diet supplementation with the appropriate elements. Treatment of low-income women in India suffering from these two conditions with riboflavin and pyridoxine showed a marked improvement in their conditions (46).

VI. INCREASED SALIVARY FLOW

Increased salivary flow (ptyalism) has been noted in pregnancy (47). This finding may be attributed to nausea and vomiting, which induces salivary flow. However, an interesting association has been observed between this condition and the craving and ingestion of unusual foods (pica), particularly starches (47). Pica can also be associated with noninfectious bilateral salivary gland swelling during pregnancy.

VII. ORAL CONTRACEPTIVES

Oral contraceptives are composed of a combination of synthetic estrogens and progestins, with current brands containing much lower levels of estrogen than earlier brands. They can therefore produce oral changes similar to those seen during pregnancy, in particular gingivitis (48,49) and pyogenic granulomata (40,50). Because oral contraceptives are used long-term, there is a potential for more severe tissue damage such as bone loss around teeth and periodontal disease (51).

REFERENCES

1. O. Coles. On the condition of the mouth and teeth during pregnancy, *Am. J. Dent. Sci. 8*:361–369, 410–419 (1874).
2. A.W. Maier and B. Orban. Gingivitis in pregnancy, *Oral Surg. 2*:334–373 (1949).
3. A.H. Arafat. Periodontal status during pregnancy, *J. Periodontol. 45*:641–643 (1974).
4. J.D. Jago, P.J. Chapman, J.F. Aitken, and T.M. McEniery. Dental status of pregnant

women attending a Brisbane maternity hospital, *Commun. Dent. Oral Epidemiol. 12*:398–401 (1984).

5. H. Loe and J. Silness, Periodontal disease in pregnancy. I. Prevalence and severity, *Acta Odontol. Scand. 21*:533–551 (1963).
6. K. Zaki, R. El Hak, and W. Amer. Salivary female sex hormone levels and gingivitis in pregnancy, *Biomed. Biochim. Acta 43*:749–754 (1984).
7. A. Hugoson. Gingival inflammation and female sex hormones, *J. Periodont. Res. Suppl. 5*:1–18 (1970).
8. A. Samant, C.P. Malik, S.K. Chabra, and P.K. Devi. Gingivitis and periodontal disease in pregnancy, *J. Periodontal. 47*:415–418 (1976).
9. K.S. Kornman and W.J. Loesche. The subgingival microbial flora during pregnancy, *J. Periodont. Res. 15*:111–122 (1980).
10. M. Albrecht, Banoczy, and E. Baranyi. Studies of dental and oral changes of pregnant diabetic women, *Acta Diabetol. Lat. 24*:1–7 (1987).
11. D. Cohen, J. Shapiro, L. Friedman, G. Kyle, and S. Franklin. A longitudinal investigation of the periodontal changes during pregnancy and fifteen months postpartum, Part II, *J. Periodontol. 47*:653–657 (1971).
12. T.C.A. O'Neil. Plasma female sex-hormone levels and gingivitis in pregnancy, *J. Periodontol. 50*:279–282 (1979).
13. Silness J. and H. Loe. Periodontal disease in pregnancy. II. Correlation with oral hygiene and periodontal condition, *Acta Odontol. Scand. 22*:121–135 (1964).
14. J. Jensen, W. Liljemark, and C. Bloomquist. The effect of female sex hormones on subgingival plaque, *J. Periodontol. 52*:599–602 (1981).
15. K.S. Kornman and W.J. Loesche. Direct interaction of estradiol and progesterone with Bacteroides melanogenicus, *J. Dent. Res. 58*:107 (abst. #58) (1979).
16. T.B. Aufdemorte and P.J. Sheridan. Nuclear uptake of sex steroids in gingiva of the baboon, *J. Periodontol. 52*:430–434 (1981).
17. J. Vittek, G.G. Gordon, S.C. Rappaport, P.R. Munnangi, and A.L. Southren. Specific progesterone receptors in rabbit gingiva, *J. Periodont. Res. 17*:657–661 (1982).
18. A.O. Ojanotko-Harri, M.P. Harri, H.M. Hurttia, and L.A. Sewon. Altered tissue jetabolism of progesterone in pregnancy gingivitis and granuloma, *J. Clin. Periodontol. 18*:262–266 (1991).
19. J. Lindhe, J. Birch, and P.I. Branemark. Vascular proliferation in pseudo-pregnant rabbits, *J. Periodontal Res. 3*:13–20 (1968).
20. A.H. Mohamed, J.P. Waterhouse, and H.H.R. Friederici. The microvasculature of the rabbit gingiva as affected by progesterone. An ultrastructural study, *J. Periodontol. 45*:50–60 (1974).
21. B. Willershausen, C. Lemmen, and G. Hamm. Modulation of glycosaminoglycan- and collagen synthesis of human gingival fibroblasts by progesterone (in German, English abstract), *Dtsch. Zahnarztl, Z. 46*:668–671 (1991).
22. D. Lundgren, B. Magnussen, and J. Lindhe. Connective tissue alterations in gingivae of rats treated with estrogens and progesterone, *Odontologisk. Revy. 24*:49–58 (1973).
23. T.M. El-Attar. Prostaglandin E2 in human gingiva in health and disease and its stimulation by female sex steroids, *Prostaglandins 11*:331–341 (1976).
24. T.M.A. El-Attar, S. Lin, and D.E. Tira, The relationship between the concentration of

female sex steroids and prostaglandin production by human gingiva in virtro, *Prostaglandins Leukot. Med. 8*:447–458 (1982).

25. N. Whitehead, F. Reyner, and J. Lindenbaum. Megaloblastic changes in the cervical epithelium: Association with oral contraceptive therapy and reversal with folic acid, *JAMA 226*:1421–1424 (1973).
26. M.E. Thomson and A.R.C. Pack. Effects of extended systemic and topical folate supplementation on gingivitis in pregnancy, *J. Clin. Periodontol. 9*:275–280 (1982).
27. R. Bulmer and K.W. Hancock. Depletion of circulating T lymphocytes in pregnancy, *Clin. Exp. Immunol. 28*:302–305 (1977).
28. L.E. Clemens, P.K. Siiteri, and Stites. Mechanism of immunosuppression of progesterone on maternal lymphocyte activation during pregnancy, *J. Immunol. 122*:1978–1985 (1979).
29. P. Stashenko, L.M. Resmini, A.D. Haffajee, and S.S. Socransky. Helper and suppressor T cells in periodontal disease, *J. Periodont. Res. 20*:515–521 (1985).
30. J.E. Raber-Dulacher, W.P. Ziejlemaker, A.A. Meinesz, and L. Abraham-Inpijn. CD4 to CD8 ratio and in vitro lymphoproliferative responses during experimental gingivitis in pregnancy and post-partum, *J. Periodontol. 62*:663–667 (1991).
31. D.E. Lopatin, K.S. Kornman, and W.J. Loesche. Modulation of immunoreactivity to periodontal disease-associated microorganisms during pregnancy, *Infect. Immunol. 28*:713–718 (1980).
32. E. Grossman, G. Reiter, O.P. Sturzenberger, M. De La Rosa, T.D. Dickinson, G.A. Ferretti, G.E. Ludlam, and A.H. Micket. Six-month study of the effects of chlorhexidine mouthrinse on gingivitis in adults, *J. Periodont. Res. 21* (Suppl. 16):33–43 (1986).
33. J.M. Gordon, I.B. Lamster, and M.C. Seiger. Efficacy of Listerine antiseptic in inhibiting the development of plaque and gingivitis, *J. Clin. Periodontol. 12*:697–704 (1985).
34. D.A. Kerr. Granuloma pyogenicum, *Oral Surg. 4*:158–176 (1951).
35. A.P. Angelopoulos. Pyogenic granuloma of the oral cavity: Statistical analysis of its clinical features, *J. Oral Surg. 29*:840-847 (1971).
36. A. Vilmann, P. Vilmann, and H. Vilmann. Pyogenic granuloma: Evaluation of oral conditions, *Br. J. Oral Max. Surg. 24*:376–382 (1986).
37. G. Shklar and I. Meyer. Vascular tumors of the mouth and jaws, *Oral Surg. 19*:335–358 (1965).
38. S.E. Mills, P.H. Cooper, and R.E. Fechner. Lobular capillary hemangioma: the underlying lesion of pyogenic granuloma, *Am. J. Surg. Pathol. 4*:471–479 (1980).
39. A. Rook. The ages of man and their dermatoses, *Textbook of Dermatology, 3rd ed.* (A. Rook, D.S. Wilkison, and F.J.G. Ebling, eds.). Blackwell Publishing, Oxford, UK, 1979, pp. 213–229.
40. N.G. Mussalli, R.M. Hopps, and N.W. Johnson. Oral pyogenic granuloma as a complication of pregnancy and the use of hormonal contraceptives, *Int. J. Gynaecol. Obstet. 14*:187–191 (1976).
41. R.L. Hilsinger, Jr., K.K. Adour, and H.E. Doty. Idiopathic facial paralysis, pregnancy, and the menstrual cycle, *Ann. Otol. Rhinol. Laryngol. 84*:433–442 (1975).
42. N.A. Falco and E. Eriksson. Idiopathic facial palsy in pregnancy and the puerperium, *Surg. Gynecol. Obstet. 169*:337–340 (1989).
43. D.L. Dorsey and W.R. Camann. Obstetric anesthesia in patients with idiopathic facial paralysis (Bell's palsy): A 10-year survey, *Anesth. Analg. 77*:81–83 (1993).

44. J.A. McGregor, A. Guberman, J. Amer, and R. Goodlin. Idiopathic facial nerve paralysis (Bell's palsy) in late pregnancy and the early puerperium, *Obstet. Gynecol. 69*:435–438 (1987).
45. J.A. Regezi and J. Sciubba. *Oral Pathology: Clinical-pathologic correlations,* 2nd ed. Saunders, Philadelphia, 1993, p. 122.
46. L. Iyengar. Oral lesions in pregnancy, *Lancet 1*:680–681 (1973).
47. F.G. Cunningham, P.C. MacDonald, and N.F. Gant, eds. *Williams Obstetrics,* 18th ed. Appleton Lange, Norwalk, CT, 1989, pp. 272, 848.
48. J. Lindhe and A.L. Bjorn. Influence of hormonal contraceptives on the giniva of women, *J. Periodont. Res. 2*:1–6 (1967).
49. G.M. El-Ashiry, A.H. El-Kafrawy, M.F. Nasr, and N. Younis. Comparative study of the influence of pregnancy and oral contraceptives on the gingivae, *Oral Surg. 30*:472–475 (1970).
50. A.Y. Kaufman. An oral contraceptive as an etiologic factor in producing hyperplastic gingivitis and a neoplasm of the pregnancy tumor type, *Oral Surg. Oral Med. Oral Pathol. 28*:666–670 (1969).
51. R.D. Zachariasen. Ovarian hormones and oral health: pregnancy gingivitis, *Compendium Contin. Educ. Dent. 10*:508–512 (1989).

7

Diseases of the Vulva in Pregnancy

Robert C. Wallach
New York University School of Medicine, New York, New York

I. INTRODUCTION

Inflammatory, traumatic, and neoplastic diseases of the vulva include a wide range of entities common to skin of other parts of the body as well as some specific to this organ. The vulva is broadly defined to include the labia majora, labia minora, clitoris, perineum, and vaginal vestibule. The changes of pregnancy lead to special consideration of the vulva.

II. INFLAMMATORY DISORDERS

A. Psoriasis

Although more frequently seen on extensor surfaces, vulvar psoriasis is occasionally the only manifestation of this disease but is usually seen with the appearance of the psoriasis elsewhere on the body. Multiple theories of etiology have been discussed. The clinical appearance of small papules that enlarge to become plaque-like elevations is well known because of the high frequency of this disease in the general population. Parakeratosis leads to the clinical appearance of gray-white plaques, and elongation of the rete pegs with intervening prominent capillaries under an otherwise thin epidermis contributes to the superficial erythema. Moisture and contact irritation on the vulva may modify the appearance of psoriasis and development of plaques is less common.

Corticoids, phototherapy, and systemic chemotherapy have been used to treat psoriasis in nonpregnant women. Chemotherapy should not be used for this indication in pregnancy which has a variable effect on the disease. Corticoids may be used with relative safety in pregnancy. Phototherapy in pregnancy is probably safe.

B. Lichen Planus

Lichen planus is another skin disease with an unestablished etiology and variable treatment. The papular lesion is generally opaque white owing to hyperkeratosis, and simulates other lesions of the vulva, requiring a histological diagnosis. The diagnosis of lichen planus requires the histological identification of a broad region filled with lymphocytes in the subcutaneous tissue. For the dermatopathologist, the clinical history and microscopic findings are sufficient for an absolute diagnosis, but I am aware of a case in which a neophyte general pathologist suggested lymphoma for this unrelated skin disease. Relatively uncommon, this disease has not provided any literature in pregnancy.

C. Behçet Syndrome

The combination of oral ulceration, ocular inflammation, and genital ulceration suggests the diagnosis of Behçet disease or syndrome (1). Infrequently seen in the United States, this entity has been attributed to viral origin, immune deficiency, or collagen disease. Arthritis and neurological symptoms are reported in advanced disease. The histological diagnosis of Behçet disease is unsure, with only vasculitis and chronic inflammatory reaction being noted. Culture techniques should be useful in the differential diagnosis with herpetic disease. As anticipated for a disease of unclear etiology with indefinite clinical course and multiple manifestations, treatment by various techniques has been suggested and includes corticosteroids, transfer factor, hormones, and antibiotics. Both the diagnosis and treatment of Behçet disease in pregnancy require conservatism, as the differential diagnosis is broad, and treatment should not include hormones or biological response modifiers.

D. Reiter Syndrome

The Reiter syndrome or disease comprises urethritis, conjunctivitis, and arthritis and should be considered when culture techniques do not yield a more specific etiology. Aside from concern for therapeutic agents that might adversely effect the fetus, no special considerations for pregnancy are reported.

E. Lipschutz Ulcer

Lipschutz ulcer has maintained an unearned place in gynecological texts for many years. Although originally used to describe a lesion in young women, this eponym has probably been used for herpetic lesions over many years prior to the availability of culture and cytological techniques and may be also confused with the vulvar lesions of Behçet disease.

F. Acanthosis Nigricans

Acanthosis nigricans, whether associated with a malignancy or not, should be considered in any patient with hyperpigmentation of the skin, although this entity is extremely rare. Occasionally seen in children, where it regresses and is unassociated with malignancy, the critical concern should be that no malignant neoplasm is missed in an adult. The diagnosis of acanthosis nigricans is occasionally applied to the increased pigmentation seen in obese patients, where it is associated with a chronic inflammation related to chafing skin surfaces, superficial epilation, long-term superficial fungal infection, and local trauma. Increased deposition of pigment with chronic dermatitis is generally an obvious clinical entity, with biopsy being available for confirmation in any questionable case. Pregnancy may increase the tendency for local inflammation but has no specific relation to acanthosis nigricans.

G. Endometriosis

The ability to make a clinical diagnosis of endometriosis of the vulva is somewhat easier than in other loci because of direct access, but confusion may exist. Symptoms may vary from none, to a mass, to chronic pain and tenderness, to cyclic pain and tenderness associated with the hormonal cycle. The lesions may be superficial or deep and vary from microscopic size up to several centimeters in diameter.

Of the various theories for the etiology of endometriosis, including hematogenous and lymphangitic spread, metaplasia, and nonspecific induction, it is a general clinical truth that endometriosis of the vulva is associated with direct implantation, which is usually clearly identified in the history. Surgery or trauma to the vulva with a break in the skin coincident with menstruation, curettage, or obstetrical delivery provides the background for implantation and the development of the emigrant endometriotic emboli. Without a secure clinical diagnosis, excisional biopsy is required, and the differential diagnosis usually includes hemangiomata but nevus or melanoma may be suspected because of retained blood pigments.

Although endometriosis is rarely recognized in episiotomy sites or vulvar lacerations, the performance of postpartum curettage increases the risk of implantation, and meticulous care for protection of the opened perineum is urged.

A health care professional with a 1-cm slightly tender, deeply pigmented, minimally raised lesion of the labium majus was told that she had a melanoma. Subsequent excisional biopsy revealed characteristic endometriosis with a small lake of dark blood responsible for the clinical appearance. She then recalled trauma to the vulva from a bicycle-riding accident at age 12 with a resultant hematoma that opened the day of her initial menses. The lesion had been slowly progressive for almost two decades.

Vulvar endometriosis should regress in pregnancy as does endometriosis in other locations under the presumed suppression of progesterone.

III. BENIGN TUMORS OF THE VULVA (2)

A. Nevus

Nevi of the vulva share with nevi of other body surfaces a potential for misdiagnosis. Junctional, intradermal, and compound nevi may be found on the skin surfaces of the labia majora as well as the labia minora. Excisional biopsy is warranted for all nevi of the vulva, especially those on the central mucous membranes both for diagnosis and as possible prophylaxis against the development of melanoma. The wide varieties of the clinical appearance of nevi are similar on the vulva to what can be seen on other parts of the body. An aggressive clinical approach with removal of vulvar nevi is urged, even in pregnancy. The hormonal effect of pregnancy may lead to increased pigmentation with difficulty in clinical diagnosis, but biopsy will resolve most questions concerning diagnosis.

B. Seborrheic Keratosis

Seborrheic keratosis is more frequently recognized on the face, trunk, and upper extremities, where it is unsightly and troublesome but not dangerous. Its appearance may provoke the use of the various topical commerical preparations available. The lesion is uncommon on the vulva. Seborrheic keratosis is well demarcated and generally slightly raised above the surrounding skin surface with a warty appearance. Its dimensions may extend to several centimeters. The color may reflect the background skin color, but frequently there is some hyperpigmentation with a brown to black color, and the superficial appearance occasionally provokes the patient to scratch, leading to superficial ulceration. Biopsy reveals hyperkeratosis surrounding a connective tissue base. Although this lesion on the vulva might be diagnosed by direct inspection, excisional biopsy is warranted because of its infrequency and the possibility of confusion with squamous carcinoma. Seborrheic keratosis on the vulva is generally seen in older women and coincidence with pregnancy must be rare.

C. Fibroepithelial Polyp

Fibroepithelial polyp, a tumor of epidermoid origin, is also known as acrochordon. Some confusion arises with the related diagnosis of squamous papilloma, which, in a majority of cases, is indistinguishable from the fibroepithelial polyp; and since the latter term is descriptive and all embracing, it is to be recommended. The fibroepithelial polyp retains the color of the surrounding skin, has a surface that is smooth or crenated, and generally has a narrow pedicle but may be broadly sessile. Fibroepithelial polyps range from a few millimeters to a few centimeters in size and probably reflect some local stimulation to a preexisting fold or protuberance of the skin, leading to a slow overgrowth of the skin with a compensatory increase in the vascularity through the base of the pedicle. These lesions are recognized more frequently with advancing age and are often noticed in individuals who have similar lesions in the axillae or elsewhere on the body. Because of the peduculated configuration, local trauma from skin contact with clothing may lead to ulceration or superficial laceration with bleeding.

Although the gross clinical diagnosis of fibroepithelial polyp is quite dependable for the experienced observer, surgical excision is recommended for histological confirmation. The fibroepithelial polyp represents a change in the surface configuration of the skin without intrinsic epithelial abnormality, and no progression to malignancy should be anticipated. Although less common in younger women, the lesion may be seen in pregnancy when vascular engorgement and edema accentuate the clinical findings.

D. Epidermal Inclusion Cyst

Epidermal inclusion cysts are related to more than one etiological origin. Direct trauma with implantation of viable surface squamous epithelium beneath the surface may lead to proliferation and desquamation and to formation of an inclusion cyst. This occurs following an episiotomy or spontaneous obstetrical vulvar laceration. A meticulous well-approximated episiotomy or obstetrical laceration scar repair with the thighs abducted may result in the burying of surface squamous epithelium when the knees are brought together. Although the eversion of skin edges is important and well understood for most repairs, there is a tendency to invert skin edges on the perineum because of the nonanatomical position during the repair. Another origin of epidermoid inclusion cysts is related to the tendency for squamous proliferation along the depths of pilosebaceous ducts with subsequent blockade of the duct lumen and continued proliferation of the squamous elements, leading to a buried tumefaction.

Epidermoid inclusion cysts may be singular or multiple and are generally slow growing and retain a spherical shape. Pressure on the basal cell layer exerted by production of skin elements leads to cessation of further proliferation when some critical size is reached. This type of cyst is rarely more than a few millimeters in size and occasionally extends to 1–2 cm. Fragments of keratin are frequently found within the inclusion cyst which is lined by squamous epithelium. Infection of these cysts may require drainage but the majority lie dormant and rarely cause symptoms. Removal for cosmetic purposes is acceptable, and progression to malignancy is unknown. Surgical treatment at the time of vaginal delivery may be convenient for both the patient and physician.

E. Pilonidal Cyst

Infrequently seen on the vulva, pilonidal cysts probably represent the same disease seen in the sacrococcygeal region. Since they are apparently more common in the periclitoral region, some clinicians think that this lesion represents a local tissue reaction to hair trapped under the epidermis, provoking a foreign-body reaction. Pain and swelling with progression to abscess formation may be expected, and complete local excision is the treatment of choice after the acute infection has been cleared by drainage and antibiotics. The histological picture is replete with inflammatory cells, necrotic material, and usually hair fragments with a prominent inflammatory reaction extending widely. Surgery at vaginal delivery may be appropriate.

F. Hidradenitis Suppurativa

Hidradenitis suppurativa is a chronic regional inflammation of the apocrine glands with superinfection by staphylococci or streptococci. Either in the axillae or on the vulva, there are multiple nodules, which may develop into small abscesses, multiple draining sinuses, irregular scarring, induration and pitting of the skin, and bright red discoloration to complete a clinical picture that generally develops after puberty. Treatment has ranged from wide surgical excision to the use of systemic corticosteroids, to surface debridement, and to the use of topical or systemic antibacterials. Patients with this disease entity generally see multiple physicians; have progressive, symptomatic, and relatively severe disease; and require major emotional support. Recently, a few patients have responded to long-term doxycycline, having failed multiple other treatment plans. The physician must be skeptical of early treatment success and the patient urged to try various treatment plans in an attempt to control this occasionally disabling disease. Exacerbation and remission may occur in pregnancy. The use of antibiotics must reflect the potential effect on the fetus.

G. Fox-Fordyce Disease

Fox-Fordyce disease is described as a widespread obstruction of the apocrine ducts with retention of apocrine secretory products. As in hidradenitis suppurativa, the vulva and the axilla are the sites of origin, and multiple treatment plans have been suggested. Because of an apparent relation to the menstrual cycle, hormonal manipulation both systemically and topically has been tried with some success, but this is not feasible in pregnancy when the disease is usually inactive.

H. Syringoma

Multiple papules representing enlarged eccrine skin appendages characterize syringoma, which is frequently asymptomatic and suspected on routine clinical examination. Although the microscopic picture has been interpreted to represent adenomatous change, an alternative interpretation might be that this is cystic dilatation of the gland systems with retention of secretory products. Since there is no malignant counterpart and progression is negligible, and since symptoms are generally minor, no treatment is necessary, although local surgery for cosmetic reasons may be requested by the patient, and this might be appropriate at vaginal delivery.

I. Hidradenoma

The hidradenoma is a benign glandular neoplasm arising in a skin appendage. Although hidradenoma can be found elsewhere, it is frequently found on the vulva and perianal skin, suggesting that its origin is related to some local effect such as a hormonal receptivity. Primarily a disease of white women, the microscopic appearance may mimic intraductal breast papilloma. The clinical manifestation is that of a small nodule, generally less than 1 cm. Central surface necrosis and umbilication may represent the pressure on the overlying skin of tight-fitting clothing against the occasionally firm tumor nodule. The microscopic appearance of hidradenoma varies from glandular proliferation with cystic spaces to a solid papillomatous mass. The busy microscopic appearance may suggest malignancy, but regularity of the cells and the regular relation to the gland spaces as well as lack of invasion confirm the benign nature of this harmless tumor. Although widely distributed over the vulva according to most reports, there may be an increased frequency of this lesion on the lateral aspect of the labia minora at the anterior third of the vulva. A malignant counterpart of hidradenoma is rarely seen. The occurrence of hidradenoma in pregnancy is unlikely.

J. Hemangiomata

1. Strawberry Hemangioma

The strawberry hemangioma, not uncommonly seen in the newborn, has been described on the vulva. Treatment for this rare location of a skin abnormality with capillary proliferation has varied over the years from hot cautery to freezing, but conservatism may be sufficient, as fibrosis and shrinkage are common with the passage of time.

2. Cavernous Hemangioma

Cavernous hemangioma, also unusual on the vulva, is generally treated because of an increase in size and the potential for hemorrhage in a larger lesion. Freezing and rarely surgical excision should be considered when treatment is necessary.

3. *Pyogenic Granuloma*

Pyogenic granuloma is probably just a variety of capillary hemangioma and may be seen on the vulva. Since it is generally well circumscribed and the clinical diagnosis may be unsure, excision leads to a good histological diagnosis and cure simultaneously. Dilated capillaries, inflammatory reaction in the loose surrounding stroma, and occasionally superficial ulceration are recognized easily by the pathologist because of the familiarity with this lesion seen in other parts of the body.

Angiokeratoma shares some qualities with the pyogenic granuloma in that dilated capillaries are the most prominent histological feature and are responsible for the clinical gross appearance. A distinction can occasionally be made by the prominence of epidermal components covering this lesion. Probably related to its larger size, thrombosis is also encountered. Spider telangiectasia, the vascular spider, is more frequently seen on the face and chest of pregnant women but may also appear on the vulva.

4. *Senile Hemangioma*

By far the most common of the hemangiomata of the vulva is the senile hemangioma, occasionally called senile telangiectasia. Although other types of hemangiomata are rarely seen on the vulva, senile hemangioma has a definite predilection for the vulva, especially in white women. The lesion is rarely seen before the fourth decade, and then it becomes increasingly frequent both in numbers of patients bearing them and in numbers of the lesions seen on individual patients. An increase in the number of lesions in individual patients is a characteristic feature. Individual senile hemangiomata rarely progress beyond 3 mm in size and are symptomatic only because they may be the source of bleeding when there is trauma to the aging thin epithelium covering them. The blue-purple color of the lesion may provoke the attention of women of northern European background, as the surrounding white skin provides an optimal contrast for detection. I have seen these lesions infrequently in light pigmented women and have never identified them in deeply pigmented vulvar skin where they may be hidden. The skin over a senile hemangioma is occasionally elevated for 1–2 mm, and minute septa have occasionally been identified clinically within these hemangiomata. Because of the increasing frequency of senile hemangioma in older women, familiarity and diagnosis by visual identification are important so that the clinician does not feel constrained to perform multiple biopsies on a lesion that has no malignant potential. This lesion would not be expected in pregnancy except for parturients in the fifth decade of life.

5. *De Morgan Spots*

De Morgan spots (cherry angiomata) are sharply demarcated 1-mm round, cherry red spots frequently seen on the face, chest, and arms of fair-skinned women with increasing frequency from the fifth decade onward. They may be seen on the abdomen and mons pubis and occasionally on the labia majora. The clinical appearance and the wide distribution with characteristic findings lead to a dependable clinical diagnosis, but an isolated lesion on the vulva would require a biopsy for confirmation. Because of an older age distribution, the lesion is rare in pregnancy.

6. Lymphangiomata

Lymphangiomata of the vulvar skin are very similar to the hemangiomata described previously, with the obvious difference of lack of blood in the vascular channels. Because the clinical appearance of the various subtypes of lymphangiomata is not characteristic, biopsy is necessary for a confident diagnosis. Because of their benign appearance and lack of symptoms, most lymphangiomata will be dismissed as minor skin abnormalities without either treatment or absolute diagnosis.

K. Fibroma

Fibroma of the vulva usually comes to the attention of a clinician when a large pedunculated tumor of the labia majora is reported by a patient or when it is seen on a screening examination. The characteristic bland histology of proliferating fibrous tissue starts as a small nodule just below the skin and with progressive growth first becomes a sessile elevated lesion and then develops a vascular pedicle with a narrow neck covered with the stretched adjoining skin covering the lesion. Once the pedicle is formed, there is probably some vascular compromise to venous and lymph return, and the skin overlying the pedunculated lesion is loose with a mildly edematous reticular component around the well-circumscribed fibroma. Because of the possibility of local trauma and bleeding, these lesions should be sharply excised, and the narrow pedicle makes this a simple procedure. Sessile or subcutaneous lesions are also encountered. An increase in size during pregnancy may be due to edema and increased vascularity.

L. Granular Cell Myoblastoma

The granular cell myoblastoma has been found on the vulva and presents as a slow-growing lesion whose clinical characteristics resemble other benign tumors of skin. Excisional biopsy is necessary for precise diagnosis according to the criteria for this lesion established for other regions of the body.

M. Leiomyoma

Leiomyomata of the vulva have a natural history, appearance, and treatment very similar to fibromata in this location, although the frequency of the former is less. The histological appearance is that of a leiomyoma anywhere, and conversion to sarcomatous malignancy is not known. Pregnancy may lead to increased benign growth potential because of early high hormone levels.

N. Lipoma

Sharing features with any lipoma found anywhere on the body, the lesion of the vulva generally comes to clinical attention when protrusion and the development of a narrow pedicle lead to a dependent growth of substantial size or when the subcutaneous mass increasingly deforms the vulva. Similar to the fibroma and leiomyoma, a narrow neck and dependent oval mass generally grow to a fair size in an older women whose attention is not focused on this region. The clinical diagnosis is generally made by the difference in palpation between this and the two solid tumor described above. The lipoma under the labia majora may increase rapidly in pregnancy, at which time surgery may be complicated by the enriched blood supply. Sessile and subcutaneous lesions are also encountered.

O. Neurofibroma

Neurofibroma, unless associated with similar lesions in other areas of the body as in von Recklinghausen disease, is a pathologist's diagnosis for a clinically bland-looking skin tumor that mimics achrocordon.

P. Vulvar Dystrophies

An extensive literature has grown on the subject of the vulvar dystrophies, which include hyperplastic dystrophy, with or without atypia, and lichen sclerosus (et atrophicus) and mixed dystrophy with or without atypia. The reader is referred to the excellent summaries available in the literature but is cautioned that diagnosis by inspection is dangerous (2). All discolored lesions of the vulva whether hyper-pigmented or hypopigmented, raised, flat, or ulcerated should have a histological diagnosis by an interested and knowledgeable dermatopathologist. An aggressive program of biopsy when these abnormalities are seen will lead to early diagnosis and reduce the risk of overlooking a malignancy. Most of the clinical presentations of vulvar dystrophy will occur in older, nonpregnant women, but they may be found from puberty onward.

Lichen sclerosus generally presents as a thin white "cigarette paper" skin lesion, frequently in a "keyhole" pattern around the vulva and anus. Pruritus is a major factor, and scratching complicates the situation. Topical preparations of testoster-one have been of some effectiveness but cannot be used in pregnancy. Occasion-ally, corticosteriods, either local or systemic, may be useful for the temporary control of itching, but the possibility of further atrophy of skin surfaces is a hazard. In previous years, chloroquine was used, but because of its potential serious side effects, it is out of favor at this time. Some students have suggested that lichen sclerosus represents an increased metabolic activity in the skin despite its bland and atrophic microscopic appearance. Inferences on the basis of radioisotope incorporation of DNA precursors have been questioned as to their validity and the microscopic appearance certainly indicates regional atrophy.

The hyperplastic dystrophies probably represent a group of reactions to systemic and local influences. Specific agents of cause or cure cannot be identified in most cases.

The relation of any of these dystrophies to the onset of cancer has been suggested, confirmed, and denied, and with current emphasis on a viral etiology for squamous carcinoma for the lower genital tract, it may be that the dystrophies serve merely as a potential nutrient soil for the growth of the carcinogenic agent.

Most patients with diagnosed vulvar dystrophies are beyond childbearing age, as symptoms and clinical recognition both usually represent long-standing disease. The incidence of these lesions in pregnancy is probably underestimated.

IV. VULVAR MALIGNANCIES

A. Carcinoma In Situ of the Vulva

Carcinoma in situ of the vulva (3) has commanded far more attention in recent years than previously. It is unclear whether the more frequent reports reflect a greater true incidence of the disease, greater awareness on the part of treating physicians, referral to specialists, more liberal use of biopsy techniques, or an increase in exposure to inducing agents such as viruses. Carcinoma in situ of the vulva has also been called by other names such as Bowen disease, erythroplasia of Queyrat, intraepithelial neoplasia, and leukoplakia.

The clinical manifestations of carcinoma in situ of the vulva may include elevation, ulceration, and induration, suggesting a full-blown invasive carcinoma, but usually the only clinical finding is color change. Every skin color change has been noted with this disease, including hyperpigmentation, hypopigmentation, melanotic, erythematous, and cyanotic coloration, and frequently a white discoloration or white plaque formation.

The diagnosis of vulvar carcinoma in situ should always elicit a scrupulous search for other involved areas and an assiduous evaluation for the possibility of invasive carcinoma on the vulva or elsewhere on the body. Multiple squamous neoplastic disease of the lower genital tract is well known, and the vagina and cervix may harbor carcinoma in situ or invasive carcinoma in these cases. Close long-term follow-up for all of these genital locations is mandatory.

The diagnosis of vulvar carcinoma in situ is made by biopsy, which should be aimed at the clinically abnormal skin area. Variations in the microscopic picture are also seen, but the usual characteristics of carcinoma in situ of squamous epithelium are recognized with loss of orderly maturation, increased mitotic activity, dyskeratosis, and nuclear hyperchromatism. Problems in the biopsy diagnosis arise when the histological abnormality extends beyond the clinically evident skin change. No good guidelines for managing the edge of the lesion diagnostically have been determined, but some investigators think that the use of toluidine blue with acetic acid wash (1% of each) may highlight the abnormal areas. Stain retention in neoplastic tissue is relatively dependable but is also seen with inflammation and superficial ulceration, and the stain may be lost where the frequently encountered hyperkeratosis is present, shielding the nucleated cells from the stain. In my experience, toluidine blue has been unequivocally positive in those cases in which direct inspection alone was adequate. The use of a dye substance as a skin diagnostic agent in a patient with suspected neoplasia and the possibility of recurrent disease requires that the process be carefully explained to the patient, especially when the stain is usually obtained from nonmedical manufacturers. Tetracycline-induced fluorescence has been used with good success by its advocates but has problems similar to the toluidine blue technique with both false-positive and false-negative responses. High clinical suspicion for invasive carcinoma, coupled with experience, and the willingness to perform multiple biopsies are necessary to rule out invasive carcinoma. The use of dyes and antibiotics for diagnosis is contraindicted in pregnancy and surgical biopsy is the choice.

Over the years, the treatment for carcinoma in situ of the vulva has become more conservative, probably because of its increased frequency of diagnosis and the difficulty in confirming progression to invasion disease. Within the last few decades, the prior recommendation for simple vulvectomy has been narrowed to wide local excision with margins usually of 0.5 cm. The problem with recommending a narrow margin is the difficulty in judging the extent of the lesion and the need for subsequent surgery. Topical 5-fluorouracil has been used, but the technique varies in effectiveness according to reported experience and should not be considered in pregnancy. The ultimate place of this very uncomfortable treatment for vulvar disease is not clearly established. Other topical agents have been used here and abroad with varying success. Since the goal of treatment is local destruction of an intraepithelial lesion, not only surgical excision but in situ ablation may be used. In addition to topical chemotherapy, cryocautery, hot cautery, and laser vaporization have been used, but with good clinical surveillance and a proven diagnosis, treatment may be deferred to the puerperium.

Vulvar carcinoma in situ is clearly a disease in which the topographic region of its location necessitates that individualization must be carefully applied in treatment planning. Complete removal of the lesion is a goal but must be weighed against cosmetic deformity and the loss of sexual function, especially when tissues adjacent to the clitoris are involved. When primary excision does not yield negative margins, the usual recommendation is for repeat excisional biopsy until negative margins are achieved, although I am unaware that any residual carcinoma in situ has been associated with progression to invasive carcinoma of the vulva. Since invasive carcinoma of the vulva frequently has a surrounding margin of carcinoma in situ, the closest surveillance of patients with known residual carcinoma in situ is mandatory and many will feel safer with wide excision.

In general, carcinoma in situ of the cervix has peak incidence some 10 years before the peak incidence of invasive carcinoma of the cervix, and the progression of the former to the latter is taught as a clinical truth. The relation of carcinoma in situ of the vulva to invasive carcinoma of the vulva, however, does not currently have the same type of supportive epidemiological or experiential data. The invasive lesion has not been noted to have increased in incidence despite the sharply rising number of cases of the in situ type. Perhaps a greater period of observation will confirm a progression of in situ lesions to invasive lesions. There seems to be a bimodal distribution of vulvar intraepithelial carcinoma (carcinoma in situ) with peaks in the third and sixth decades of life. Scrutiny for this disease in young women and in pregnant women is strongly advised.

B. Squamous Carcinoma of the Vulva (4,5)

Primarily a disease of women in the sixth and seventh decades of life, epidermoid or squamous carcinoma of the vulva has been ascribed to numerous possible etiologies, including estrogen deficit, poor hygiene, chemical carcinogens, and viral exposure. The disease has a similar biology, age distribution, and treatment response in developing countries with poor nutrition and hygiene as well as in more affluent societies. Relation to preexisting carcinoma in situ is suggested by the frequent finding of severe dysplastic epithelium around an invasive vulvar carcinoma, although progression from the former to the latter has not been proved. The relationship of known viral diseases of the vulva to subsequent carcinoma of the vulva has also been suggested but not demonstrated.

Invasive carcinoma of the vulva is generally a disease of older women and may grow slowly, permitting its victim to become acclimated to a lesion of impressive size when first seen. Diminished attention to the vulva by some older women and their sexual partners, institutional or celibate life styles, and many other factors frequently lead to a delay in the reporting of symptoms, generally itching, burning, or awareness of a mass or ulceration. Unfortunately, when first reported, these symptoms may not provoke an adequate physical examination and many such patients are treated without the physician viewing the lesion. Antipruritics are frequently prescribed and, of course, are useless for the management of the disease. Especially depressing is physician delay in achieving a biopsy diagnosis and referral to a physician equipped for appropriate treatment of the disease. Any elevated or ulcerated lesion must be suspect for carcinoma, and early biopsy is urged. With confirmation of the diagnosis of invasive carcinoma of the vulva, staging and treatment should be executed rapidly. Despite the advanced age and frequent coincident medical problems of women with invasive carcinoma of the vulva, the majority of these lesions should be treated by aggressive surgery. For the occasional very early microinvasive lesion of limited extent, radical vulvectomy or less extensive surgery may be sufficient, as spread to lymph nodes is not anticipated. But for most invasive lesions without distant spread, the treatment of choice is radical vulvectomy with bilateral groin lymphadenectomy. The addition of deep pelvic lymphadenectomy may give better prognostic information but will not necessarily achieve a greater cure rate. Radiation therapy to the deep pelvic or higher level lymph nodes can be effective, but the primary lesion is best treated by radical surgery. Without spread to the groin lymph nodes, 5-year survival approaches 90%, and with lymph node involvement, the 5-year survival will drop by about one-half. Spread to pelvic lymph nodes worsens the prognosis, as does fixation to bone, involvement of the urinary or intestinal tract, and distant spread. Radiation therapy *alone* for carcinoma of the vulva is disappointing both in low control rate and serious morbidity from treatment, and it must be considered a very weak choice in its management except for the node-bearing areas. Chemotherapy and immunotherapy await advances that have not yet been seen. In eastern Europe, a major clinic with extensive experience has documented an outstanding record of treatment of carcinoma of the vulva with ablative liquid nitrogen cryotherapy to the primary lesion and radiation therapy to the lymph nodes. In selected cases treated here, similar good results have been achieved (6).

With its slow-growing behavior and accessibility to a good cancer operation, and with a high 5-year survival for early cases, this disease deserves greater attention in order to achieve the benefits of many years of study and improved treatment planning.

Although vulvar carcinoma is primarily a disease of older women, it is also seen in women in the third decade of life and in pregnancy. As an uncommon pregnancy condition, this disease may not attract appropriate attention and biopsy diagnosis may be delayed as it frequently is in older women. Treatment for vulvar carcinoma in pregnancy must be highly individualized with regard both to the patient and her offspring. The surgical operation may be staged or deferred. Vaginal delivery will be contraindicated when the potential for tumor hemorrhage or dispersal exists. When vulvar carcinoma is seen in younger or pregnant women, compromised immune surveillance must be suspected and acquired immunodeficiency syndrome (AIDS) should be considered.

C. Paget Disease of the Vulva

Paget disease of the vulva (extramammary Paget disease) is a disease of theories and guilt by association. Paget disease of the nipple, which shares with the vulvar lesion the microscopic appearance of epidermal Paget cells, is always associated with an underlying ductal carcinoma. Histological similarity, however, does not lead to the analogy of an underlying carcinoma in all vulvar cases. The literature suggests that up to 20% of vulvar cases are associated with an underlying carcinoma, generally of the skin appendages such as an aporcrine gland carcinoma, but it must be remembered that the negative association would rarely be considered worthy of being published, so many such cases go unreported. The true figure for underlying carcinoma is probably under 10%. The association of extramammary Paget disease with other carcinoma has also attracted attention; but since this disease usually occurs in older women, since no consistent pattern has emerged, and since the mechanism is unclear, it must be concluded that the present evidence suggests only a temporal, not a causal, relationship with a more distant carcinoma. Because the milk lines extend to the vulva and because, phylogenetically, the breast is a modified sweat gland, the appearance of Paget disease of the vulva might suggest the possibility of an underlying carcinoma of an aberrant island of breast tissue, but this is not a clinical event.

The clinical presentation of Paget disease of the vulva is generally pruritic, well-demarcated erythematous areas with scattered hyperkeratosis noticed visibly as white patches. The appearance, however, is widely variable and should never be the basis of diagnosis. These lesions are frequently described as appearing moist owing to light reflection, but they are only occasionally wet as a result of superficial ulceration and bleeding.

Biopsy reveals scattered Paget cells in the epidermis with clear cytoplasm and a nucleus retracted from the cell walls. The nuclei are variable in size and shape, may be hyperchromatic, and rarely demonstrate mitoses. The Paget cells can be found in skin appendages and must be scrutinized to see whether these are examples of invasion or merely extension down the lining of the skin appendages. Although the hematoxylin and eosin preparation is usually diagnostic, mucicarmine-positive and PAS-positive–diastase-resistant material makes for colorful slides to confirm the diagnosis and rule out an occasional suspected melanoma or an unusual squamous carcinoma in situ. The diagnosis of Paget disease requires a careful clinical evaluation for the possibility of an underlying carcinoma of the skin appendages as well as a screening for malignancy elsewhere, especially in the colon, bladder/urethra, breasts, and upper genital tract.

Vulvectomy has been recommended for the treatment of Paget disease because of the frequently noted skip areas and multicentric nature of the disease. But, without proof of an underlying carcinoma and without biological evidence of progression, wide local excision may be advocated analogously to squamous carcinoma in situ.

Other local ablative techniques to treat Paget disease may be considered. The problem of residual disease at excisional margins is also most troublesome. Limited knowledge of the biology of Paget disease precludes a scientific basis for advising patients, and great stress must be placed on patient awareness of the limited predictability for the long-term outcome of residual disease. Most women with vulvar Paget disease are well beyond the capability of pregnancy.

D. Basal Cell Carcinoma

Although relatively near the top of the frequency list of vulvar neoplasms, basal cell carcinoma is only 2–3% as common as invasive squamous cell carcinoma in this region and shares with it a distribution mostly in the sixth and seventh decades of life. This tumor is more often a problem of the face and upper torso but must be considered on the vulva, where it is uncommon and not a real consideration in most pregnancies.

Central ulceration is frequently seen in basal cell carcinoma, and it is this characteristic that is responsible for the appelation of "rodent ulcer." If permitted to progress without treatment, this tumor advances locally and will invade the subcutaneous tissues and eventually bone. Infection of advanced lesions is common and metastasis has been reported rarely.

The microscopic picture of basal cell carcinoma is that of a tumor composed of cells resembling the basal cell of the normal epidermis. The lesion is occasionally mixed with a squamous cell carcinoma. For the basal cell tumor, wide local excision is the treatment of choice with a visible margin of normal tissue at the skin edges and at the depth of the resection. Residual tumor will continue to grow and become a clinical problem, and recurrence is usually a result of overly conservative initial treatment.

The excised lesion should be carefully evaluated for the possibility of extension to the surgical margin or the possible coincidence of invasive squamous carcinoma whose treatment must be far more aggressive and radical.

E. Melanoma

Although the sun worshippers of Queensland, Australia, seem to achieve an increased incidence of melanoma for other body sites, it is hard to understand why the vulva with about 1% of body skin is the seat of 3–4% of the malignant melanomas worldwide, since even the most flexible heliophile will have limited actinic radiation to this part of the body. Localized melanoma of the vulva may be treated with radical vulvectomy and lymphadenectomy, but the survival is not as good as for squamous carcinoma, and secondary treatment is still experimental in most centers (7,8). Coincidence of vulvar melanoma and pregnancy must be exceedingly rare.

F. Other Malignancies

Hidradenocarcinoma of skin appendages and carcinoma of Bartholin gland are most unusual and in early stages respond to radical surgery as treatment. Sarcomas of varying behaviors can be found on the vulva, and treatment is tied to histological diagnosis.

V. INFECTIOUS DISEASES

A. Candidiasis/Moniliasis

Monilial infections are common enough apart from pregnancy and are somewhat more frequently seen in pregnant women. Whether this is related to the change in hormonal levels or other factors of the physiological changes of pregnancy is a less important issue than the need for getting clinical relief for frequently troubling pruritus. Although the diagnosis is frequently obvious on direct inspection with erythema and edema at the vestibule, occasionally spreading to the labia majora, and a cheesy-white discharge, it is most important to be diagnostically specific. A wet smear microscopic examination with saline or KOH is frequently sufficient to make a definitive diagnosis. Laboratory culture studies will be helpful when the wet smear is unrevealing. Treatment has two goals: (a) to reduce the *Monilia* infection and (b) to reduce the symptoms. Miconazole, clotrimazole, and related agents have been most popular in recent years in the treatment of *Monilia/Candida* infections. Nystatin is still available and has the advantage of long years of experience, although possibly somewhat less potent. All of these agents are deemed safe as local applications in the vagina during pregnancy. Topical gentian violet is no longer popular and would best be avoided in pregnancy because of the potential for absorption through occasionally fragile tissues. Symptomatic relief is generally achieved with topical hydrocortisone 0.25, 0.50, or 1.0%, and even with some local absorption, this agent is safe in pregnancy. More expensive analogues of hydrocortisone are available but are frequently troublesome because of very small packages whose use is limited. Screening for diabetes should always be considered when the presence of *Monilia/Candida* is noted. Transmission of *Candida* to the newborn may be responsible for oropharyngeal disease of the newborn (thrush).

B. Trichomoniasis

Trichomoniasis, infestation of the lower genital tract with *Trichomonas vaginalis*, can be a source of an irritating vaginal discharge leading to vulvar irritation with burning and itching. Topical or systemic metronidazole is highly effective in the treatment of trichomonas, but the systemic agent should be avoided in pregnancy unless the indication is for some other infectious problem. Many clinicians will defer the treatment of trichomoniasis until the pregnancy is completed. Passage to the newborn is a consideration but has not become a clinical problem.

C. Gardnerella

Gardnerella vulvovaginitis is occasionally troublesome in pregnancy. It is characterized by a foul-smelling vaginal discharge. Metronidazole is very effective in treating this infection, which is not threatening to the pregnancy. The treatment may be deferred until after delivery.

D. Gonorrhea

Gonorrhea of the lower genital tract is a continuing problem despite the availability of potent antibiotics for its treatment. Infection of the urethra, Skene glands, and Bartholin glands and ducts can be seen in pregnancy as well as at other times in the life cycle. Diagnostic techniques have been improved, so that rapid laboratory reports can be made leading to effective treatment.

E. Chancroid

Chancroid, infection with *Haemophilis ducreyi*, as a source of vulvar disease has been on the rise in recent years and has been increasingly reported in some of the southern United States. The characeristic tender and painful soft ulcer might be confused on visual examination alone with the primary lesion of syphilis, and this differential diagnosis should be considered. Early diagnosis and effective antibiotic treatment are obviously in the patient's best interest in pregnancy as at other times.

F. Miscellaneous Bacterial Infections

Streptococcal vulvovaginitis carries a special importance in pregnancy. Although symptoms may be minor with some vaginal discharge and vulvar itching, group B streptococci pose a potential threat for the exposed newborn. Discretion calls for vaginal cultures when vulvar symptoms occur during pregnancy. Of the various streptococci that may normally be found in the lower genital tract, it is important to determine which are present and to treat either the mother or the newborn, depending on the organism isolated. Staphylococcal infections of the vulva are uncommon in pregnancy but may be troublesome when changes in the skin secretions may provide a nidus from which furunculitis may lead to abscess formation. Laboratory evaluation of the organism for antibiotic sensitivities will be valuable in determining treatment. Dicloxacillin is usually effective but cannot be used in penicillin-allergic women.

Escherichia coli may be responsible for some vulvovaginal problems during pregnancy, but the organism is quite commonly found even in the absence of symptoms or clinical manifestations. Local sulfonamide treatments may be useful for reducing the levels of this bacterium.

Multiple other organisms are responsible for vulvovaginal complaints, and when cultures verify their presence, specific therapy can be used. Fusospirochetosis, an infection caused by a combination of *Borrelia* and *Fusobacterium* organisms, represents a problem more frequently found in the oral cavity and is rarely a problem in the lower genital tract. *Pseudomonas* and *Proteus* species are occasionally found as well as *Corynebacterium*, *Nocardia*, and *Leptothrix* species. Tuberculosis of the lower genital tract is a rarity, but the various stages of syphilis may be found in the vulvar tissues.

G. Viral Diseases

The viral diseases of the skin have become more prominent in clinical practice and in the literature in recent years, possibly associated with changes in social and sexual habits and are certainly related to AIDS. Condylomata accuminata result from infection with the human papilloma virus (HPV). The characteristic nodules and masses of the viral warts with their irregular surface, gray-brown color, and lack of surrounding edema or erythema make a clinical diagnosis relatively simple. A biopsy diagnosis is needed if the lesion is at all atypical, or if the clinician considers the possiblity of a carcinoma. Treatment for condylomata reflects the availability of the various options for treatment. Electrocautery, cryosurgery, laser vaporization, direct surgical removal, and other techniques are effective in pregnant as well as nonpregnant individuals. Trichloroacetic acid (TCA) or bichloroacetic acid is another option, and the use of these agents requires special care because of their extremely corrosive nature. Podophyllin should not be used during pregnancy because of the potential for absorption in the rich vascular beds of the lower genital tract and surrounding tissues. Although most physicians and clinics are not prepared to use this agent, liquid nitrogen is an inexpensive and effective agent which achieves ablation of the lesions with minimal effort. Treatment of conydylomata in pregnancy must be carefully considered with regard to the increased vascularity of the region at risk. Identification of the HPV viral type responsible for condylomata is relatively expensive but easily available. There is a special importance in pregnancy to identify those patients who are harboring HPV-11, which may be transmitted to the newborn and lead to laryngeal or trachael viral-induced warts. Although this is an infrequent problem, it is potentially a very serious disease in childhood. When HPV-11 is identified, close surveillance for control of the disease throughout the pregnancy is mandatory, ablation of all lesions should be achieved, and in the absence of a clean, cured lower genital tract, consideration should be made for delivery by cesarean section prior to rupture of membranes.

Herpes genitalis, herpes virus hominis, is a common vulvar problem and pregnant women are not spared. Although some types of this virus show predilection for the oral cavity and others for the genital tract, overlap is well known in their manifestations. The initial viral infection of the vulva may be quite severe with urinary retention due to pain and involvement of the lower urinary tract. Bacterial superinfection is common, and many of these patients will require hospitalization. Secondary attacks are generally sharply circumscribed, which are known by the patient in advance of the visible lesion and require little attention in many cases. Acyclovir, either systemically or topically, has been used before and after pregnancy to reduce the severity of attacks and to reduce the frequency of attacks, but questions exist as to its ultimate efficacy and cure is unlikely. Acyclovir is not teratogenic in standard animal studies, but it has been reported to be responsible for chromosome breaks at high concentrations. The use of this drug in pregnancy probably carries some potential risk for the fetus, and the risks and benefits should be carefully considered before prescribing the drug in pregnancy.

Cytomegalovirus, herpes zoster, and vaccinia infections do not usually involve the vulva and are rarely of clinical importance in pregnancy.

H. Molluscum

Molluscum contagiosum with its characteristic small umbilicated raised lesions has no special predisposition for pregnancy, but it may be seen in pregnant women from time to time. Local ablation of the lesion is important, as autoinoculation is frequent. Various mechanical and other techniques for destruction of small skin lesions have been used depending on physician preference. Freezing, TCA, and local curettage are options, but podophyllin should be avoided in pregnancy.

The name *lymphogranuloma venereum* used for a vulvar lesion has given way to chlamydia, but more importantly, laboratory diagnosis is now rapid and secure. Effective treatment is easily administered and should forestall progression to the deforming and destructive picture of advanced disease.

I. Arthropod-Induced Diseases

The arthropod-induced diseases of the vulva include infestations with *Phthirus pubis* (pediculosis pubis, crab lice), *Sarcoptes scabiei* (scabies), *Eutrombicula* (chiggers), *Cimex* (bedbugs), *Pulex* (fleas), ticks, and mosquitoes. The characteristic appearance and generally easy identification of these organisms will lead to effective treatment. Multiple topical agents are available, and patients should be cautioned not to exceed the recommended number of applications or dose. The potential for systemic absorption should be considered during pregnancy.

Although not usually the site of attachment for the offending tick, the vulva might rarely be the host to the ticks responsible for Rocky Mountain spotted fever and related rickettsial diseases as well as Lyme disease.

The rashes of the rickettsial diseases and the local reaction to the deer tick bite for Lyme disease are usually seen on the lower extremity and the coincidence of pregnancy and these skin lesions on the vulva must be very rare.

Treatment for the infectious diseases, venereal and others, of the vulva is continually evolving, and the reader is referred to standard sources for the current recommendations (9,10).

VI. TRAUMA

The physiological increase in blood supply and stasis edema of the vulva as well as the limitations in freedom of motion as the pregnancy advances lead to an increased risk of trauma to the vulva. The edematous tissues are at increased risk for surface trauma, and the subcutaneous tissues can be the site for rapidly growing hematomas which may require surgical treatment after comparatively minor external force has been applied. Trauma related to sexual activity may lead to vulvar damage, especially with unconventional or forced participation. Clinicians should always be attuned to occasionally subtle clues to problems of this type. Screening for infectious and venereal diseases is mandatory. Pregnancy confers no immunity to sexual abuse.

VII. CHEMICAL AGENTS

In the last two decades, a host of chemical agents has been aimed at the vulva for various purposes. Body perfumes, scented toilet paper, antiperspirants, and deodorant preparations have all achieved wide popularity but occasionally are responsible for severe local symptoms and signs such as pruritus, erythema, and edema. Withdrawal of the agent and a topical corticosteroid are generally sufficient. Prolonged local inflammation in pregnancy is common, and continued topical steroid treatment will usually suffice.

VIII. CONCLUSION

There are many diseases of the vulvar skin and, although some of these are more commonly seen in older women when pregnancy is no longer possible, the many inflammatory, neoplastic, infectious, and traumatic disorders of this organ require attention and care, with special considerations for the changes induced by pregnancy.

REFERENCES

1. N. Dilsen, M. Konice, and C. Ovul eds. Behçet's disease: *Proceedings of an International Symposium on Behçet's Disease.* Istanbul, 29–30 September, 1977. Exerpta Medica, Amsterdam, 1979, pp. 1–306.
2. H. Gardner and R. Kaufman. *Benign Diseases of the Vulva and Vagina*, 2nd ed. Boston, Hall, 1981 pp. 1–505.
3. J. H. Shepherd and J. M. Monaghan eds. *Clinical Gynaecological Oncology*. Oxford, UK, Blackwell, 1985, pp. 35–53.
4. F. Rutledge, R. C. Boronow, and J. T. Wharton. *Gynecologic Oncology*. Wiley, New York, 1976, pp. 213–224.
5. S. Way. *Malignant Disease of the Vulva*. Churchill Livingstone, Edinburgh, 1982, pp. 1–76.
6. R. C. Wallach. Cryosurgery of advanced carcinoma of the vulva, *Obstet. Gynecol. 47*:454–458 (1976).
7. R. C. Wallach and R. N. Taub. Adjuvant immunotherapy for vulvar malignant melanoma, *Mt. Sinai J. Med. 46*:161–162 (1979).
8. J. U. Gutterman and H. I. Scher. Melanoma, *Cancer Medicine* (J.F. Holland and E. Frei, III, eds.). Lea & Febiger, Philadelphia, 1982, pp. 2109–2140.
9. G. R. G. Monif. *Infectious Disease in Obstetrics and Gynecology*. Philadelphia, Harper & Row, 1982.
10. Centers for Disease Control and Prevention: 1993 Sexually transmitted diseases treatment guidelines. *MMWR* 42 (No. RR-14): i–102 (1993).

8

Genital Infections of Perinatal Importance

Susan M. Forster and Michael John Hare
Hinchingbrooke Hospital, Huntingdon, Cambridgeshire, England

I. INTRODUCTION

Genital infections are of particular importance to the pregnant woman, as they not only may be the cause of significant symptoms and long-term complications if untreated, but they may also be associated with an increased risk of premature labor, premature rupture of the membranes, postnatal complications for the mother, and infection or congenital malformation of the baby.

Many genital infections are sexually transmitted, and it is therefore essential to ensure that current sexual partners are also treated to prevent reinfection. The presence of one sexually transmitted disease greatly increases the risk of others being present, and asymptomatic infection should be looked for in those at greatest risk.

It is well known that many infections are exacerbated by pregnancy (1). The immune response may be impaired, perhaps associated with mechanisms to prevent rejection of the fetus, but there is little evidence to confirm this (2). Hormonal and physical changes are also important.

Treatment options are often limited, as care must be taken to avoid drugs potentially harmful to the fetus. Time must be taken to discuss screening tests and their implications at length with the patient to allay unwarranted anxiety.

In this chapter, we address the relevant aspects of clinical presentation, diagnosis, and treatment of each genital infection of perinatal importance with particular reference to the pregnant woman.

II. CHLAMYDIA TRACHOMATIS

Chlamydia trachomatis is a small intracellular bacterium that can cause ocular, pulmonary, genital, and enteric infections. There are 17 different immunotypes of this organism, of which L1, L2, and L3 are associated with lymphogranuloma venereum, and D, E, F, G, H, I, J, and K are associated with a variety of genital infections, conjunctivitis, and pneumonia in the newborn. The relatively inactive extracellular form of *Chlamydia*, the elementary body, attaches to the host cell and is absorbed and converted to the more active reticulate form, which replicates within an enlarging phagosome or "inclusion," protected in some way from the normal defense mechanisms of the host cell. Eventually the cell ruptures releasing infectious elementary bodies.

The target cell is usually columnar epithelium, with infection involving the conjunctiva, urethra, endocervix, endometrium, and fallopian tubes. Batholinitis and perihepatitis may also occur. Acute infection produces a polymorphic response, but reinfection or prolonged untreated infection produces a chronic inflammatory response with a predominence of mononuclear cell infiltration. The subsequent fibrosis and scarring causes considerable morbidity, including infertility and chronic pelvic pain.

Women present primarily with dysuria, frequency, mucopurulent vaginal discharge, pelvic pain, dyspareunia, or abnormal bleeding. Chlamydial urethritis is an important cause of urinary symptoms in a patient with a normal midstream urine or sterile pyuria. Canalicular spread from the cervix may result in pelvic inflammatory disease (3), with an important complication of this being infertility (4). In pregnancy, the fetal membranes provide a protective barrier against canalicular spread of infection (although such spread may be facilitated by procedures such as chorionic villus sampling), with chorioamnionitis being the more common complication. Involvement of the endometrium and fallopian tubes may be asymptomatic (5); in fact, the incidence of asymptomatic chlamydial infection is generally high, and these women may be at more risk of developing long-term sequelae of their infection.

A number of investigators have found an association between cervical chlamydial infection and an increased risk of preterm delivery, premature rupture of the membranes, and perinatal mortality (6–10), with the risk of low birth weight or prematurity being correlated with the presence of chlamydial immunoglobulin (IgM) antibodies (11,12), suggesting that recently acquired or more extensive infection may be associated with a higher risk of such complications (13), and this may explain the inconsistency of some studies. Patients may present several weeks after delivery with a chlamydial metritis, causing fever, bleeding, discharge, and pain (14). A number of studies suggest that treatment during pregnancy may be beneficial (15–17).

Up to 50% of babies born to mothers with a chlamydial cervicitis are infected (11), and a number of these babies will develop conjunctivitis and/or pneumonia. The respiratory problems may not develop until the baby is several weeks old, and their onset may be insidious with a dry cough, nasal discharge, and diffuse interstitial infiltrates on the chest x-ray. Although the mortality rate is low, the infection can have a prolonged course and possibly lead to an increased risk of chronic lung and eye problems (11,18).

A. Diagnosis

On examination there may be a mucopurulent discharge coming from the cervix rather than the vagina associated with a hypertrophic ectopy or cervicitis with contact bleeding, edema, and erythema. Charateristic follicular cervicitis has been described on colposcopy (19). However, in adolescence and pregnancy, these findings can be less reliable (20). On microscopy of a Gram stain of the cervical secretions, the presence of more than 30 polymorphs per high-power field strongly supports the diagnosis of either a chlamydial or a nonspecific cervicitis.

Occasionally, a purulent discharge will be seen from an inflamed urethra. Taking samples from the urethra as well as the cervix to look for chlamydiae will increase the pickup rate by 20–25% even in those who have no urethral symptoms.

1. Culture

To culture for the presence of *C. trachomatis* is the most sensitive and specific diagnostic method, but the cost and expertise required limit its usefulness in routine screening programs. It remains the gold standard for research, difficult clinical cases, and any case with medicolegal implications.

Correctly taking the specimens greatly increases the chance of a positive result. Swabs should have thin wire shafts (not wood), either Dacron or cotton. More recently, certain types of cytobrushes have been used (21). The cervix must be cleaned first to remove vaginal secretions, which may have an inhibitory effect, and studies have demonstrated that if sequential samples are taken, the last is most likely to be positive (22). The appropriate transport medium should be used and samples refrigerated or frozen if they will not reach the laboratory in 24 hr.

2. Enzyme-Linked Immunosorbent Assays

Chlamydial antigens eluted from swabs taken as described above are detected by an enzyme-linked immunosorbent assay (ELISA) (23,24). This method is ideal for processing large numbers of specimens and is not subject to observer error, but it is significantly less sensitive and specific than culture. The false-positive rate is largely due to cross reactivity with organisms such as those seen in bacterial vaginosis, and to some extent these problems have been overcome by utilizing blocking antibodies. When testing low-risk populations, the positive predictive value of these assays may be disturbingly low (25), and the possibility of false positivity should always be considered when the clinical result is unexpected.

3. Direct Immunofluorescence

Fluorescein-conjugated monoclonal antibodies can be used to detect elementary bodies in cervical or other smears, and in expert hands it can be as sensitive as culture (26). Direct immunofluorescence (IF) may be even more sensitive than culture for detecting chlamydiae in endometrial or tubal specimens (27). The success of this method is determined by the expertise of the technician reading the slides. IF is not suitable for processing large numbers of specimens rapidly.

4. Serology

In cervical chlamydial infection, serological assays are usually positive with a higher titer than in some other infections; for example, in men with urethritis. It is rare to see a rising titer, and positive serology can occur in women without evidence of active genital chlamydial infection, so the use of this test is very limited. In cases of diagnostic doubt, a negative serology makes any active infection unlikely (28). The main use for chlamydial serology is in the diagnosis of neonatal pneumonia where specific IgM antibodies are present.

B. Management of Genital Chlamydial Infection During Pregnancy

The patient should be screened for any other coincident sexually transmitted infection and any recent or current sexual partners seen, screened, and offered treatment regardless of the results of their tests. It should be clearly explained to the patient how important it is to complete the course of treatment. The patient should be told not to resume intercourse with their partner until they both have been fully treated to prevent reinfection.

The tetracyclines are the most widely used antibiotics for chlamydial infection, but these are absolutely contraindicated in pregnant women, breastfeeding women, or children under the age of 12 years, because the tetracyclines are deposited in growing bones and teeth and cause persistent yellow discoloration and hypoplasia of the dental enamel. Erythromycin is the drug of choice in pregnancy, but not the estolate form of the drug, because it has been associated with hepatotoxicity. The standard dose of 500 mg four times daily for 1 week produces gastrointestinal side effects in many patients resulting in poor compliance. Doses of 500 mg twice daily for 1 week may be inadequate (29), and if this dosage is used, it should be given for 2 weeks. Alternatively, amoxicillin has been shown to be almost as effective as erythromycin with fewer instances of gastrointestinal upset (30). Azithromycin is a possible future treatment (31). Screening for chlamydiae should be repeated in the third trimester to ensure that reinfection has not occurred.

C. Reiter Syndrome

Rarely a woman with chlamydial genital infection will present with a reactive arthritis, usually in the knees, ankles, and feet with associated sacroiliitis, tendinitis, and plantar fasciitis. Chlamydial elementary bodies have been demonstrated in these joints (32) but not viable replicating organisms. Animal studies have indicated that cell-mediated immunity may have an important role in the pathogenesis of the disease.

The classic triad of the Reiter syndrome (arthritis, urethritis, and conjunctivitis) form only part of the spectrum of this disorder. Women may suffer from an erosive vulvitis which is the equivalent of the circinate balinitis seen in men. Skin manifestations are common. Keratoderma blenorrhagica, erythematous macules that enlarge to hyperkeratotic papules, occurs characteristically on the soles of the feet, and a more extensive rash indistinguishable from that of psoriasis may be seen. Painless shallow ulcers are found on the buccal mucosa, and the nails are thickened and discolored. In severe cases, the patient can be systemically unwell with a fever, anorexia, and weight loss. Less common are cardiological conduction defects, pericarditis, aortitis, pneumonitis, and neurological complications. The Reiter syndrome is associated with a number of other infections including human immunodeficiency virus (HIV) infection.

III. NEISSERIA GONORRHOEAE

As with chlamydial infection, women with gonorrhea usually present with a purulent vaginal discharge, dysuria, pain, and dyspareunia or abnormal bleeding. The cervix is the commonest site of infection, although coincident infection of the urethra occurs in most women, and occasionally is the only source of *N. gonorrhoeae*. Oral and rectal infection may be more common in pregnancy (33). Gonorrhea is an important cause of pelvic inflammatory disease (again, this is less likely to occur in pregnancy), preterm labor, premature rupture of the membranes, chorioamnionitis, puerperal endometritis, or with neonatal complications, including a scalp abscess at the site of fetal scalp electrode insertion, ophthalmia neonatorum, or disseminated infection.

A. Clinical Diagnosis

Physical examination may be completely normal in a gonococcal infection. A mucopurulent cervical discharge associated with an inflamed, edematous cervix, and contact bleeding is the commonest finding in gonorrhea. Pus can be expressed from the urethra, periurethral glands, or Bartholin gland, and there may be a Bartholin abscess. The perianal area should be examined for evidence of irritation, erythema, discharge, or bleeding and the pharynx and tonsils for inflammation. A bimanual examination of the pelvis identifies any localized pelvic infection.

Disseminated gonococcal infection is more common in pregnancy. The dermatitis-tenosynovitis syndrome presents with a rash, bacteremia with a mild fever, rigors and general malaise, polyarthralgias, and tenosynovitis. Skin lesions are predominantly on the arms and legs, occurring as painful necrotic papules, pustules, vesicles, macules, or ecchymoses. More than one type of lesion may be present at any one time, and the lesions tend to occur in crops, usually less than 30 in total, perhaps only 1–10 at any one time, and are associated with fever. The lesions often lie over affected joints. The knees, ankles, wrists, elbows, and small joints of the hands are mainly involved. Rarely, endocarditis and meningitis can complicate disseminated disease.

The septic arthritis syndrome usually is a monoarthritis with purulent joint fluid growing *Neisseria* gonnococci in up to 50% of cases. An adult gonococcal ophthalmia is rarely seen as a result of direct inoculation.

B. Laboratory Diagnosis

Swabs taken from the cervix and urethra can be rolled gently onto a microscope slide and examined by Gram stain with a light microscope for the presence of typical pink intracellular gram-negative diplococci that occur in pairs shaped like two kidney beans facing each other. The sensitivity and specificity of the Gram stain varies depending on the site from which the specimens are taken. It is most sensitive in men with symptomatic urethritis (over 90%), although this falls in asymptomatic men and in women regardless of symptoms to between 50 and 70%. In experienced hands, this technique can give an immediate diagnosis and allow treatment to be started without having to wait for the cultures to be completed. However, cultures should always be performed to confirm the diagnosis and allow antibiotic sensitivity tests to be performed.

Samples should be taken from the endocervix, urethra, and rectum. If the patient is asymptomatic, the rectal swab can be taken blindly without proctoscopy. Gram stains are not routinely performed on pharyngeal or rectal swabs, as other organisms present at these sites, for example, *N. meningitidis* and partly digested staphylococci and streptococci, which can cause confusion. If there is a history of pharyngeal symptoms or oral sex, throat swabs should be taken for culture. Regardless of the history, taking rectal and urethral swabs increases the chance of gaining a positive culture by 5–10%. The swabs must not be allowed to dry out and should be inoculated immediately onto culture plates containing the correct media, usually a form of chocolate agar containing antibiotics to prevent overgrowth of other organisms. The plates must be incubated at 35–37°C in a 5% CO_2 atmosphere. If direct inoculation is not possible, the swabs can be placed in transport medium, but they must be plated out within 24 hr. In a patient with disseminated gonorrhea, blood cultures may be diagnostic, although the other sites should always be tested. Aspirated joint fluid is more likely to give a positive Gram stain and culture in a septic monoarthritis (34,35).

C. Treatment

Sexual contacts of infected patients must be seen and treated to prevent reinfection. The patient must be screened for other sexually transmitted diseases, and the occurrence of *Chlamydia* in patients with proven gonococcal infection is so common the majority of clinicians routinely treat such patients with antichlamydial therapy (see Section II. B; in the pregnant patient, usually erythromycin is the first line of therapy).

Patients should be advised to refrain from intercourse until they have been confirmed as negative for gonococcal infection on two sets of cultures usually 7 days apart following treatment. Where possible, single-dose regimens are preferred because of the problems of compliance.

The two main forms of drug resistance (36) are discussed below.

1. *Chromosomal Resistance*

Patients who have a strain of gonorrhea with a particularly high MIC have a much higher treatment failure rate. This is due to a chromosomal mutation and tends to be associated with resistance to other antibiotics; for example, tetracyclines and erythromycin. Mutations at some loci will produce resistance to a single antibiotic; at other loci, resistance to several antibiotics may result. Penicillin resistance is thought to occur because of a reduction in the affinity for penicillin in the cell membrane binding proteins (37). This form of resistance tends to develop slowly but relentlessly to most of the antibiotics that have been introduced.

2. *Plasmid-Mediated Resistance*

A number of beta-lactamase encoding plasmids have been described in *Neisseria gonorrhoeae*, which require a further plasmid to allow their transfer between strains of the organism (38). Strains that possess this plasmid produce penicillinase and penicillinase producing *Neisseria gonorrhoeae* (PPNG) seem to have originated in the Far East or West Africa. This form of resistance develops relatively rapidly.

Where resistant strains are known to be rare, and the patient is thought to be relatively reliable and will therefore be available for follow-up, or if the source of the infection and its sensitivities are known, the standard regimen of ampicillin 3.5 g and probenecid 1.0 g can be safely used in pregnancy as one stat oral dose. Where there is penicillin allergy, or the risk of resistance is significant, intramuscular spectinomycin 2 g should be used again as a stat dose. Another alternative in areas of greater resistance is intramuscular ceftriaxone 125–250 mg.

Patients with disseminated infection should be hospitalised and treated with longer courses of antibiotics. Pharyngeal infection should be treated with ceftriaxone.

IV. TRICHOMONAS VAGINALIS

Trichomonas vaginalis is a protozoon with a posterior flagellum attached to an undulating membrane which propels the organism. It causes infection primarily of the stratified squamous epithelium of the vagina (cf. *Chlamydia* [Section II] and *Neisseria* gonorrhoeae [Section III], which prefer columnar epithelium) and the urethra. Controversy raged for many years as to the role of sexual transmission in trichomoniasis, but there is now unequivocal evidence that this is the source of the infection in the majority of cases. Trichomoniasis has been associated with an increased incidence of premature labor and low birth weight (39,40), although other studies have not confirmed this. Five percent of babies born to mothers with untreated *T. vaginalis* infection acquire the infection perinatally, but this seems to be transient in most cases (42,43).

A. Presentation

Patients classically present with a copious, frothy, yellow or green vaginal discharge that is often malodorous and causes severe soreness. On examination, the vulva is often red, excoriated, and edematous. The vaginal wall and cervix are inflamed with the typical strawberry pattern seen particularly well by colposcopy. The inguinal lymph nodes may be enlarged and painful, occasionally extending to the pelvic nodes, although pelvic pain usually indicates the presence of another infection. Trichomoniasis is also sometimes asymptomatic or associated with only vaginal discharge or minimal irritation.

B. Diagnosis

If a specimen of discharge is taken from the vaginal fornices with a swab or loop and suspended in normal saline on a microscope slide, the jerky swaying motion of the motile protozoa can be seen and are diagnostic. Using phase contrast or darkfield illumination makes this easier. A Gram stain of the vaginal secretions will not identify the organisms, but it usually shows large numbers of polymorphonuclear neutrophils. A significant number of cases are missed if wet smears alone are relied on, and taking specimens for culture increases the diagnosis. Other slide staining techniques may be used, including Gram stain with a safranine counterstain, Giemsa stain, and acridine orange using a fluorescent microscope. The vaginal secretions have a high pH. Trichomoniasis may be reported on a cervival smear taken for cytology as part of a screening program for dyskaryosis; however, the diagnosis should always be confirmed by light microscopy or culture.

C. Treatment

The treatment of choice for trichomoniasis is metronidazole, but this is contraindicated in the first trimester of pregnancy, as animal studies have demonstrated carcinogenicity in rats and mutagenicity in bacteria; however, no apparent problems have developed in the babies of a large numbers of women who have received the drug in early pregnancy (44). Treatment with topical agents is not ideal, as involvement of extravaginal tissue is known to occur. Providone-iodine topically is contraindicated in pregnancy, as enough iodine can be absorbed to affect the baby's thyroid gland. In general, if the patient can be supported during the first few weeks with symptomatic topical therapy such as clotrimazole pessaries, vaginal vinegar douches, and acetic acid pessaries (Aci-Jel), metronidazole therapy can then be considered in the second trimester. Several regimens have been shown to be effective: metronidazole 400 mg twice daily for 5–7 days is probably the most reliable. If the patient is unlikely to comply with this, 2 g of metronidazole can be given as a stat dose, but this may produce more gastrointestinal side effects. Alcohol must be avoided until the drug is out of the patient's system. Partners of infected patients should be treated, and intercourse should be avoided (or condoms used) until metronidazole has been given and the infection cleared. Rarely, resistance to metronidazole can occur. If the organism persists and reinfection has been ruled out, malabsorption, inactivation by other vaginal organisms, and rarely zinc deficiency may all be responsible.

V. MYCOPLASMAS

Mycoplasmas are the smallest free living organisms. There are many different species; the two main ones isolated from the genital tract are *Mycoplasma hominis*, and *Ureaplasma urealyticum* (the latter form a distinct subgroup owing to their ability to hydrolyze urea). *Mycoplasma genitalium* was first described in 1981, but difficulties in culturing the organism have limited clinical studies. The emergence of the polymerase chain reaction (PCR) has revived interest recently, and it certainly seems to be implicated in some genital infections; for example, male nongonococcal urethritis (46). Many women are asymptomatically colonized with these organisms, and the incidence of this increases with number of sexual partners and may also be associated with race, contraceptive use (increased in intrauterine contraceptive device [IUCD] users and in those on a contraceptive pill), and low socioeconomic status. The organisms are isolated more frequently in association with other sexually transmitted diseases such as gonorrhea and *Chlamydia tracho-*

matis infection, as well as in patients with bacterial vaginosis. Treatment of these conditions produces symptomatic relief and eradication of the mycoplasmas even when the antibiotic used has no antimycoplasmal action. Presumably, the mycoplasmas can thrive in the abnormal vaginal environment produced by these infections.

It is difficult to determine to what extent the organisms can themselves produce disease. They are certainly the cause of some cases of pelvic inflammatory disease, having been isolated from the fallopian tubes of 8% of cases in one study (45), which is an area not normally colonized. Antimycoplasmal antibody responses and animal studies have also confirmed this association. The role of mycoplasmas in producing problems in pregnancy is more complicated. Studies have suggested that ureaplasmas are isolated more frequently from the endometrium of women who have had repeated spontaneous abortions (47), and fetuses have been shown to be infected after stillbirth or spontaneous abortion (48). Blanco et al. (49) found that mycoplasmas were isolated significantly more frequently from patients with intra-amniotic infection than from controls, and Lamont (50) found that a high percentage of women admitted with preterm labor had infection with *M. hominis* and *U. urealyticum* as well as *C. trachomatis*. Treatment with tetracyclines or erythromycin has produced an improvement in birth weight and reduced the spontaneous miscarriage rate, but this may be due to other factors predisposing to mycoplasma carriage rather than to eradication of the organism itself (15,51). A further problem is that treatment with erythromycin may only eradicate the organism temporarily, with recolonization being common. Although the organisms seem to have a role at least in the etiology of preterm labor, identifying those patients at risk may not be easy. The Vaginal Infections and Prematurity Study Group has published convincing data that treating women colonized with *U. urealyticum* with erythromycin does not reduce the risk of preterm labor or low birth weight babies or eradicate the organism, and that the association described between preterm labor and its complications with *U. urealyticum* is removed when other risk factors, for example, associated sexually transmitted diseases or smoking, are taken into account (52,53). So whereas isolation of these organisms from the upper genital tract would seem to be associated with preterm labor and low birth weight, their isolation from the lower genital tract is no good at predicting who will develop problems. *M. hominis* is definitely associated with postpartum fever in some patients, and the organism can be isolated from the blood and from the joints of some patients with postpartum arthritis (54). Transient colonization of the newborn can occur, but the role of these organisms in neonatal respiratory disease again is unclear (55). They are a very rare cause of meningitis.

It is therefore not routine practice to screen for mycoplasmas at present; however, any pregnant women presenting with sepsis should be treated with an antibiotic regimen that will cover these organisms also, and if available, the relevant cultures should be performed.

VI. BACTERIAL VAGINOSIS

Bacterial vaginosis is the most common cause in the developed world of vaginal discharge originating from the vagina rather than the cervix. It is a syndrome diagnosed by the presence of certain symptoms, signs, and microbiological abnormalities rather than the presence of one specific organism. Bacterial vaginosis often coexists with other genital infections and improves when they are treated. The infection appears to result from a change in the vaginal environment, although the etiology is not known. As with vaginal candidiasis, hormonal changes, sexual activity, and hypersensitivity may all play a part in the development of bacterial vaginosis.

In the past, bacterial vaginosis has been dismissed as a relatively trivial problem. In fact, as well as causing distressing symptoms, bacterial vaginosis has been associated with an increased risk of pelvic inflammatory disease, postoperative infection following hysterectomy (and therefore possibly other gynecological procedures), and postpartum and post–cesarian section endometritis (56,57). Recent work has suggested a link with premature rupture of the membranes and prematurity (58), possibly as a result of disruption of the cervicovaginal mucosa by microbiologically produced enzymes such as mucinase and sialidase. It has also been reported that women with bacterial vaginosis and related conditions are more likely to have female offspring (59)!

A. Diagnosis

Women with bacterial vaginosis present with a history of malodorous discharge, gray, cream, or white in color, which occasionally causes irritation. The presence of other symptoms such as dysuria or pain should always suggest the presence of another infection.

On examination, the cervix and vagina are not inflamed; indeed a feature of the condition is the lack of an inflammatory response on vaginal smears. The pH of the discharge can be easily tested using appropriate litmus papers, and it is usually high (5 or more). The pH may be falsely high if cervical mucus is sampled in error, the patient is bleeding, or there is semen present. If a drop of 10% potassium hydroxide solution is added to a drop of discharge on a slide, a characteristic odor is released. This is called the amine test; amines produced by the abnormal microbial flora cause the "fishy" odor. If a smear is made of the discharge and Gram stained, the normal lactobacilli are seen to be depleted or completely absent, being replaced by a mixed group of organisms, including *Gardnerella vaginalis* (a gram-negative or gram-variable coccobacillus), mobiluncus (poorly staining gram-negative curved bacilli), *Bacteroides* (small gram-negative bacilli), and *Mycoplasma hominis*. Some epithelial cells are completely covered with adherent bacteria, so that their margins are obscured, the "clue cell." Several investigators have attempted to define criteria for the diagnosis of bacterial vaginosis (60,61).

Clue cells may also be demonstrated in a "wet prep," where a drop of discharge is mixed with a drop of normal saline on a microscope slide. A raised pH is very sensitive but not very specific, as it can be raised for many other reasons. The presence of clue cells are specific but not as sensitive. Where possible, a Gram stain should always be performed, as this is the "gold standard" to confirm the diagnosis. A scoring system for reading Gram stains has also been developed (62).

Bacterial cultures can be performed but are not usually helpful. *G. vaginalis* and *M. hominis* are often present in the normal vagina, although very high concentrations of the organisms are more likely to be associated with disease.

B. Treatment

The treatment of choice for bacterial vaginosis is metronidazole 400 or 500 mg twice daily for 7 days, topical clindamycin cream 2 g intravaginally at night for 7 days, or oral clindamycin 300 mg twice daily for 7 days. Metronidazole is contraindicated in the first trimester of pregnancy; topical clindamycin cream does not yet have a licence for use in pregnancy but is a possible alternative treatment. As with *Trichomonas vaginalis*, if the patient is symptomatic and wishes treatment, this may be offered to her in the second and third trimesters. It is not current practice to treat sexual partners of patients with bacterial vaginosis, although it may be wise to screen them for other sexually transmitted diseases. In women with recurrent bacterial vaginosis, partners are often treated coincidentally in an attempt to reduce the rate of recurrence, but controlled studies have not shown this to be effective. Traditionally, treatment of bacterial vaginosis was only offered to symptomatic patients, but in view of the increasing evidence that vaginosis may be associated with other complications, it is becoming more widespread to offer treatment to anyone with the diagnosis of this infection regardless of their symptoms. Certainly patients who have been diagnosed as having bacterial vaginosis on routine screening should at least be informed of this. A recent study indicates that the ideal time to diagnose and treat the infection would be early in the second trimester (63), but as yet, no studies have clearly demonstrated that such treatment will reduce the risk of complications in pregnancy developing.

VII. CANDIDIASIS

The majority of cases of genital candidiasis are due to *Candida albicans*; however, occasionally other organisms, in particular *Torulopsis glabrata*, are isolated. *C. albicans* is a dimorphic organism, existing as a yeast form and as a fungal form, which forms mycelia and is generally considered to be more pathogenic. Studies have demonstrated that the mycelial form is more resistant to phagocytosis and more adherent to vaginal epithelial cells.

C. albicans, particularly in its yeast form, can certainly be carried asymptomatically, and it is found in the mouth or gastrointestinal tract of 10–30% of the population and in the genital tract of 5–10% of women. This rises to 20–40% of women in pregnancy (64,65).

It has been supposed that the increased risk of candidiasis in pregnancy is associated with an increase in the number of large glycogen-containing cells in the vagina owing to hormonal stimulation (66). Certainly glucose produced as a result of cytolysis of those cells would form a substrate for the candidal organisms, and it is well recognized that there is an increased risk of candidiasis in diabetes. Segal showed that the ability of the organisms to bind to the vaginal epithelial cells was enhanced in pregnancy (67), and Witkin has suggested that hormones may have a direct ability to enhance transition from the yeast form to the more pathogenic fungal form (68). Whatever the cause of candidiasis, the problem becomes more severe as the pregnancy progresses, and it is worse during the third trimester.

Obviously symptomatic women should be treated, but it is unclear at present how important it is to treat asymptomatic carriers. Systemic candidiasis in a previously healthy woman is a very rare complication. Potasman (69) reviewed eight cases, and the majority had a predisposing factor; for example, the presence of an IUCD or a urinary catheter. Again, infection in utero fortunately seems to occur rarely, either producing fetal death or delivery of a baby with disseminated candidiasis at birth. Johnson (70) reviewed 29 cases and could not elucidate any maternal risk factor that could have predicted the outcome. The main complication of candidiasis is neonatal infection usually associated with low birth weight babies. This follows two patterns, relatively early presentation mainly due to *C. albicans* infection, and probably related to transmission of the organisms from an infected mother at delivery (64); and infection occurring later when other organisms such as *C. parapsilosis* may be found more commonly as a result of nosocomial transmission (e.g., from the hands of a nurse). Once the baby is colonized, development of systemic disease is related to the procedures and treatments often necessary for any premature baby; for example, the use of intravenous or urinary catheters, total patenteral nutrition, aminophylline, steroids, or antibiotics (71).

A. Presentation

Genital candidiasis presents with an itchy, white, curdlike discharge, associated with dysuria, superfical dyspareunia, and painful excoriation of the vulva, which is often red, inflamed, and edematous in severe cases. In milder cases, however, itch may be the only symptom, but this can cause considerable distress and embarrassment. A maculopapular rash may be seen perianally and periorally as well as the vulvar area, and occasionally it spreads onto the inner thighs.

Neonatal infection also usually presents with a perioral or perianal rash or oral candidiasis. The rash may be localized to an intravenous or other catheter site, and it may spread to become a diffuse pustular or desquamative eruption. Disseminated infection is associated with fever, respiratory symptoms, abdominal distention, lethargy, endocarditis, meningitis, or endophthalmitis.

B. Diagnosis

C. albicans may be seen on microscopy of either a normal saline or 20% potassium hydroxide preparation of discharge taken with a swab from the vaginal wall. The organisms will also be demonstrated on a Gram stain preparation used for the diagnosis of bacterial vaginosis or on a cervical smear for cytology. The most sensitive method of detection of *C. albicans* is culture using the necessary transport and culture media, of vaginal discharge in genital infection, throat swabs in oral candidiasis, or blood cultures in neonatal or disseminated infection.

C. Treatment

The treatment of choice for candidiasis in pregnancy is topical clotrimazole in the form of vaginal pessaries, 100 mg every night for 1 week, 200 mg every night for 3 days, or 500 mg for 1 night. Clotrimazole cream should be applied twice daily for a week extensively to the entire vulvar area, including perianally.

VIII. STREPTOCOCCI

Streptococci are gram-positive organisms with a somewhat confusing nomenclature. Historically, they were divided by their action when cultured on blood agar into nonhemolytic, alpha-haemolytic, and beta-haemolytic organisms. However, the classification dependent on certain cell wall antigens, the Lancefield group antigens, bears more correlation with their pathogenic behavior. Thus, *Streptococcus agalactiae* bear Group B antigens and are beta-hemolytic, although other beta-hemolytic streptococci cause disease in animals, and some of these bear group B antigens.

The rate of asymptomatic colonization with group B streptococci in the genital area varies with different populations from 2.3 to 28% (72), and it is now recognized as the second most common cause of death in neonates as a result of bacterial sepsis (exceeded only be *Escherichia coli*) and of life-threatening systemic illness in adults. Infection rates are higher in those attending sexually transmitted disease clinics. Group B streptococci are isolated from up to half of babies born to mothers with positive vaginal cultures. Easmon et al. (73) found 37 of the babies of 95 mothers infected with group B streptococci were colonized, and in 17 of these cases, the maternal colonization was "light." Only a small number of these babies will go on to develop disease, usually in preterm infants, or following premature rupture of the membranes or intrapartum fever. There is an increased risk of neonatal illness where there has been a previous baby suffering from group B streptococcal disease (72,74).

There is still some debate as to the role of group B streptococci in actually precipitating preterm labor or premature rupture of the membranes. Group B streptococcal colonization of mothers (75) and women with a positive urine culture are at an increased risk of these complications (76), and treatment may significantly reduce this rate (67), but treatment of both mothers and their partners during pregnancy has not been successful in completely eradicating the organism, as recolonization occurs. Treatment at term may reduce the risk of neonatal disease (78), but this would involve treating large numbers of women not at risk, who may suffer problems; for example, penicillin allergy.

To further complicate the issue, cultures may only be intermittently positive from the vagina and may also be positive from the urethra, perianal area, and upper respiratory tract.

A. Clinical Presentation

Genital infection with group B streptococci is usually asymptomatic. Neonatal infection follows two distinct patterns. Early-onset disease may present within a few hours (or occasionally be a cause of stillbirth) certainly within 5 or 7 days, and is usually associated with maternal vaginal colonization. These babies have septicemia, respiratory symptoms, and occasionally meningitis. The late-onset disease is usually a purulent meningitis and is not associated with maternal carriage. The babies with late-onset disease are generally of normal birth weight and full term, whereas the early-onset babies are usually low in birth weight, often premature, and follow complicated labor with premature rupture of the membranes.

Group B streptococci may cause puerperal fever, and particularly in those with an underlying condition such a diabetes mellitus or following a gynecological procedure, can cause, for example, septicemia, endocarditis, and purulent meningitis.

B. Diagnosis and Treatment

Culture of group B streptococci takes 24–48 hr. Rapid diagnostic tests are currently being developed (80,81). Urinary antibodies may prove to be better at picking out those at risk than cultures (82), but the role of screening is still being investigated (83). Ampicillin either orally or intravenously is the drug of choice in most group B streptococcal infections, with the addition of gentamicin in severe cases.

IX. HERPES SIMPLEX VIRUS

All of the herpesviruses produce latent infection in which the virus lives within the host cell but is not completely expressed and does not produce infectious virus. In herpes simplex infection, the virus enters the body through a mucocutaneous surface and then moves centripetally along the axonal vascular or lymphatic vessels to the sensory ganglia, where it can remain latent (84). When reactivation occurs, the virus is thought to travel back down the nerve producing clinical symptoms and viral shedding at the point of first entry or other sites supplied by the same nerve ganglion.

The majority of genital infections are caused by herpes simplex virus (HSV) type 2; however, a significant number of infections occur as a result of HSV-1 infection, usually following orogenital contact. The most severe clinical picture occurs in those patients who have had no previous exposure to either HSV-1 or HSV-2, a "primary HSV attack," where serology to both HSV strains is initially negative. In a number of patients claiming to have their first clinical attack of genital herpes, there is serological evidence of previous exposure to HSV-1, which usually results in the clinical picture being less severe. There may also be evidence of previous exposure to HSV-2, presumably because the true primary attack was asymptomatic. These patients are referred to as "nonprimary initial infection."

If the first clinical episode occurs during pregnancy, it may result in spontaneous abortion or preterm labor. Those women who are actually shedding virus at the time of delivery may infect their babies. Cervical shedding occurs in up to 13% of women with a vulvar recurrence at term (85,86), but the greatest risk of neonatal disease is in those mothers suffering a primary attack at the time of delivery. Unfortunately, asymptomatic shedding of the virus is possible, and as most clinicians are aware of the dangers of delivering a baby vaginally in the presence of clinical genital herpes, the majority of babies born with neonatal herpes have mothers with no clinical lesions. However, Whitley (87) showed that a third of these cases may have a history of previous genital herpes or a partner with HSV infection. Brown et al. (88) studied 15,923 pregnant women and found that 0.35% of these were asymptomatically shedding the virus at term. Those with an asymptomatic primary infection were more likely to infect their babies (33%) compared with those with recurrent infection (3%). The use of fetal scalp electrodes was associated with an increased risk of transmission.

A. Presentation

Primary attacks of HSV infection are often severe, with fever, headache, malaise, and myalgia. The mucocutaneous lesions may be preceded by localized tingling or other abnormal sensations in the skin. Vesicles form which soon develop into painful ulcers that crust over and then heal. Nonspecific symptoms such as dysuria, vaginal discharge, pain, and dyspareunia will accompany involvement of the urethra or the cervix. The symptoms resolve in the second week, although in a true primary infection, they last longer. Localized tender lymphadenopathy is common and persists after resolution of the other symptoms. Acute infection may be complicated by radiculomyopathy producing urinary retention, aseptic meningitis, and psychological disturbance (89), and this can precipitate erythema multiforme. Much less commonly in the otherwise well adult, serious disseminated and neurological disease occurs. The lesions can be spread, and patients should be warned about scratching and local hygiene. Extragenital lesions are seen; in particular infection of the eyes can be serious.

Neonatal disease of the skin, eyes, and mouth has a similar picture; however, disseminated, or neurological, involvement is common and has a very high mortality. One of the problems is making the diagnosis in the absence of typical mucocutaneous lesions either on the child or the mother (see below).

B. Diagnosis

HSV serology is only helpful in those patients who have a primary first HSV infection where seroconversion can be demonstrated. In other situations, a rise in antibody titer is not usually demonstrated. Consequently, it is not routinely used. Most infections are diagnosed clinically and confirmed by cell culture, which can take 7–10 days. Swabs should be taken from the base of fresh moist ulcers or from the fluid from new vesicles. Once the lesion has begun to dry, the culture is much less likely to be positive. Cultures should also be taken from the cervix, particularly if there is a clinical cervicitis. The chance of growing the virus is greatest during the first attack, and is less for recurrences, and a negative culture does not rule out the diagnosis. Antigen detection assays are currently being evaluated for the more rapid diagnosis of HSV infection.

C. Treatment

True primary attacks of HSV infection can be very distressing and rest, adequate analgesia, and occasionally hospitalization are needed. Acyclovir is used in non-pregnant women to treat all primary attacks and in severe recurrences when it can be given soon enough to make its use worthwhile. In patients with severe frequent recurrences, maintenance treatment with acyclovir may now be used, usually for a period of 6 months or 1 year in the first instance, although it has been used for 3 or more years without any problems (90). Fortunately, resistance to acyclovir is rare and drug sensitivity tests are not routinely performed. It can be used in high doses intravenously in more severe disease.

Acyclovir is not currently licensed for use in pregnancy, although animal studies have not demonstrated any teratogenicity and when it has been used major problems have not occurred (91). No studies have yet demonstrated that treating primary attacks of HSV infection in pregnancy reduces the risk of complications such as preterm labor. Women with clinical disease at term should be offered a cesarian section. Serial HSV cultures performed during the last trimester may help indicate patients likely to secrete the virus asymptomatically who have a history of recurrent disease, and they can also be offered cesarian section. Unfortunately, the problem is mainly one of primary attacks at term, particularly in those with no previous antibody protection, and the only means of preventing this at present is by educating patients antenatally about the importance of avoiding unprotected intercourse with new partners during pregnancy. Because of the high risk to the baby in true primary attacks of HSV infection during the third trimester, some experts are now recommending treatment with acyclovir (92). In the future, it may be possible to vaccinate women before pregnancy to reduce this risk.

X. CYTOMEGALOVIRUS

Cytomegalovirus (CMV) is a herpesvirus which is found in saliva, urine, semen, cervical and vaginal secretions, breast milk, and blood. It is transmitted by intimate contact, mainly from mother to child, child to child or indeed child to parent, blood transfusions or organ donations, and in adulthood as a sexually transmitted disease. A number of studies have shown how important sexual transmission is for those who have escaped infection by puberty (93,94). In developing countries or low socioeconomic groups, virtually the entire community has been infected by adulthood. In the West, however, particularly in more middle class areas, the incidence of exposure to the virus may be as low as 40%.

A. Clinical Presentation

Most adults with CMV infection are asymptomatic when they acquire the infection or develop a glandular fever–like illness with fever, myalgia, headache, hepatitis, and general malaise. A sore throat, lymphadenopathy, and atypical lymphocytosis occur but less frequently than in Epstein-Barr virus infection. Serious neurological and disseminated disease is rare in the healthy adult.

In the region of 1% of neonates are born with the infection, but again in many this is asymptomatic. About one-fifth of these infected neonates will develop complications. The severe disseminated infection with neurological involvement, hepatosplenomegaly, jaundice, and eye disease has a high mortality, and those that survive have a high risk of permanent neurological disease, mental impairment, or deafness.

B. Diagnosis

Recent infection with CMV can be diagnosed by demonstrating serological seroconversion (a fourfold rise in titer over a period of a few weeks), and the presence of immunoglobulin M (IgM) antibodies suggests this is primary infection (these antibodies can persist for some months). Patients with CMV infection often secrete virus that can be cultured, and they continue to excrete virus for many months or even years. Episodic recurrent shedding of CMV also occurs. Viral cultures may take 10 days or even several weeks in low titers and are expensive to perform. Neither diagnostic method has a very high sensitivity.

C. Treatment

Gancyclovir (a DNA polymerase inhibitor related to acyclovir) and Foscarnet (phosphonoformate) are used in the treatment of life-threatening CMV infection, usually in the immunosuppressed patient. Unfortunately, there is no treatment that will prevent viral excretion that can be given safely to pregnant women.

D. Reducing the Risk of Maternal Transmission

Fowler has demonstrated (95) that the majority of serious congenital CMV infection results from primary infection during pregnancy rather than viral shedding as a result of reactivation of old disease or reinfection, presumably as a result of a protective effect of maternal antibody. Routine screening of pregnant women is not generally performed at present. However, those at high risk of contracting CMV infection at work, for example, health care workers dealing with patients with acquired immunodeficiency syndrome (AIDS), nursery school workers (babies born with asymptomatic CMV infection can continue to excrete virus for many months), or pediatric nurses could be screened for CMV antibodies, and should they be negative advised to avoid contact with babies under 1 year old or infected patients (96). All pregnant women and adolescents in particular should be warned of the importance of avoiding unprotected casual sex during pregnancy. Unfortunately, should a pregnant woman contract primary CMV infection, there is no treatment at present to prevent her passing this on to her child. In the future as with HSV infection, a vaccination may be available prenatally for those found to be serologically negative.

XI. HUMAN PAPILLOMAVIRUS

More than 70 types of human papillomavirus (HPV) infection have been identified by DNA hybridization, but only a certain number of these types are associated with genital disease and are considered to be sexually transmitted in the majority of cases. Two-thirds of the male partners of women with genital warts have significant lesions themselves (97). Warts often recur, or existing warts progress with pregnancy. Large vulval or vaginal lesions can bleed or cause obstruction during labor. There is also a risk of transferring the virus to the baby and causing infection of the respiratory tract and producing laryngeal papillomatosis. The risk of this is very low, so the presence of vulval warts is not in itself an indication for cesarian section; indeed the virus may be transmitted to the baby in the absence of any clinical maternal disease and despite cesarian section (98).

Topical podophyllin and 5-fluorouracil cream are both contraindicated in pregnancy. Cryotherapy is the treatment of choice for HPV infection; the entire lesion should be frozen including 1–2 mm of surrounding tissue for at least 20 sec. Local anesthetic creams can be used prior to treatment to reduce the discomfort of cryotherapy. Trichloroacetic acid may be applied with care, avoiding normal skin, but it should not be given to the patients to use themselves. Repeated treatments are usually required. Severe or unresponsive lesions can be treated with diathermy or laser. Certain strains of HPV infection have been associated with cervical cancer (99) (although the majority of clinical genital warts are not due to these strains), and cervical smears should be performed annually in all women with genital warts to exclude dyskaryosis until viral typing is routinely available to identify those at most risk. The entire lower genital tract should be examined preferably with a colposcope to exclude any small lesions on the cervix or vagina which will be a source of recurrence if untreated, and many centers now routinely give all women with warts a colposcopic examination to exclude clinical evidence of premalignant disease, although the benefit of this has not yet been fully established.

XII. SYPHILIS

Syphilis remains a serious problem in most of the developing world. Seroprevalence studies may be difficult to interpret owing to endemic nonvenereal treponemal disease. Studies such as that by Hira et al. in 1986 (100) show that 12.5% of those presenting for health care in Zambia have positive serology for syphilis, and in Swaziland over 30% of those presenting for antenatal care had a positive TPHA/FTA (*Treponema pallidum* hemagglutination assay-fluorescent treponemal antibody) (101). There has also been a recent increase in the occurrence of syphilis in the West, particularly in the United States. This was initially found mainly in homosexual men, but since the late 1980s, there has been a startling rise in the number of heterosexual cases, including congenital syphilis. This is thought to be linked to drug misuse (102), and it correlates with the increase in chancroid and HIV infection seen in the same areas.

Virtually all of the babies carried by women with primary or secondary syphilis are affected by the infection, which causes spontaneous abortion, preterm labor, perinatal death, or neonatal infection. Routine screening is still therefore performed in most countries at antenatal clinics, and the U.S. Centers for Disease Control recommend screening at presentation, at term, and in high-risk women also screening at 28 weeks. Even in areas of very low risk, screening has been shown to be cost effective (103).

A. Clinical Presentation

The first sign of syphilis is the chancre, which occurs at the site of entry of the etiological organism, *Treponema pallidum*. The chancre is most commonly found in the genital area (including the cervix) but can occur anywhere on the body or mucous membranes. The lesion is a red, painless papule which develops into a well-defined ulcer often with an indurated edge and is associated with nontender rubbery local lymphadenopathy.

The chancre gradually heals, but in a third of patients presenting with secondary syphilis, evidence of the original chancre may still be found. Most patients have headache, fever and malaise, and a rash, usually maculopapular and symmetrical and affecting the palms and soles. White-gray patches occur on the mucous membranes, and condylomata lata may be confused with veneral warts. Patchy alopecia and nail disease, hepatosplenomegaly, and neurological abnormalities, including meningitis, deafness, iritis, and optic neuritis are seen.

Babies born with congenital syphilis are usually asymptomatic at birth but within a few weeks develop failure to thrive, mucocutaneous lesions similar to those seen in adult secondary syphilis, nasal discharge and ulceration, hepatosplenomegaly and lymphadenopathy, and skeletal and hematological abnormalities. Some infected children, however, develop late congenital syphilis, which may not be detected until puberty. (For a full review of the clinical presentation of early and late syphilis see Ref. 104.)

B. Diagnosis

Ideally, a dark ground examination for the *T. pallidum* should be performed on serum exuded from the skin lesions. Histology may be needed. A number of serological tests are used to both diagnose and monitor the treatment of syphilis. These may be nonspecific; for example, the Venereal Research Disease Laboratory (VDRL) test in which antilipoidal antibodies produced in response to an antigen "cardiolipin" are detected. Low levels of this substance are also detected in a number of acute and chronic inflammatory conditions resulting in false-positive reactions. A positive VDRL is always confirmed by a specific antigen test, usually the *Treponema pallidum* hemagglutination assay (TPHA), fluorescent treponemal antibody (FTA) test, or the *Treponema pallidum Inhibition* (TPI) test; the latter test is now not used routinely, as it is time consuming and requires the use of live organisms. The FTA is the first to become positive in primary syphilis.

Neonatal infection should be diagnosed where possible by dark ground examination of suitable specimens, including nasal discharge. IgM levels may help in differentiating serological abnormalities from passive transfer of maternal antibodies. In both the infected adult and child, the VDRL titer is useful in monitoring response to therapy, and a rising titer indicates reinfection or reemergence of infection. In a baby, a failure in the titer to fall indicates active infection.

C. Treatment

Penicillin is the treatment of choice for syphilis. Tetracyclines are contraindicated in pregnancy. If there is a very clear history of penicillin allergy, skin testing and desensitization may be considered. The alternative is to treat the infection with erythromycin, but we know that infected babies have been born to mothers apparently adequately treated with this drug (105). If erythromycin is used, the baby should be treated at birth with penicillin. Women with syphilis in their third trimester may be at risk of premature labor as a result of a Jaresch-Herxheimer reaction. Ideally, they should be hospitalized for treatment, or they should at least be warned to seek help if they experience any contractions or change in fetal movements.

XIII. HUMAN IMMUNODEFICIENCY VIRUS INFECTION

Many women with HIV infection are first diagnosed when they become pregnant, and they require considerable support. Although pregnancy does not seem to increase the risk of disease progression in the mother as was once thought, the treatment of opportunistic disease is more difficult, and many of the drugs used are potentially toxic to the fetus. However, it is the rate of maternofetal transmission of HIV and the devastating pediatric disease that results which are the main problems. The reported risk of transmission varies widely in different studies, with 12.9% being recorded in Europe, but much higher rates are seen in developing countries. HIV infection can occur as early as 15 weeks of gestation (106) but usually occurs perinatally. Factors associated with an increased risk of HIV infection in the mother are a low CD4 count, increased viral load as assessed by P24 antigenemia, anemia, and the presence of chorioamnionitis (107). Villari (108) combined the results of a number of studies and drew the conclusion that cesarian section would reduce the risk of perinatal transmission, and the European Collaborative Study data support this view (109). However, the small reduction in the cases of transmission of HIV must be weighed against the risk of surgery. In the baby, scalp electrodes and other invasive procedures should be avoided, all secretions should be washed off as soon as possible, and breastfeeding should be avoided where a reasonable alternative exists. A recent placebo-controlled trial of the use of zidovudine in the last trimester of pregnancy, administered to the mother during labor intravenously and postnatally to the baby, demonstrated a reduction in the transmission HIV from 25.5 to 8.3% (110). Long-term follow-up is required to see what harm, if any, the drug has done to the othewise healthy children, but at present no major problems have occurred. Other strategies such as passive immunotherapy or active immunization of the mother are being studied, as the presence of maternal neutralizing antibodies has been shown to reduce the risk of transmission of HIV (111).

Pregnant women may present with a HIV-related illness. At the time of seroconversion, a few weeks after contracting the infection, an acute illness with fever, malaise, lymphadenopathy, sore throat, rashes, mucosal ulceration, and occasionally severe pulmonary and neurological manifestations may be seen. These symptoms usually resolve spontaneously, and the patient enters the latent asymptomatic phase of the illness, with no abnormality except for perhaps some persistent generalized lymphadenopathy. Much later (usually many years), immunosuppression occurs, and a whole range of opportunist diseases may develop (112).

As so many women with HIV infection are asymptomatic, the question of antenatal screening as is routinely performed by many countries for syphilis arises. At present, most areas offer HIV testing only to those considered to be at risk. However, many studies have indicated that this will miss a number of cases, particularly as the infection spreads into the heterosexual community. Barbacci (113) reported that universal testing of all pregnant women raised the detection rate from 57 to 87%. Routine testing of all women will reduce the stigma attached to the test, and the problems with, for example, life insurance companies, but it may deter some women who are afraid to be tested from attending antenatal clinics. The increased cost of universal testing with proper pretest counseling may be prohibitive and not justifiable in areas of relatively low prevalence. The subject of HIV infection should at least be discussed with every pregnant woman by an informed professional.

A. Diagnosis

Although HIV can be isolated in tissue culture from blood and most body fluids, it is expensive and time consuming. Most screening is performed using an enzyme-linked immunosorbent assay (ELISA) to detect anti-HIV antibodies. False negatives may occur during the window period between infection and seroconversion, usually no more than 2–3 months, but occasionally longer. False-positive tests are due to cross reaction of other antibodies; for example, after multiple blood transfusions, in autoimmune diseases, and in women who have had multiple pregnancies. Tests are usually confirmed by performing a Western blot, but even then occasional problem sera may be difficult to interpret and tests need to be repeated by different laboratories over a period of time, perhaps with culture or radioimmunoprecipitation assays (RIPA).

In babies, serological diagnosis is a problem because of placental transfer of the IgG antibodies, which may persist for a year. A few HIV-infected babies will be unable to synthesize their own IgG at that time and may become falsely negative. Unfortunately, IgM is unreliable as many babies do not make it. As with the P24 antigen assay and HIV culture, a negative result does not mean that the baby is not infected. Anti-HIV IgA is not transmitted across the placenta, and this along with PCR (polymerase chain reaction) may have a role in the diagnosis of HIV infection in the future.

Because of the poor prognosis of children born with HIV infection, women are still encouraged not to get pregnant, and many who fall pregnant accidentally will choose to have a termination, particularly if they already have a family.

XIV. HEPATITIS B

Hepatitis B is a DNA virus transmitted by injection (e.g., drug abuse, blood transfusion, needlestick injury), sexual transmission, vertical transmission from mother to child, and horizontal transmission usually within families from parent to child or between siblings. In parts of Asia and Africa, more than 90% of the population have serological evidence of past or current hepatitis B infection. In the West, hepatitis B infection is much less common and tends to be seen in high-risk groups.

Most hepatitis B infections are self-limiting and many are asymptomatic. Acute hepatitis is preceded by fever, maculopapular rash, arthralgias, and migratory arthritis in a number of patients. Less than 1% of infected patients develop fulminant hepatocellular disease and may die as a result, but about 5% develop chronic antigenemia with a risk of chronic active hepatitis and cirrhosis, although a more benign persistent viral hepatitis is more common. Asymptomatic patients with acute infection or who have persistent antigenemia and are therefore still infectious can only be detected by antenatal screening, either universally if the prevalence warrants it or of high-risk groups.

Maternofetal transmission does occur in utero, but most hepatitis B infections are transmitted perinatally. Administering hepatitis B vaccine and hepatitis B–specific immunoglobulin greatly reduces the risk of the baby being infected if they are given within 12 hr of birth.

A. Diagnosis

The detection of anti–hepatitis B core antibodies (anti-HBc) is the usual screening test, and if it is negative, the infection has been effectively excluded; unless the patient is seen very early after an acute exposure, in which case the antibodies may not have developed.

If the anti-HBc is positive, the presence of surface antigen (HBsAg) indicates infectivity, and IgM antibodies will determine if this is acute or chronic. The presence of e antigens indicates increased infectivity, conversely the loss of these antigens and the development of anti-e antibodies may indicate resolution of hepatocellular disease. If hepatitis B surface antigens are not detectable, the presence of surface antibodies confirms that the patient is now immune to further infection. Women who are found to be seronegative for hepatitis B infection but whose lifestyle is putting them at risk should be encouraged to be vaccinated postnatally.

XV. THE ROLE OF INFECTION IN PRETERM LABOR

Many different factors contribute to the etiology of preterm labor (spontaneous labor prior to 37 weeks' gestation). In some cases, for example, multiple pregnancy,

Müllerian abnormality, or preeclampsia, there is an obvious predisposing cause. Certain epidemiological associations have been recognized; for example: high maternal age, low socioeconomic status, an unskilled or unemployed father, a single mother, and certain racial characteristics. It is not clear how the presence of these factors produce their effect. There is increasing evidence that infection contributes not only to the increased maternal and neonatal morbidity following premature rupture of the membranes but is actually a cause of membrane rupture and of preterm labor (PTL). Sexually transmitted diseases are important in the cause of PTL, but in many cases, the organisms associated with PTL are those previously considered to be of low virulence and are often found in the genital area of healthy women.

Hillier et al. (114) showed that patients with premature delivery were five times more likely to have histological chorioamnionitis, and Russell et al. demonstrated that the presence of a chorioamnionitis is associated with neonatal sepsis and death particularly in preterm infants (115). Premature rupture of the membranes is similarly associated with neonatal sepsis (66,67), and two patterns have been described, that occurring early, possibly reflecting infection initiating the process; and that occurring later, being due to ascending infection from the vagina complicating the rupture. Of course, both patterns may coexist, particularly if a sexually acquired infection is then complicated by colonization with vaginal organisms.

The argument is supported by work suggesting that bacteria produce proteases and other enzymes which may both damage the cervical mucous plug and reduce chorioamniotic membrane strength. The associated activation of the immune system may result in the production of prostaglandins and other substances which can directly stimulate the onset of labor (58,117,118).

Diagnosing chorioamnionitis prior to the onset of preterm labor is difficult. Abdominal pain and vaginal discharge occur relatively late. The presence of a fever with a maternal or fetal tachycardia should always arouse suspicion. A leuokocytosis or very raised C-reactive protein may confirm this (121). Once labor has begun, treatment with broad-spectrum antibiotics until the results of the infection screen are available may reduce the risk of complications. This is widely practiced in premature rupture of the membranes, but the role of broad-spectrum antibiotics in preterm labor with intact membranes is still not clear.

Studies that have attempted to elucidate the role of coitus in PTL have shown conflicting results (91,119,120), but this may reflect concern with the frequency of sex with one partner, postulating that factors such as the presence of proteolytic enzymes in semen may damage cervical mucus, rather than concentrating on the incidence of unprotected sex with different partners or indeed having sex with a regular partner who is having other partners.

The appropriateness of antenatal screening for infection depends not only on the risk of exposure of the mother to infection but also the prevalence of the infection in the population being studied, the sensitivity, specificity, and suitability of the screening tests and any confirnatory tests available, the likelihood of transmission to the fetus, and the risk of serious disease as a result (122). Certainly, it would seem that an important function in any antenatal clinic would be skillful history taking to identify those patients at risk of infection so that they may be adequately screened and counseling all women about the importance of avoiding unprotected sex with new partners.

REFERENCES

1. B.J. Brabin. Epidemiology of infection in pregnancy, *Rev. Infect. Dis. 7*:579–603 (1985).
2. C.A. Hart. Pregnancy host resistance, *Baillieres Clin. Immunol. Allergy 2*: 735–757 (1988).
3. P.A. Munday, C.M. Stacey, C.A. Ison, et al. Clinical and microbiological investigation of women with acute salpingitis and their consorts, *Br.J.Obstet. Gynaecol. 94*: 281–2 (1987).
4. P.A. Mardh. Ascending chlamydial infection in the female genital tract, *Chlamydial Infections*, (D. Oriel, et al., eds.). Cambridge, UK, Cambridge University Press, 1986, pp. 173–184.
5. J.W. Sellors, J.B. Mahoney, M.A. Chernesky, and D.J. Rath. Tubal infertility: An assocition with prior chlamydial infection and asymptomatic salpingitis, *Fertil. Steril. 49*: 451–457 (1988).
6. J. Schacter, J. Grossman, R.L. Sweet, et al. Prospective study of perinatal transmission of chlamydia trachomatis, *JAMA 255*: 337A (1986).
7. L.S. Alger, J.D. Lovchik, J.R. Hebel, et al. The association of Chlamydia trachomatis, Neisseria gonorrhoeae and group B streptococci with preterm rupture of the membranes and pregnancy outcome, *Am. J. Obstet Gynecol. 159*: 397–404 (1988).
8. M.G. Gravett, H.P. Nelson, T. DeRouen, et al. Independent association of bacterial vaginosis and Chlamydia trachomatis infection with adverse pregnancy outcome, *JAMA 256*: 1899–1903 (1986).
9. J. Martius, M.A. Krohn, S.L. Hillier, et al. Relationships of vaginal lactobacillus species, cervical Chlamydia trachomatis and bacterial vaginosis to preterm birth, *Obstet. Gynecol. 71*: 89–95 (1988).
10. D.H. Martin, L. Koutsky, D.A. Eschenbach, et al. Prematurity and perinatal mortality in pregnancies complicated by maternal Chlamydia trachomatis infection, *JAMA 247*: 1585–1588 (1982).
11. H.R. Harrison. Chlamydial infections in neonates and children, *Chlamydial Infections* (D. Oriel, et al., eds.). Cambridge, UK, Cambridge University Press, 1986.
12. S.M. Berman, H.R. Harrison, W.T. Boyce, et al. Low birth weight, prematurity and postpartum endometritis. Association with prenatal cervical Mycoplasma hominis and Chlamydia trachomatis infection, *JAMA 257*: 1189–1194 (1987).
13. J.A. McGregor and J.I. French. Chlamydia trachomatis infection during pregnancy, *Am. J. Obstet. Gynecol. 164*: 1782–789 (1991).
14. U.B. Hoyme, N. Kiviat, and D.A. Eschenbach. The microbiology and treatment of late postpartum endometritis, *Obstet. Gynecol. 68*: 226–232 (1986).

15. H.A. Elder, B.A.G. Santamaria, S. Smith, and E.H. Kass. The natural history of asymptomatic bacteriuria during pregnancy: The effect of tetracycline on the clinical course and outcome of pregnancy, *Am. J. Obstet. Gynecol. 111*: 441–462.
16. I. Cohen, J.C. Veilla, and B.M. Calkus. Improved pregnancy outcome following successful treatment of chlamydial infection, *JAMA 263*: 3160–3163 (1990).
17. G.M. Ryan, T.M. Abdulla, S.G. McNeeley, et al. Chlamydia trachomatis infection in pregnancy and the effect of treatment on outcome, *Am. J. Obstet. Gynecol. 162*: 34 (1989).
18. K. Steinberg and P.A. Mardh. Persistent neonatal chlamydial infection in a 6 year old girl. *Lancet 2*: 1278–1279 (1986).
19. M.J. Hare, E. Toone, D. Taylor Robinson, et al. Follicular cervicitis-colposcopic appearances and association with chlamydia trachomatis, *Br. J. Obstet. Gynaecol. 88*: 174–189 (1981).
20. R.C. Brunham, J. Paavonen, C.E. Stevens, et al. Mucopurulent cervicitis. The ignored counterpart of urethritis in men, *N. Eng. J. Med. 311*: 1 (1984).
21. D. Taylor Robinson. Genital chlamydial infection: Clinical aspects, diagnosis treatment and prevention, *Recent Advances in Sexually Transmitted Diseases and AIDS*, No. 4 (J.R.W. Harris and S.M. Forster, eds.). Edinburgh, Churchill Livingstone, 1991, pp. 219–262.
22. R.C. Barnes. Laboratory diagnosis of human chlamydial infections, *Clin. Microbiol. Rev. 2*: 119 (1989).
23. G. Mumtaz, B.J. Mellars, G.L. Ridgway, and J.D. Oriel. Enzyme immunoassay for the detection of Chlamydia trachomatis antigen in urethral and endocervical swabs, *J. Clin. Pathol. 38*: 740–742 (1985).
24. D. Taylor Robinson, B.J. Thomas, and M.F. Osborn. Evaluation of enzyme immunoassay (Chlamydiazyme) for detecting Chlamydia trachomatis if genital tract specimens, *J. Clin. Pathol. 40*: 194–199.
25. J. Lefebvre, H. Laperriere, H. Rousseau, and R. Masse. Comparison of three techniques for detection of Chlamydia trachomatis in endocervical specimens from asympsomatic women, *J. Clin. Microbiol. 26*: 726–731 (1988).
26. B.J. Thomas, R.T. Evans, D.A. Hawkins, and D. Taylor Robinson. Sensitivity in detecting Chlamydia trachomatis elementary bodies in smears by use of a fluoroscein labelled monoclonal antibody comparison with conventional chlamydial isolation. *J. Clin. Pathol. 37*: 812–816 (1984).
27. N.B. Kiviat, P. Wolner Hansson, M. Petersen, et al. Localization of Chlamydia trachomatis infection by direct immunofluorescence and culture in pelvic inflammatory disease, *Am. J. Obstet. Gynecol. 154*: 865–873 (1986).
28. P.A. Csango, B. Sarov, H. Scholtz, I. Sarov. Comparison between cell culture and serology for detecting Chlamydia trachomatis infection in women seeking abortion, *J. Clin. Pathol. 41*: 89–92 (1988).
29. C.C. Linneman, C.L. Heaton, and M. Ritchey. Treatment of Chlamydia trachomatis infections. Comparison of 1 and 2 gram doses of erythromycin daily for 7 days. *Sex. Transm. Dis.* 14: 102–106 (1987).
30. N.S. Silverman, M. Sullivan, M. Hochman, et al. A randomized prospective trial comparing amoxycillin and erythromycin for the treatment of Chlamydia trachomatis in pregnancy, *Am. J. Obstet. Gynecol. 170*: 829–32 (1994).

31. M.R. Bush and C. Rosa. Azithromycin and erythromycin in the treatment of cervical chlamydial infection during pregnancy, *Obstet. Gynecol. 84*: 61–63 (1994).
32. A. Keat, B.J. Thomas, J. Dixey, et al. Chlamydia trachomatis and reactive arthritis: the missing link, *Lancet 1*: 72–74 (1987).
33. S.A. Al Suleiman, E.M. Grimes, and H.S. Jones. Disseminated gonococcal infections, *Obstet. Gynecol. 61*: 48–51 (1983).
34. D.C. William, et al. *Sex. Transm. Dis. 8*: 16 (1981).
35. R.J. Thin and E.J. Shaw. Diagnosis of gonorrhoea in women, *Br. J. Vener. Dis. 55*: 10–13 (1979).
36. C.A. Ison and C. S. Easmon. Epidemiology of penicilin resistant Neisseria gonorrhoeae, *G.U. Medicine 67*: 307 (1991).
37. A.G. Barbour. Properties of penicillin binding proteins in Neisseria gonorrhoeae, *Antimicrob. Agents Chemother. 19*: 316–322 (1981).
38. J. Brunton, M. Meier, N. Ehrman, et al. Origin of small beta-lactamase specifying plasmids in Haemophilus species and Neisseria gonorrhoeae, *J. Bacteriol. 168*: 374–379 (1986).
39. H. Minkoff, A.N. Grunebaum, R.H. Schwarz, et al. Risk factors for prematurity and premature rupture of the membranes. A prospective study of the vaginal flora in pregnancy, *Am. J. Obstet. Gynecol. 150*: 965–972 (1984).
40. M. Bromley. Study of female babies of women entering confinement with vaginal trichomoniasis, *Br. J. Vener. Dis. 52*: 58–62 (1976).
41. P.H. Hardy, E.E. Nell, M.R. Spence, et al. Prevelance of six sexually transmitted diseases among pregnant inner city adolescents and pregnancy outcomes, *Lancet 2*: 333–337 (1984).
42. J.G. Lossick. Treatment of sexually transmitted vaginitis/vaginosis, *Rev. Infect. Dis. 12* (Suppl. 6): 5665–5681 (1990).
43. P.J. Wendel and G.D. Wendel. Sexually transmitted diseases, *Semin. Perinatol. 17*: 443–451 (1993).
44. F.W. Rosa, C. Baum, and M. Shaw. Pregnancy outcomes after first trimester vaginitis drug therapy, *Obstet. Gynecol. 69*: 751–755 (1987).
45. P.A. Mardh, and L. Westrom. Tubal and cervical cultures in acute salpingitis with special reference to Mycoplasma hominis and T strain mycoplasmas, *Br. J. Vener. Dis.* 179–186 (1970).
46. D. Taylor Robinson, C.B. Gilroy, and P.E. Hay. Occurrence of Mycoplasma genitalium in different populations and its clinical significance, *Clin. Infect. Dis. 17* (Suppl. 1): 66–68 (1993).
47. B. Stray Pedersen, J. Eng, T.M. Reikvam, and T. Utenne. Mycoplasma colonisation in reproductive failure, *Am. J. Obstet. Gynecol. 130*: 307–311 (1978).
48. P.A. Quinn, J. Butany, M. Chipman, et al. A prospective study of microbial infection in stillbirths and early neonatal death, *Am. J. Obstet. Gynecol.* 151: 238–249 (1985).
49. J.D. Blanco, R.S. Gibbs, H. Malkerke, et al. A controlled study of genital mycoplasmas in amniotic fluid from patients with intra-amniotic infection, *J. Infect. Dis. 147*: 650–653 (1983).
50. R.F. Lamont, D. Taylor Robinson, J.S. Wigglesworth, et al. The role of mycoplasmas, ureaplasmas and chlamydia in the genital tract of women presenting in spontaneous early preterm labour, *J. Med. Microbiol. 24*: 253–257 (1987).

51. E.H. Kass, W. McCormack, J.S. Lin, and B. Rosner. Genital mycoplasmas as a hitherto unsuspected cause of excess premature delivery in the underprivileged, *Clin. Res. 29*: 575A (1981).
52. C. Carey, W.C. Blackwelder, R.P. Nugent, et al. Vaginal infections and prematurity study group. Antepartum cultures for Ureaplasma urealyticum are not useful in predicting pregnancy outcome, *Am. J. Obstet. Gynecol. 164*: 728–737 (1991).
53. D.A. Eschenbach. Ureaplasma urealyticum and premature birth, *Clin. Infect. Dis. 17* (Suppl. 1) S100–106 (1993).
54. D.G.R. Verinder. Septic arthritis due to Mycoplasma hominis. A case report and review of the literature, *J. Bone Joint Surg. 60*: 224 (1978).
55. P.T. Rudd, K.B. Waites, L.B. Duffy, et al. Ureaplasma urealyticum and its possible role in pneumonia during the neonatal period and infancy, *Paediat. Infect. Dis. 5* (Suppl.): 288–291 (1986).
56. P. Larsson, J. Platz-Christensen, U. Forsum, and C. Pahlson. Clue cells in predicting infections after abdominal hysterectomy, *Obstet. Gynecol. 77*: 450–452 (1991).
57. D.H. Watts, M.A. Krohn, S.L. Hillier, and D.A. Eschenbach. Bacterial vaginosis as a risk factor for postcesarian section endometritis, *Obstet. Gynecol. 75*: 52–58 (1990).
58. J.A. McGregor, J. French, W. Jones, et al. Bacterial is associated with prematurity and vaginal fluid mucinase and sialidase. Results of a controlled trial of topical clindamycin creamvaginosis, *Am. J. Obstet. Gynecol. 94*: 170 1048–1059 (1994).
59. H. Minkoff, A. Grunebaum, W.M., McCormack, and H. Schwartz. Relationship of vaginitis to the sex of conceptuses, *Am. J. Obstet. Gynecol. 137*: 432–438 (1985).
60. R. Amsell, P.A. Totta, C.A. Spiegel, et al. Nonspecific vaginitis diagnostic criteria and microbial and epidemiological associations, *Am. J. Med. 74*: 14–22 (1983).
61. D.A. Eschenbach, S.L. Hillier, C.W. Critchlow, et al. Diagnosis and clinical features associated with bacterial vaginosis, *Am. J. Obstet. Gynecol. 158*: 819–828 (1988).
62. R.P. Nugent, M.A. Krohn, and S.L. Hillier. Reliability of diagnosing bacterial vaginosis is improved by a standardized method of Gram stain interpretation, *J. Clin. Microbiol. 29*: 297–301 (1991).
63. P.E. Hay, D.J. Morgan, C.A. Ison, et al. A longitudinal study of bacterial vaginosis during pregnancy, *Br. J. Obstet. Gynecol. 101*: 1048–1053 (1994).
64. J.D. Schnell. Epidemiology and prevention of periportal mycoses, *Chemotherapy 28* (Suppl. 1): 66–72 (1982).
65. S. Haberman, E. Mendel, D.K. Hall, and L. Ramsey. The incidence of Staphylococcus aureus and Candida albicans in pregnant women, *Obstet. Gynecol. 20*: 639–644 (1962).
66. J.D. Schnell. Investigations into the pathophysiology and diagnosis of vaginal mycoses, *Chemotherapy 28* (Suppl. 1): 14–21 (1982).
67. E. Segal, A. Soroka, and A. Schechter. Correlative relationship between adherence of Candida albicans to human vaginal epithelial cells in vitro and candidal vaginitis, *J. Med. Vet. Mycol. 22*: 191–200 (1984).
68. S.S. Witkin. Immunological factors influencing susceptability to recurrent candidal vaginitis, *Clin. Obstet. Gynecol. 34*: 662–668 (1991).
69. I. Potasman, Z. Leibovitz, and M. Sharf. Candida sepsis in pregnancy and the postpartum period, *Rev. Infect. Dis. 13*: 146–149 (1991).
70. D.E. Johnson, T.R. Thompson, and P. Ferrieri. Congenital candidiasis, *Am. J. Dis. Child. 134*: 273–275.

71. D.E. Weese-Mayer, D.W. Fondriest, R.T. Brouillette, and S.T. Schulman. Risk factors associated with candidemia in the neonatal intensive care unit. A case control study, *Pediatr. Infect. Dis. 6*: 190–196 (1987).
72. J.A. Regan, M.A. Klebanoff, and R.P. Nugent. The epidemiology of group B streptococcal colonization in pregnancy, *Obstet. Gynecol. 77*: 604–610 (1991).
73. C.S.F. Easmon, M.J. Hastings, A.J. Clare, et al. Nosocomial transmission of group B streptococci, *Br. Med. J. 283*: 459–461.
74. C.J. Baker. Summary of the workshop on perinatal infections due to group B streptococcus, *J. Infect. Dis. 136*: 137–152.
75. J.A. Regan, S. Chao, and L.S. James. Premature rupture of the membranes, preterm delivery and group B streptococcal colonization of mothers, *Am. J. Obstet. Gynecol. 141*: 184–186 (1981).
76. M. Moller, A.C. Thompson, K. Borch, et al. Rupture of the foetal membranes and premature delivery associated with group B streptococci in urine of pregnant women, *Lancet 2*: 67–70 (1984).
77. A.C. Thomsen, L. Morup, and K.B. Hansen. Antibiotic elimination of group B streptococcus in urine in prevention of preterm labour, *Lancet 1*: 591–593 (1987).
78. K.M. Boyer and S.P. Gotoff. Prevention of early onset neonatal group B streptococcal disease with selective intrapartum chemoprphylaxis, *N. Engl. J. Med. 314*: 1665–1669 (1986).
79. G.B. Merenstein, W.A. Todd, G. Brown, et al. Group B beta-haemolytic streptococci: randomized controlled treatment study at term, *Obstet. Gynecol. 55*: 315–318.
80. M.K. Yancey, T. Armer, and P. Clark. Assessment of rapid identification tests of genital carriage of group B streptococci, *Obstet. Gynecol. 80*: 1038–1047 (1992).
81. W.J. Morales and D. Lim. Reduction of group B streptococcal maternal and neonatal infections in preterm pregnancies with premature rupture of the membranes through a rapid identification test, *Am. J. Obstet. Gynecol. 157*: 13–16 (1987).
82. H. McKenzie, M. Louise Donnet, P.W. Howie, et al. Risk of preterm delivery in pregnant women with group B streptococcal urinary infections or urinary antibodies to group B streptococcal and E. Coli antigens, *Br. J. Obstet. Gynaecol. 101*: 107–113 (1994).
83. Neonatal group B streptococcal infection, *J.R. Soc. Med. 86*: 712–715 (1993).
84. J.J. Sasadeusz and S.L. Sacks. Herpes latency, meningitis, radiculomyelopathy and disseminated infection, *GUM 70*: 369–377 (1994).
85. J.H. Harger, A.J. Amortegui, M.P. Meyer, et al. Characteristics of recurrent genital herpes simplex infections in pregnant women, *Obstet. Gynecol. 73*: 367–372 (1989).
86. A.E. Wittek, A.S. Yeager, D.S. Au, P.A. Hensleigh. Asymptomatic shedding of herpes simplex virus from the cervix and lesion site during pregnancy: Correlation of antepartum shedding with shedding at delivery, *Am. J. Dis. Child. 138*: 439–442 (1984).
87. R. Whitley, A. Arvin, C. Proben, et al. Predictors of morbidity and mortality in neonates with herpes simplex virus infection, *N. Engl. J. Med. 4*: 324–350 (1991).
88. Z.A. Brown, J. Benedetti, R. Ashley, et al. Neonatal Herpes simplex infection in relation to asymptomatic maternal infection at the time of labor, *N. Engl. J. Med. 324*: 1247–1252.

89. O. Carney, E. Ross, C. Bunker, et al. A prospective study of the psychological impact on patients with a first episode of genital herpes, *GUM 70*: 40–45 (1994).
90. L.G. Kaplowitz, D.A. Baker, L. Gelb, et al. Prolonged continuous acyclovir treatment of adults with frequently occurring genital Herpes simplex virus infection, *JAMA 265*: 747–751 (1991).
91. E.B. Andrews, B.C. Yankaskas, J.F. Cordero, et al. Acyclovir in pregnancy registry; Six years experience. *Obstet. Gynecol. 79*: 7–13 (1992).
92. C. Chazotte, F. Anderson, and W.R. Coren. Disseminated Herpes simplex infection in an immunocompromised pregnancy: treatment with intravenous acyclovir, *Am. J. Perinatol. 4*: 363–364 (1987).
93. Y.M. Sohn, M.K. Oh, K.B. Balcarek, et al. Cytomegalovirus in sexually active adolescents, *J. Infect. Dis. 163*: 460–463.
94. A.C. Collier, H.H. Handsfield, P.L. Roberts, et al. Cytomegalovirus in women attending a sexually transmitted diseases clinic, *J. Infect. Dis. 162*: 46–51 (1990).
95. K.B. Fowler, S. Stagno, R.F. Pass, et al. The outcome of congenital cytomegalovirus infection in relation to maternal antibody status, *N. Engl. J. Med. 326*: 663–667 (1992).
96. S.P. Adler. Cytomegalovirus and child day care. Risk factors for maternal infection, *Pediatr. Infect. Dis. J. 10*: 590–594 (1991).
97. R. Barrasso, J. Debrux, O. Croissant, and G. Orth. High prevalence of papillomavirus-associated penile intraepithelial neoplasia in sexual partners of women with cervical intraepithelial neoplasia, *N. Engl. J. Med. 317*: 916–923 (1987).
98. E.M. Smith, S.R. Johnson, T.P. Cape, et al. Perinatal veritical transmission of human papillomavirus and subsequent development of respiratory tract papillomatosis, *Ann. Otol. Rhinol. Laryngol. 100*: 479–483 1991.
99. M.H. Schiffman. Recent progress in defining the epidemiology of human papillomavirus infection and cervical neoplasia, *J. Natl. Cancer Inst. 84*: 394–398 (1992).
100. S.K. Hira, G.J. Bhat, A. Ratnam, and C. Chintu. Maternal and congenital syphilis in Zambia—some epidemiological aspects, *Afr. J. Sex. Trans. Dis. 3*: 3–6 (1987).
101. A. Meheus, F. Friedman, E. Van Dyck, and T. Guyver. Genital infections in prenatal and family planning attendants in Swaziland, *East Afr. Med. J. 57*: 212–217 (1980).
102. H.L. Minkoff, S. McCalla, I. Delke, et al. The relationship of cocaine use to syphilis and human immunodeficiency virus infections among inner city parturient women, *Am. J. Obstet. Gynecol. 163*: 521–526.
103. B. Stray Pedersen. Economic evaluation of material screenign to prevent congenital syphilis, *Sex. Transm. Dis. 10*: 167–172 (1983).
104. K.K. Holmes, et al., eds. *Sexually Transmitted Diseases* (2nd ed.). McGraw-Hill, New York, 1990.
105. L.J. Fenton and I.J. Light, Congenital syphilis after maternal treatment with erythromycin, *Obstet. Gynecol. 47*: 492–494 (1976).
106. J. Falloon, T. Eddy, L. Wiener, and P. Pizzo. Human Immunodeficiency virus infection in children, *J. Pediatr. 114*: 1–30 (1989).
107. M.E. St. Louis, M. Kamenga, C. Brown, et al. Risk of perinatal HIV transmission according to maternal immunological, virological and placental factors, *JAMA 269*: 2853–2859 (1993).
108. P. Villari, C. Sprio, T.C. Chalmers, et al. Cesarian section to reduce perinatal

transmission of human immunodeficiency virus. A Metanalysis, *Online J. Curr. Clin. Trials 74*: 930708 (1993).

109. The European Collaborative Study. Caesarian section and risk of vertical transmission of HIV infection, *Lancet 343*: 1464–1467 (1994).
110. Centers for Disease Control and Prevention. Zidovudine in the prevention of HIV transmission from mother to infant, *MMWR 43*: 285–287 (1994).
111. G. Scarlatti, J. Albert, P. Rossi, et al. Mother to child transmission of HIV type 1: Correlation with neutralizing antibodies against primary isolates, *J. Infect. Dis. 168*: 207–210 (1993).
112. M.A. Sande and P.A. Volberding, eds. *The Medical Management of AIDS*, 3rd ed. Saunders, Philadelphia, 1992.
113. M. Barbacci, F.T. Rephe, and R.E. Chausson. Routine prenatal screening for HIV infection, *Lancet 337*: 709–711 (1991).
114. S.L. Hillier, J. Martius, M. Krohn, et al. A case control study of chorioamnionic infection and histological chorioamnionitis in prematurity, *N. Engl. J. Med. 319*: 972–978 (1988).
115. P. Russell. Inflammatory lesions of the human placenta. 1. Clinical significance of acute chorioamnionitis, *Am. J. Diagn. Gynecol. Obstet. 1*: 127–137 (1979).
116. L.L. Cederquist, I.A. Zerroudakis, L.C. Ewool, et al. The relationship between prematurely ruptured membranes and fetal immunoglobulin production, *Am. J. Obstet. Gynecol. 134*: 784–788 (1974).
117. R. Romero, N. Kadar, J.C. Hobbins, et al. Infection and labour: the detection of endotoxin in amniotic fluid, *Am. J. Stet. Gynecol. 157*: 815–819 (1987).
118. R.F. Lamont, D. Taylor Robinson, M. Newman, and J. Wigglesworth. Spontaneous early preterm labour associated with abnormal genital bacterial colonisation. *Br. J. Obstet. Gynecol. 93*: 804–810 (1986).
119. R. Naeye. Coitus and associated amniotic fluid infections. *N. Engl. J. Med. 301*: 1198–1200 (1979).
120. W.E. Pugh and N. A. Fernandez. Coitus in late pregnancy, *Obstet. Gynecol. 2*: 636–642 (1953).
121. N.M. Fisk, J. Fysh, A.G. Child, et al. Is C reactive protein really useful in preterm premature rupture of the membranes?, *Br. J. Obstet. Gynaecol. 94*: 1159– (1987).
122. G.L. Gilbert. Routine antenatal screening and prenatal diagnosis of vertically transmissable infection, *Baillieres Clin. Obstet. Gynecol. 7*: 1–93 (1993).

9

Dermatological Therapy During Pregnancy and Lactation

Denis Sasseville
McGill University, Montreal, Quebec, Canada

I. INTRODUCTION

Gone are the days when the only solace a skin disease sufferer could obtain was some sympathetic words and innocuous salves or poultices. The modern dermatological armamentarium comes equipped with potent drugs that may occasionally cause undesirable results and effects in those using them and give rise to significant systemic toxicity.

This problem is further compounded when drugs are used during pregnancy, a situation in which two patients are in fact being treated. The toxicity of pharmacological agents on the rapidly developing but still immature fetus may be markedly different from what is seen in the mother (1).

Pregnancy is a state of altered physiology which may elicit the appearance of specific dermatoses or the exacerbation of preexisting entities (2–5). In the treatment of these disorders, the dermatologist must choose drugs with favorable maternal and fetal safety profiles. It is especially important to rule out pregnancy and to emphasize contraception before prescribing a potentially fetotoxic drug to a woman of childbearing age.

Unfortunately, standard pharmacology textbooks and common sources of information such as the *Physicians' Desk Reference* (Medical Economics, Oradell, NJ) either do not mention or are overcautious on the subject of drug safety during pregnancy and lactation. This lack of information is bound to entertain a nihilistic approach to therapy and result in denial of effective treatment. In many cases, such an attitude will be more detrimental to the mother and her unborn child than the alleged risks of pharmacological agents.

A. Maternal Pharmacokinetics

The four basic processes that govern the ultimate action of a drug are absorption, distribution, biotransformation, and excretion (6). The physiological changes that occur throughout pregnancy may considerably alter these fundamental functions.

High levels of progesterone in pregnancy are responsible for delayed gastric emptying, decreased gastrointestinal motility, and hyperemesis gravidarum. The normally rapid absorption of lipophilic drugs is not modified, but slowly transferred, ionized and hydrophilic drugs are more completely absorbed and display a greater toxicity (7).

The extracellular volume increases by up to 50% in the latter half of pregnancy, an expansion which directly affects the distribution of most drugs. Thus, larger loading doses are usually required to achieve similar plasma levels than in the nonpregnant state. Protein binding decreases, however, so that at equilibrium concentrations of pharmacologically active free drug may be higher (8).

Hepatic blood flow is unmodified by pregnancy, but progesterone increases the activity of hepatic microsomal enzymes, which causes the faster inactivation of many drugs (7).

Cardiac output and glomerular filtration rates increase by 30–50% during pregnancy. In the absence of toxemia and fluid retention, drugs which are eliminated by the renal route will be cleared more rapidly and have a shorter half-life.

B. Transplacental Drug Transfer and Metabolism

The placenta effectively segregates the maternal from the fetal circulation, whereby allowing exchange of gases, nutrients, antibodies, and waste products. Most drugs freely cross the placenta by passive diffusion proportionally to the maternal-fetal gradient (8). Nonionized and lipophilic drugs with a molecular weight under 600 D are easily transported across the placental membrane.

It was formerly thought that the fetus was a passive recipient of maternally administered drugs. It is now known that the placenta can metabolize and inactivate various steroid hormones (9). Furthermore, active enzymatic biotransformation of drugs has been demonstrated in the fetal liver as early as the eighth week of pregnancy (8). The generation of reactive metabolites may increase the carcinogenic, mutagenic, or teratogenic properties of many drugs.

The overall activity of hepatic metabolism remains, however, lower in the fetus than in the adult, with resultant slower detoxification of most pharmacological agents. Furthermore, drugs are excreted more slowly in the fetus, as their clearance involves retrograde transfer to the mother through the placental unit. Some drugs may be sequestered in the amniotic fluid after renal excretion or be partially reabsorbed with the swallowing movements of the fetus (7).

C. Fetal Development and Teratology

Congenital malformations occur in 2–7% of all infants, but only 5% of these anomalies can be blamed on the activity of a teratogenic drug (1,8). Drugs may produce noxious effects during any of the four recognized stages of fetal development.

1. Implantation Stage

The first stage, or implantation period, of development extends from conception to day 17 of pregnancy. At this stage, all cells are pluripotential and are either unaffected or completely killed by maternal administration of therapeutic agents. Toxic drugs therefore induce spontaneous abortion without causing congenital defects (1).

2. Embryonic Stage

The embryonic phase of development lasts from the second to the eighth week after conception. Organogenesis takes place during this period, and it is during this critical timeframe that teratogenic agents exert their adverse effects. The period of maximal susceptibility appears to be the third week of gestation, when the first menstrual period is missed and while the patient may not yet be aware of her pregnancy (9).

3. Fetal Stage

The fetal phase of development extends from the eighth week of pregnancy to near the time of parturition. Organogenesis is complete and this period is characterized by intense growth and functional maturation. Deleterious effects of drugs administered during this period will be manifested by delayed growth and psychomotor retardation, as the blood-brain barrier remains highly permeable until late in pregnancy, and because the central nervous system achieves full maturation only during the third trimester. It is also during this period that hormonal agents may adversely affect the normal differentiation of the genitalia.

4. Perinatal Stage

During the perinatal period, drugs no longer induce congenital defects or growth retardation, but their pharmacological activity may lead to side effects such as, for example, hypotonia, sedation, respiratory depression, agitation or withdrawal symptoms, jaundice, and hemorrhagic disorders.

D. Pharmacokinetics of Lactation

The passage of drugs into breast milk obeys the law of passive diffusion, and it is influenced by the same drug characteristics that facilitate transplacental transfer; namely, low molecular weight, liposolubility, and absence of ionization (10). Weak bases are less ionized in plasma than in the more acidic breast milk, where they tend to remain trapped and become concentrated (8). Because drugs passively follow concentration gradients, most of them leave milk and are excreted back into the mother's circulation as plasma levels fall.

Most drugs that reach milk have been partially metabolized by maternal liver enzymes, and further biotransformation will occur following absorption by the neonate. Drugs that are present in milk in significant amounts may fail to reach pharmacological serum levels in the nursing child despite copious feedings. Some drugs with poor gastrointestinal absorption will be secreted into breast milk when parenterally administered to the mother. Even if they fail to be absorbed, such drugs (e.g., aminoglycoside antibiotics) may cause side effects from their actions in the infant's gut.

E. Principles of Drug Therapy

Preexisting disease or new conditions that arise during pregnancy may require pharmacological therapy. Whenever the use of a potentially fetotoxic drug is contemplated, it is the responsibility of the prescribing physician to ascertain the absence of pregnancy and make sure that adequate contraception is implemented.

When pregnancy is already present, a careful assessment of the need to treat the associated disorders should be carried out, balancing the potential benefits with the risks of the proposed therapy. This assessment should also take into account the possible maternal and fetal consequences of withholding treatment. Only the safest drugs should be used, and in those life-threatening conditions in which less toxic alternatives may not be available, the issues should be discussed with the patient and informed consent obtained.

The use of drugs during lactation is somewhat less problematic, as teratogenicity is no longer a concern during this period. When a woman requires the administration of a drug which is contraindicated in the nursing child, it is usually possible to suppress lactation if it is not already established. In a fully lactating mother, milk should be pumped and discarded until the drug is stopped (10). The compatibility of drugs with breast-feeding has been extensively studied by a committee of the American Academy of Pediatrics (11,12).

This chapter summarizes the available information concerning the safety of most drugs commonly or occasionally prescribed by dermatologists during pregnancy and lactation. In the United States, the Food and Drug Administration (FDA) has devised a useful classification which rates the potential fetomaternal toxicity of drugs according to the following five categories:

Category A: Controlled studies in women fail to show a risk to the fetus in the first trimester, and there is no evidence of a risk in later trimesters.
Category B: Animal studies have not demonstrated a risk but controlled studies in women are lacking, *or* adverse effects in animals were not confirmed by controlled studies in women.
Category C: Animal studies have revealed adverse effects and there are no controlled studies in women, *or* animal and human studies are lacking.
Category D: There is evidence of human fetal risk. The potential benefits may outweigh the risks in certain circumstances (e.g., life-threatening disease).
Category X: Fetal abnormalities have been noted in animals and humans. The risks clearly outweigh the benefits. The drug is contraindicated in pregnancy.

II. SYSTEMIC THERAPY

A. Antimicrobial Agents

1. *Penicillins* (FDA class B)

The penicillins form a family of natural or semisynthetic antibiotics whose basic structural unit is the beta-lactam ring. They exert a bactericidal effect through interference with bacterial cell wall synthesis. Their antimicrobial activity is greatest against gram-positive cocci, treponemes, meningococci, and gonococci, although the newer members of the group possess extended activity against gram-negative bacilli.

Penicillins have been used extensively in pregnancy and are devoid of any teratogenic potential (13). All penicillins cross the placenta to some extent, and therapeutic fetal levels can be obtained except during the first trimester of pregnancy (14). Penicillins which bind strongly to serum proteins, such as cloxacillin or dicloxacillin, will reach much lower fetal serum levels than ampicillin or methicillin, which are more loosely bound (15).

Breast milk concentrations of most penicillins usually fall within the range of 2–20% of maternal serum levels (15). Penicillins are considered safe for breast-feeding, although the exposed infant may incur the risk of developing hypersensitivity reactions.

2. *Cephalosporins* (FDA class B)

Cephalosporins are bactericidal antibiotics which share with penicillins a similar chemical structure developed around the beta-lactam ring. Susceptible bacteria are destroyed by cell wall synthesis inhibition. All members of the cephalosporin family possess good to excellent antimicrobial activity against staphylococci and some activity against enterobacteria. Newer agents are effective against *Pseudomonas* and *Bacteroides* organisms. Cephalosporins are more resistant to inhibition by beta-lactamase than penicillins, but the latter drugs are usually more effective against susceptible organisms, and cephalosporins are rarely first-line agents for any given infection. The exception is gonorrhea, for which ceftriaxone is now the agent of choice.

Cephalosporins are nonteratogenic (16). In the pregnant state, cephalosporins and penicillins exhibit a similar pharmacokinetic profile (14). Most of these agents, including ceftriaxone, have been used in pregnancy (17). Transplacental transfer is negligible during the first trimester and becomes progressively higher near term.

Small amounts of cephalosporins are secreted into breast milk. These antibiotics are safe for breast-feeding.

3. Erythromycin (FDA class B)

Erythromycin is a macrolide antibiotic which inhibits bacterial protein synthesis when it reversibly binds to 50S ribosomal subunits (18). Its dermatological indications include acne vulgaris, staphylococcal or streptococcal pyodermas, erythrasma, syphilis, gonorrhea, borreliosis, and bacillary angiomatosis associated with acquired immunodeficiency syndrome (AIDS). Erythromycin absorption is erratic in pregnant women and transplacental passage of a single dose is poor, resulting in subtherapeutic levels in the fetus (19). Repeated doses lead to fetal liver accumulation and the obtention of higher levels, which, however, may still remain too low for effective eradication of fetal syphilis.

Erythromycin is not fetotoxic and has not been associated with the production of congenital abnormalities (13). Erythromycin base and succinate have been used extensively during pregnancy without adverse effect on mother or fetus. Erythromycin estolate, however, is contraindicated during pregnancy, because this salt has caused reversible hepatotoxicity in 10–15% of women who received it for more than 3 weeks (20). The phenomenon appears to be a hypersensitivity reaction and is manifested by a rise in aspartate aminotransferase (AST) and gamma- glutamyltranspeptidase (γ-GT). Hepatotoxicity is usually subclinical, but in some instances it presents with fever, jaundice, and abdominal pain mimicking cholecystitis (14).

Erythromycin is excreted in breast milk in amounts equivalent to 50% of maternal serum levels. This antibiotic is compatible with breast-feeding (12).

4. Clindamyin (FDA class B)

Clindamycin is a lincosamide antibiotic. Like erythromycin and chloramphenicol, it inhibits bacterial protein synthesis by binding to 50S ribosomal units. It possesses the same spectrum of activity as erythromycin, but it is also effective against a wide range of anaerobic pathogens. Dermatological indications of systemic clindamycin appear limited to rare cases of bacterial synergistic or gas gangrene. A rare but serious side effect of systemic clindamycin administration is the development of pseudomembranous colitis.

Clindamycin is not teratogenic or fetotoxic. Transplacental transfer is in the range of 50%, and therapeutic levels can be obtained in the fetus after systemic maternal administration (21). Clindamycin is excreted into breast milk, where concentrations can reach 10–20% of maternal serum levels (14). Despite the potential risk of pseudomembranous colitis in the child, clindamycin is considered compatible with breast-feeding (12).

5. *Sulfonamides and Sulfones* (FDA class A [dapsone], B [sulfonamides], and D [sulfonamides, near term])

Sulfonamides and sulfones are structural analogues of para-amino-benzoic acid (PABA). They are bacteriostatic for microorganisms that require PABA for the synthesis of folic acid (18). Although the popularity of sulfonamides as antibacterial agents has decreased since the advent of more potent drugs, dapsone has retained a preeminent place in the treatment of leprosy. Dapsone and sulfapyridine are commonly used by dermatologists because of their beneficial activity in selected dermatoses with a neutrophil-rich infiltrate such as dermatitis herpetiformis, subcorneal pustulosis, and leucocytoclastic vasculitis. A renewed interest for the use of sulfasalazine in the treatment of psoriasis and atrophie blanche has been seen in recent years.

Sulfonamides cross the placental barrier. Teratogenic effects have been reported in some animal species, but monitoring of large numbers of expectant women treated with sulfonamides at various stages of pregnancy did not reveal an increased incidence of congenital malformations (13). Likewise, the safety of dapsone in pregnancy has been established (22,23).

Sulfonamides are slowly excreted by the neonate. Administration of these agents near term can increase the risk of neonatal hyperbilirubinemia and kernicterus, as they displace bilirubin from plasma albumin (24). Premature infants are more vulnerable to this complication. Hemolytic anemia has been reported in two newborns whose mothers received sulfonamides. Glucose-6-phosphate dehydrogenase (G6PD)–deficient fetuses are more prone to this potentially lethal side effect. Avoidance of sulfonamides or sulfones near term is therefore recommended.

These agents are excreted in breast milk in small amounts and are considered compatible with breast-feeding by the American Academy of Pediatrics; with the exception of sulfasalazine, which has caused bloody diarrhea in an infant (12). A case report has described mild hemolytic anemia in the nursing child of a mother treated for dermatitis herpetiformis with dapsone in daily doses of 50 mg. Milk concentrations of dapsone were higher than maternal serum levels (25). Other investigators have found traces of sulfonamides in the urine of breast-fed infants after maternal administration of dapsone. It appears wise to discourage breast-feeding in sulfone-treated mothers.

6. *Aminoglycosides* (FDA class C or D)

Members of this group of antibiotics include amikacin, gentamicin, neomycin, and netilmycin (FDA class C) and kanamycin, streptomycin, and tobramycin (FDA class D). These agents disrupt protein synthesis at the level of the 30S ribosomal unit and are bactericidal against aerobic, gram-negative bacilli. Streptomycin has an extended spectrum which makes it invaluable in the treatment of tuberculosis, some infections with atypical mycobacteria, tularemia, all forms of plague, and in combination therapy for some cases of mycetoma. Streptomycin is thus the aminoglycoside most likely to be used by dermatologists.

Aminoglycosides are rapidly transported across the placenta and fetal concentrations are roughly 30–60% of maternal serum levels (14). No reports linking congenital defects with the prepartum administration of amikacin, kanamycin, neomycin, and tobramycin have been published. Streptomycin has been more extensively studied and found devoid of teratogenicity by Lowe (26), as well as by Heinonen and collaborators (13).

Congenital eighth nerve damage with deafness has been described after maternal therapy with streptomycin, and this can theoretically occur following administration of other aminoglycosides. Although the incidence of this complication remains low, some investigators recommend avoidance of aminoglycosides during pregnancy, or if they cannot be withheld, careful monitoring of maternal serum levels to minimize overexposure (14). A point to remember is that aminoglycoside ototoxicity is independent of embryogenesis and therefore can occur after exposure anytime in pregnancy.

Aminoglycosides diffuse into breast milk in significant amounts. However, oral absorption of these compounds is extremely poor, and their use is compatible with breast-feeding (12).

7. *Tetracyclines* (FDA class D)

Tetracyclines are bacteriostatic antibiotics extracted from strains of *Streptomyces* or semisynthetically elaborated. They reversibly bind to bacterial 30S ribosomes to inhibit protein synthesis (27). Because of its safety and effectiveness, tetracycline has gained wide acceptance in the systemic therapy of acne. Therefore, a large number of women of childbearing age, many of whom may not be practicing contraception, are potentially exposed to this drug. Furthermore, tetracycline can reduce serum levels of oral contraceptives, thereby decreasing their efficacy.

Fatty liver of pregnancy, or obstetrical acute yellow atrophy, refers to a rare but potentially fatal complication of pregnancy. The syndrome is characterized by headache, nausea, vomiting, and abdominal pain of acute onset in the third trimester of pregnancy. It is associated with jaundice, azotemia, marked electrolyte imbalance, and occasional progression to shock, coma, and death. Acute pancreatitis is almost invariably present in cases with a fatal outcome. Autopsy findings show a diffuse, foamy vacuolization of hepatocytes, focal renal cortical necrosis and tubular fat vacuolization, fat emboli in the brain, and focal or diffuse pancreatic necrosis. Although the precise etiology of the syndrome remains controversial, approximately 50% of the reported cases have occurred following parenteral tetracycline administration in the third trimester of pregnancy, most commonly for the treatment of pyelonephritis (28). However, fatty liver of pregnancy has also been attributed to oral tetracycline ingestion prior to conception (29).

Tetracycline crosses the placenta and 50% of maternal doses are retrieved in cord blood. The drug binds strongly with calcium orthophosphate, and it is actively deposited in bones and teeth undergoing calcification. In teeth, this deposition is permanent, as remodeling and calcium turnover do not occur after calcification is completed (16). Deciduous teeth calcification begins in mid pregnancy and continues 6 months postpartum, whereas permanent teeth formation occurs between the ages of 4 months and 12 years (30). Thus, the deciduous teeth of a child exposed to tetracycline in utero after the twentieth week of gestation will exhibit a yellowish staining with a green fluorescence under ultraviolet light. Over the years, as a result of photo-oxidation, the stains become brownish and the fluorescence decreases. Earlier reports of enamel hypoplasia have not been confirmed by prospective studies (31,32).

Deposition of tetracycline in fetal bone after maternal ingestion has been documented (33). These same investigators also reported growth retardation in a litter of rats given tetracycline during gestation, as well as a 40% reduction of fibula growth in human premature infants treated with tetracycline. The study by Genot and colleagues found no differences in skeletal development between children exposed in utero and age-matched controls (32). However, the effects on fetal weight and growth of chronic tetracycline administration in pregnancy remain unknown.

In 1964, a single report described the possible association of maternal tetracycline intake with the development of cataracts in eight children (34). Since these findings were not confirmed by subsequent studies, the association remains speculative.

Teratological studies have shown that tetracycline can elicit abnormalities of skeletal development in chick embryos. In human lymphocyte cultures, the addition of tetracycline produces chromosomal aberrations (27). The association of tetracycline with the production of human malformations is supported by only three case reports. In 1962, Wilson described a child, who having been exposed to tetracycline at day 33 of pregnancy was born with absent and webbed fingers (35). The second case, published by Corcoran and Castles in 1977, concerned a boy exposed to tetracycline in utero during the first 6 weeks after conception: He weighed 1928 g and displayed low-set ears, micrognathia, deformed scapulae, arthrogryphosis, cardiomegaly, genital hypoplasia, and clubbed feet (36). The third case presented with hypomelia, hypotrichosis, and a facial hemangioma (37). In spite of these reports, however, two prospective studies have failed to show an increased risk of congenital malformations in children exposed to tetracycline in utero (27).

In conclusion, tetracyclines do not appear to be major teratogens when administered in the first trimester of pregnancy. With later administration, there is a risk of fatty liver atrophy in the mother and deciduous dental staining in the offspring. Tetracyclines should not be prescribed during pregnancy, and ongoing treatment should be discontinued as soon as pregnancy is diagnosed or suspected.

Tetracyclines are excreted into breast milk in small amounts. However, these drugs remained undetectable in the serum of breast-fed infants, probably because strong binding to milk calcium reduces their bioavailability (16). Tetracyclines are compatible with breast-feeding (12).

8. *Quinolones* (FDA class C)

The newer quinolones are derived from nalidixic acid by the addition of a fluorine atom, a modification which has greatly enhanced antibacterial activity. Ciprofloxacin, norfloxacin, and ofloxacin are representative members of this family, and other quinolone compounds are being developed. They inhibit DNA gyrase and thus interfere with DNA replication. Fluoroquinolones are active against gram-positive and gram-negative bacteria. They can be administered orally and are useful in the treatment of pyodermas, gonorrhea, and possibly chancroid (38).

Embryotoxicity and teratogenicity studies of quinolones in various animal species have shown no adverse effects. Quinolones, however, can damage growing cartilage, and arthropathy has been demonstrated in some animals and in children following their long-term use (39). This side effects and potential DNA alteration contraindicate the use of all quinolones in pregnancy and childhood.

Quinolones are excreted into breast milk, and women receiving these drugs should not breast-feed.

9. *Antituberculous Agents*

a. Isoniazid (FDA class C). This hydrazide of isonicotinic acid, isoniazid, is the primary drug for the chemotherapy and prophylaxis of tuberculosis (18). The drug has been used extensively during pregnancy, and most reviews have failed to demonstrate an increased rate of malformations in the offspring of women taking isoniazid (15,40).

There is a theoretical risk of convulsions and neurotoxicity in the fetus, associated with isoniazid, which are potentially preventable by the concomitant administration of vitamin B_6 (41). In addition, pregnant women may face a greater risk of hepatic damage from isoniazid than nonpregnant individuals. Therefore, even though isoniazid is safe for the treatment of active disease in the pregnant state, some investigators recommend postponing prophylaxis until the postpartum period (14).

Isoniazid is excreted in breast milk, but it is considered safe for breast-feeding.

b. Rifampin (FDA class C). Rifampin is a complex macrocyclic antibiotic which is bactericidal against most gram-positive and many gram-negative bacteria. It has replaced streptomycin as a first-line agent in triple-drug antituberculosis regimens, and it is used with dapsone to treat all forms of leprosy. Rifampin has some antiprotozoal activity, and it has been combined with sodium stibogluconate in the treatment of leishmaniasis.

Transplacental transfer of rifampin is high (14). The drug has shown some teratogenic potential in certain animal species (42). The number of rifampin-exposed pregnancies remains too small to draw any firm conclusion, but the drug appears acceptably safe. A survey of 442 exposed pregnancies has detected 14 miscellaneous abnormalities, including limb reduction and central nervous system lesions (40). In addition, Eggermont and coworkers, as well as Pagani, have shown that rifampin can increase the risk of hypoprothrombinemia and hemorrhage in the newborn (42,43).

Rifampin is excreted into breast milk in amounts considered too low to be harmful (44).

c. Ethambutol (FDA class B). Ethambutol is an ethylenediamine derivative which exerts a specific antibacterial activity against mycobacteria through an unknown mechanism of action. It has replaced para-aminosalicylic acid in antituberculous regimens because of its low toxicity. The major side effect of ethambutol is reversible optic neuritis (18).

Although ethambutol crosses the placenta and has produced cleft palate in animal pregnancies, no teratogenicity has been reported in humans (40,41).

Levels in breast milk are considered too small to be harmful, and the drug is compatible with breast-feeding (12,44).

10. Antilepromatous Agents

a. Clofazimine (FDA class C). Clofazimine is a phenazine red dye. Its tricyclic core has a structure similar to anthracene, being capable of intercalating into DNA chains (45). Clofazimine is active against *Mycobacterium leprae*, and it remains the only drug against which bacterial resistance has not yet developed. It is also highly effective against *Mycobacterium ulcerans* and variably effective against other atypical mycobacteria. Clofazimine exhibits anti-inflammatory properties which have proven useful in the treatment of erythema nodosum leprosum reactions and reversal reactions in borderline leprosy (46).

Clofazimine accumulates in body tissues and is slowly excreted. Its major side effect is a brownish red cutaneous discoloration, which may be distressing to fair-skinned individuals. The drug crosses the placental barrier. Compounds which bind to DNA may be teratogens or mutagens, but no such effect has been demonstrated to be associated with clofazimine in human pregnancies (45,46). Reports of normal offspring in clofazimine-treated mothers have been published, although cutaneous discoloration has occasionally been observed in the neonate (47).

Clofazimine is secreted into breast milk. Other than skin pigmentation, no untoward effect has been reported in the nursing infant.

B. Antifungal Agents

1. *Amphotericin B* (FDA class B)

Amphotericin B, extracted from *Streptomyces nodosus*, is a polyene fungicidal agent which binds to ergosterol, which is an essential constituent of fungal cell membranes. This binding causes the formation of pores in the cell membranes with subsequent leakage of cytosolic molecules (18). Because of poor absorption from the gastrointestinal tract, the drug is usually administered intravenously. Amphotericin B produces a wide range of adverse effects, such as nephrotoxicity, thrombocytopenia, fever, anorexia, and anemia. Its use is therefore restricted to the treatment of severe or systemic mycoses.

Amphotericin B crosses the placenta (48). In spite of its high toxicity, the drug is surprisingly devoid of embryotoxic and teratogenic potential. A number of reports have described the use of amphotericin B in pregnancy without ill effect in the offspring (16).

No data are available concerning the secretion of amphotericin B into breast milk. Inasmuch as the drug is poorly absorbed orally, untoward effects would be unlikely in the nursing infant.

2. *Flucytosine* (FDA class C)

Flucytosine is a fluorinated pyrimidine whose fungicidal activity is effected by prior conversion within susceptible microorganisms to 5-fluorouracil (5-FU) and subsequent inhibition of nucleic acid synthesis (18). Because of the rapid emergence of resistant strains, flucytosine is used in combination regimens in the treatment of cryptococcosis, disseminated candidiasis, and chromoblastomycosis.

Flucytosine is teratogenic in rats, an effect attributable to its major metabolite, 5-FU. In humans, 4% of an oral dose of flucytosine is transformed by intestinal bacteria into 5-FU (49). Data about the use of flucytosine in pregnancy are scarce, and Briggs could locate only three reports documenting its administration in the second and third trimesters: no ill effects were observed in the newborns (16). The safety of flucytosine during the first trimester of pregnancy is unknown, and there is no information about its pharmacokinetics in lactation.

3. *Griseofulvin* (FDA class C)

Griseofulvin is a metabolic product of some species of *Penicillium*. It is fungistatic against dermatophytes by arresting cellular division in metaphase through disruption of the mitotic spindle (50). This mode of action, shared by *Vinca* alkaloids and colchicine, may contribute to the recognized anti-inflammatory properties of griseofulvin.

Griseofulvin has the advantage of being orally effective, even though its gastrointestinal absorption is slow and incomplete. Serum levels in pregnant patients are lower than in the nonpregnant state, but the drug was shown to cross the placental barrier (51). High doses have caused fetal wastage and polysystemic congenital anomalies in rats and cats (52,53). Furthermore, griseofulvin has also produced hepatocarcinomas and thyroid tumors in rodents (50). The treatment of dermatophyte infections with griseofulvin should be avoided during pregnancy. No data are available concerning breast milk excretion and the safety of griseofulvin during lactation (16).

4. *Imidazoles and Triazoles* (FDA class C)

Ketoconazole is a substituted imidazole, active against dermatophytes, yeasts, and dimorphic fungi. Some activity has been demonstrated against protozoa such as *Leishmania braziliensis*, *Entamoeba histolytica*, *Trypanosoma cruzi*, and *Plasmodium falciparum*. Its fungicidal effect is achieved through inhibition of the synthesis of ergosterol, which is an essential constituent of fungal cell membranes. Ketoconazole is well absorbed after oral administration, as are the triazoles fluconazole and itraconazole. The latter drugs are generally more effective, have a wider spectrum of activity, and are less hepatotoxic than ketoconazole.

The pharmacokinetics of imidazoles in pregnancy are poorly known. Transplacental absorption in animal studies has been shown to represent approximately 0.8% of an administered dose of ketoconazole (54). High doses, however, have been teratogenic and embryotoxic in rats (55). Furthermore, ketoconazole is a known inhibitor of androgen synthesis, and prolonged administration in pregnancy carries the risk of sexual ambiguity in the male fetus. Therefore, it is recommended to avoid all imidazoles in pregnancy unless safer alternatives are unavailable. Little is known to date about the safety of the newer triazoles in pregnancy: itraconazole has produced dose-related teratogenic effects in mice and rats.

All imidazoles are secreted into breast milk. Maternal ketoconazole administration exposes the nursing child to potential hepatotoxicity. Although itraconazole is safer, it is also excreted in milk, and its manufacturer, Janssen Pharmaceutica, advises against its use during lactation.

5. *Allylamines*

Allylamines are a novel class of antifungal agents that block squalene epoxidase, which is an enzyme that mediates an early step in ergosterol synthesis (56). Terbinafine (FDA class B) is the only orally active allylamine. The drug is endowed with excellent activity against dermatophytes, but it is less effective against dematiaceous and dimorphic fungi, molds, and yeasts (57). Terbinafine is a highly lipophilic chemical which is well absorbed, diffuses widely, and concentrates in sebum and stratum corneum (58).

Terbinafine has been found devoid of embryotoxic effects in rats and rabbits. Furthermore, it is not a mutagen in the Ames test (57). Nevertheless, its use in human pregnancy is not recommended, as data about its safety are lacking. The drug is excreted in milk and is therefore contraindicated in breast-feeding pending further information about its innocuousness.

6. *Potassium Iodide* (FDA class D)

Oral administration of a saturated solution of potassium iodide (SSKI, 1 g/ml) is the time-honored treatment for lymphocutaneous sporotrichosis. In addition, the immunosuppressive properties of potassium iodide have been helpful in the management of erythema nodosum and other panniculitides. The successful control of these conditions often requires weeks to months of continuous therapy.

Iodides rapidly cross the placenta. Prolonged administration anytime in pregnancy leads to inhibition of fetal thyroid function and goiter formation. These goiters may be large enough to cause death through tracheal compression (59). Near term, even short courses of iodides may cause transient neonatal hypothyroidism. For these reasons, pregnancy contraindicates the use of potassium iodide.

Potassium iodide is secreted into breast milk, where it is highly concentrated. The high doses of SSKI required in the treatment of dermatological disorders expose the nursing infant to a significant risk of thyroid suppression. Potassium iodide should be avoided during lactation even though the American Academy of Pediatrics considers it compatible with breast-feeding (12).

C. Antiviral Agents

1. *Acyclovir* (FDA class C)

Acyclovir is a guanosine analogue, effective against viruses of the herpes and varicella-zoster groups. Once phosphorylated within infected cells, acyclovir selectively inactivates viral DNA polymerase, whereas sparing normal cellular replication. Because the drug is incorporated into growing DNA chains, concerns have been expressed about its potential mutagenicity. Chromosomal damage and teratogenicity were not observed in animals or humans given doses of acyclovir within the normal range. Chromosome breaks occurred in 3 of 25 animal studies with doses in excess of 400 times peak human plasma levels (60).

The use of acyclovir in pregnancy is not approved by the FDA, and is not recommended by its manufacturer, Burroughs-Wellcome. Nevertheless, scattered reports published during the past 10 years have demonstrated the absence of fetal toxicity following treatment of pregnant women with disseminated herpes simplex virus infections (61–63). In addition, Burroughs-Wellcome has established a registry to monitor the outcome of acyclovir-exposed pregnancies. As of September 1987, 112 pregnancies had been prospectively screened: 83 infants were normal, 2 were born with congenital abnormalities deemed unrelated to acyclovir, 8 pregnancies ended in spontaneous abortions, and 19 were electively terminated (64). The number of reported cases remains too small to allow extrapolations about the safety of acyclovir in pregnancy, particularly during the critical first trimester. Until this issue is settled, the use of acyclovir in pregnancy should be restricted to severe, disseminated infections.

Acyclovir is concentrated into breast milk, but its use is not incompatible with breast-feeding (12).

2. *Miscellaneous Agents*

a. Vidarabine (FDA class C). An analogue of adenosine, vidarabine is used parenterally for the treatment of herpes simplex encephalitis and topically for herpetic keratoconjunctivitis. It inhibits DNA replication by blockade of viral DNA polymerase (18). Vidarabine is teratogenic in animal species after systemic and topical administration (16). Its use in pregnancy should be restricted to life-threatening conditions. The pharmacokinetics of vidarabine during lactation are unknown.

b. Zidovudine (FDA class C). Formerly called azidothymidine (AZT), this antiretroviral dideoxynucleoside is used in the treatment of patients infected with the human immunodeficiency virus (HIV). It prevents viral replication by inhibiting reverse transcriptase. Major side effects of zidovudine are neutropenia and anemia. The drug crosses the placenta and has been shown to afford significant protection to the fetus (65). Animal studies have not demonstrated mutagenic or teratogenic effects (66). Although its safety in pregnancy remains largely unknown, zidovudine therapy should not be withheld if it is clearly indicated.

c. Didanosine. Dideoxyadenosine, or didanosine, shares with zidovudine a similar mechanism of action against retroviral reverse transcriptase. It is a second-line agent in the management of AIDS. It is not myelotoxic but can cause severe pancreatitis and peripheral neuropathy. Animal studies have shown no teratogenic effects in rats and rabbits, but the safety of didanosine in human pregnancy is unknown. It should therefore be used only if clearly indicated. Didanosine excretion in breast milk is unknown and breast-feeding should be discouraged.

d. Zalcitabine. Dideoxycytidine, or zalcitabine, is a pyrimidine analogue whose mode of action and toxicity profile are similar to didanosine. It causes neuropathy more often and pancreatitis less often than its congener. Teratogenic effects have been demonstrated in rats at doses of zalcitabine in excess of 2142 times the maximum human dose. Its safety in human pregnancy and its rate of transfer into breast milk are unknown.

e. Ganciclovir (FDA class C). 9-(1,3-dihydroxy-2-propoxymethyl)guanine, or DHTG, is an analogue of acyclovir which is active against cytomegalovirus (CMV). It is indicated for CMV chorioretinitis and may be useful in gastrointestinal and central nervous system infections. Animal studies have shown ganciclovir to be mutagenic, embryotoxic, and teratogenic. Malformations range from brachygnathism, cleft palate, and microphthalmia to hydrocephalus and aplasia of the kidney and pancreas. Pregnancy is contraindicated during ganciclovir therapy, and its manufacturer, Syntex, recommends that contraception be maintained for 3 months after the last dose. Ganciclovir excretion in breast milk is unknown but its manufacturer states that breast-feeding can be resumed 72 hours after the last dose.

D. Parasiticides

1. Antimalarials

a. Chloroquine and Hydroxychloroquine (FDA class C). Chloroquine and hydroxychloroquine are substituted 4-aminoquinolines which are used in the prophylaxis and treatment of acute attacks of malaria. Dermatologists, however, rely on the anti-inflammatory properties of these drugs in the management of lupus erythematosus, dermatomyositis, photosensitive dermatoses, sarcoidosis, and prophyria cutanea tarda. Their mechanism of action is poorly understood but may involve light filtration, inhibition of prostaglandin synthesis, stabilization of lysosomal membranes, chemotaxis inhibition, and interference with immune complex formation (67). In addition, chloroquine and hydroxychloroquine have been shown to intercalate between base pairs of double-stranded DNA.

Both chloroquine and hydroxychloroquine are water soluble and their gastrointestinal absorption is rapid and complete. They are stored in body tissues in concentrations that exceed plasma levels by as much as 20,000 times (67). Melanized tissues have a strong affinity for aminoquinolines, and clearance of the drugs from these sites may require months to years. Chloroquine and hydroxychloroquine easily cross the placental barrier.

Drugs that interact with DNA are potential teratogens or mutagens, and chloroquine has induced chromosomal abnormalities in patients with rheumatoid arthritis (68). On the other hand, animal studies have failed to demonstrate the suspected teratogenicity of chloroquine and hydroxychloroquine (69). Wolfe and Cordero studied a cohort of 169 women treated with chloroquine base 300 mg once weekly throughout pregnancy for malaria prophylaxis and compared the incidence of congenital malformations with that of a control group of 454 nonexposed women. No statistical difference was found between the two groups, but the small size of the sample could not exclude a risk lower than a 5.7-fold increase in the incidence of birth defects (69). Other studies have emphasized the benefits of malaria prophylaxis with standard doses of chloroquine in pregnant patients (70).

The doses of 4-aminoquinolines used in the treatment of collagen vascular diseases are usually higher than in malaria and can therefore be associated with more serious fetal toxicity. Reports have appeared describing the normal outcome of pregnancies in women treated with daily doses of chloroquine or hydroxychloroquine for lupus erythematosus (71,72). Yet, Paufique and Magnard have found retinal degeneration in two children born to a mother treated with a daily dose of 200–300 mg base chloroquine throughout pregnancy (73). Hart and Naunton, in 1964, reported the outcome of seven pregnancies in a woman intermittently treated with chloroquine for lupus erythematosus: the woman produced normal children when she was off therapy, whereas abnormalities were noted during the four exposed pregnancies. Two children were ataxic and deaf with severe cochleovestibular dysfunction (74). Histopathological studies have demonstrated near complete destruction of the organ of Corti and its supporting cells (75) to be associated with chloroquine.

From these reports, most investigators consider the higher dosage of antimalarials, as used in the treatment of collagenoses, to be contraindicated in pregnancy (67,71). Parke (72), however, takes exception with this approach, and she states:

> Despite the recommendation of others, we advise our patients with systemic lupus erythematosus to continue antimalarial therapy throughout pregnancy. Based on a retrospective study of eight patients with systemic lupus erythematosus who took antimalarial drugs continuously throughout at least one pregnancy, we now believe that the risk for precipitating a flare of the disease outweighs the possible teratogenic effects of chloroquine and hydroxychloroquine.

If such an approach appears reasonable in the face of severe systemic illness, sound medical judgment condemns the use of antimalarials in pregnant patients with cutaneous involvement only.

Chloroquine and hydroxychloroquine are excreted in breast milk in significant amounts (44). Still both drugs are considered compatible with breast-feeding (12).

b. Trimethoprim and Pyrimethamine (FDA class C). Trimethoprim and pyrimethamine are diaminopyrimidines, which are strong but selective inhibitors of dihydrofolate reductase in lower organisms. Whereas trimethoprim possesses antibacterial and antiparasitic activities, pyrimethamine is only effective against *Toxoplasma gondii* and some strains of *Plasmodium*. These drugs can be used singly or, more commonly, in association with sulfonamides or sulfones. In combinations, they act synergistically by sequential blockade of two different steps in folic acid synthesis (18).

Trimethoprim and pyrimethamine are small molecules which freely cross the placenta. Like other antifolates, they have exhibited teratogenicity in some animal species, and concern has been voiced about their use in human pregnancy (76). Prospective studies, however, have found both drugs to be safe during pregnancy as long as folic acid supplementation is concomitantly administered (13).

Some investigators advocate a more cautious approach in the use of these agents in pregnancy and recommend their avoidance in early pregnancy and in the last trimester if they are associated with long-acting sulfonamides (14). Alternatives to trimethoprim-sulfamethoxazole are numerous, and spiramycin is probably safer for the treatment of toxoplasmosis in pregnancy. However, malaria is associated with a high rate of fetal wastage and pyrimethamine-sulfadiazoxine (Fansidar) should not be withheld if it is clearly indicated.

Both compounds are excreted in breast milk but no ill effects have been reported in nursing children. The American Academy of Pediatrics considers trimethoprim and pyrimethamine safe for breast-feeding (12).

2. *Antiprotozoals*

a. Metronidazole (FDA class B). This nitroimidazole derivative is highly toxic against anaerobic bacteria and protozoa, including *Bacteroides fragilis, Clostridium perfringens, Gardnerella vaginalis, Trichomonas vaginalis, Entamoeba histolytica*, and *Giardia lamblia*. Susceptible organisms reduce the nitro group of metronidazole and generate toxic metabolites which bind to DNA and interfere with its synthesis, thus killing the host (77). Apart from cutaneous amebiasis and cases of vaginitis and cellulitis caused by susceptible pathogens, the dermatological applications of systemic metronidazole are restricted. However, the drug is highly effective in acne rosacea, and topical formulations are widely used for this indication.

Because of its low molecular weight, metronidazole is almost completely absorbed after oral intake, and it distributes throughout the organism. Metronidazole freely crosses the placental barrier at any time during pregnancy. The drug has been found to be mutagenic in the Ames test and in mice. Carcinogenicity associated with metronidazole use has also been reported in mice and rats (78). Although this potential for carcinogenicity has not been demonstrated in humans, long-term follow-up is lacking.

Metronidazole is not a teratogen in animal experiments (79). Several studies, including one large series, have concluded that metronidazole is safe for use in human pregnancy (80,81). Other reports have documented a possible association with congenital malformations (16). Because of these conflicting reports, most investigators recommend avoidance of metronidazole in the first trimester of pregnancy (14,15).

Breast milk concentrations are equal to maternal serum levels. Neonatal clearance of metronidazole may be delayed owing to hepatic and renal immaturity. Therefore, nursing mothers should not be given metronidazole unless a single dose is required, in which case breast-feeding should be discontinued for 24 hr (12).

b. Sodium Stibogluconate and Meglumine Antimonate. These two parenterally administered pentavalent antimony compounds represent the first line of treatment for chronic cutaneous, mucocutaneous, and visceral leishmaniasis. Their mechanism of action involves inhibition of glycolytic pathways with resultant decreased production of ATP and GTP. According to Kubba and Al-Gindan, their use is contraindicated in pregnancy (82).

For the pregnant patient, alternative treatment would include amphotericin B and rifampin, which are safe, or pentamidine and nifurtimox, for which safety is not yet clearly established.

c. Pentamidine (FDA class C). This member of the diamidine family exhibits antiprotozoal activity which makes it useful as a second-line agent in the treatment of leishmaniasis. It is also effective in the management of *Pneumocystis carinii* pneumonia either systemically for trimethoprim-sulfamethoxazole failures or via aerosol nebulization for prophylaxis. Its precise mode of action is unknown but probably involves inhibition of kinetoplast DNA replication (18). Serious toxicity may occur after parenteral administration of pentamidine, such as hypertension, renal dysfunction, hypoglycemia, and diabetes. The safety of pentamidine in pregnancy has not been established and the *Medical Letter on Drugs and Therapeutics* cautions that its use be restricted to "strong clinical indication in absence of suitable alternative" (83).

3. Anthelmintics

a. Thiabendazole (FDA class C). Thiabendazole is indicated for the treatment of strongyloidiasis (larva currens), cutaneous larva migrans, and trichinosis. Its mechanism of action is unknown but probably involves inhibition of helminthic microtubules and the enzymes fumarate reductase and malate dehydrogenase (84). Thiabendazole is significantly absorbed after oral administration (85). The drug has shown no teratogenic or embryopathic effects in rodents, pigs, cows, and goats. No toxicity is known from its use in human pregnancy, but the safety of thiabendazole is not clearly established (14,83). Thiabendazole has been measured in cow's milk and could likewise be excreted into human milk.

b. Albendazole. This newer benzimidazole has a much lower incidence of side effects than its parent compound, thiabendazole. It is equally effective in the treatment of cutaneous larva migrans (84). However, albendazole has proved to be teratogenic and embryotoxic in rats and rabbits and is thus contraindicated in pregnancy (86).

c. Ivermectin. This relatively new addition to the antiparasitic armamentarium is derived from avermectin-B, a compound produced by *Streptomyces avermitilis*. It has become the drug of choice for onchocerciasis and has been used to treat strongyloidiasis and cutaneous larva migrans (86). Ivermectin interacts with parasitic gamma-aminobutyric acid (GABA), causing motor neuron paralysis (87). No information is available documenting the safety of ivermectin in pregnancy (85).

d. Diethylcarbamazine. This filaricidal drug is effective against *Onchocerca volvulus*, *Wuchereria bancrofti*, *Brugia malayi*, and *Loa loa*, although its specific mode of action is unknown. Diethylcarbamazine rapidly kills microfilariae, which may cause severe Jarisch-Herxheimer–like reactions in the host. Its manufacturer, Lederle, does not warn against its use in pregnancy, and Ellis mentions that diethylcarbamazine can be used in standard doses for severe ocular onchocerciasis during pregnancy (85).

e. Suramin. Suramin is a polyanion with binding properties, which effectively kills filariae. It is used in the treatment of onchocerciasis after a course of diethylcarbamazine. The administration of suramin may be associated with a wide range of toxic reactions, such as vomiting, loss of consciousness, seizures, acute renal failure, and optic atrophy. Suramin is teratogenic in mice and should be used with caution in pregnancy (83).

f. Praziquantel (FDA class B). This pyrazinoisoquinoline is effective against all three species of *Schistosoma* which are infective to humans. It increases membrane permeability to calcium ions and tetanizes the parasite's musculature. Praziquantal has not been shown to cause teratogenicity, embryotoxicity, or mutagenesis, and it is probably safe in pregnancy (14,85).

g. Nifurtimox. The specific target of this nitrofuran compound is *Trypanosoma cruzi*, the agent of Chagas disease. The trypanosomal activity of this drug results from the formation of toxic oxygen radicals (87). The safety of nifurtimox in pregnancy is not established, although Rollo states that there are no absolute contraindications to its use (18).

E. Antineoplastics and Immunosuppressants

1. Alkylating Agents

a. Cyclophosphamide (FDA class D). Cyclophosphamide, a synthetic derivative of mechlorethamine, is an alkylating agent with strong cytostatic and immunosuppressant properties, particularly on B cells (88). Used alone or with systemic corticosteroids, it can induce remissions in Wegener granulomatosis, intractable cases of systemic lupus erythematosus, pemphigus vulgaris, cicatricial pemphigoid, or pyoderma gangrenosum.

The embryotoxicity of cyclophosphamide has been demonstrated in experimental animal studies (89). Alkylating agents can theoretically produce severe toxicity when administered during pregnancy, when fetal cellular turnover is rapid. In practice, however, embryopathic effects are difficult to assess from the few published case reports. Some pregancies have had a normal outcome despite maternal ingestion of cyclophosphamide, but others have resulted in congenital anomalies that have included hypoplastic or absent digits, cleft palate, single coronary artery, and anal imperforation (16,90–92). In addition to cyclophosphamide, most of these patients had also been exposed to radiation therapy or to other antineoplastic agents.

The risk of congenital defects from cyclophosphamide administration after the first trimester of pregnancy appears negligible (93). However, children exposed to the drug can present with growth retardation and bone marrow suppression.

Cyclophosphamide diffuses into breast milk and has caused reversible neutropenia in the offspring of a nursing mother (94). The American Academy of Pediatrics considers the use of cyclophosphamide contraindicated during breast-feeding (12).

b. Dacarbazine (FDA class C). Dacarbazine is a triazene derivative that was initially thought to be an antimetabolite but is now known to operate through alkylation (18). Its major indication is the palliative treatment of metastatic melanoma. Dacarbazine is teratogenic in experimental animals. No data are available concerning its safety during human pregnancy and lactation.

c. Chlorambucil (FDA class D). Similar to cyclophosphamide, chlorambucil is a nitrogen mustard–derived alkylating agent and therefore is dependent on the presence of a bis-(2-chloroethyl) grouping for cytotoxic activity (18). It has a low toxicity profile and is used mostly in the management of chronic lymphocytic leukemia. Dermatological conditions that have been treated with chlorambucil include mycosis fungoides and the Sézary syndrome, systemic lupus erythematosus and scleroderma, Wegener granulomatosis, sarcoidosis, pyoderma gangrenosum, and generalized granuloma annulare.

Chlorambucil is teratogenic, mutagenic, and carcinogenic. It should not be used in pregnancy unless it is deemed essential, and such treatment should ideally be deferred until the third trimester. Chlorambucil is contraindicated during breast-feeding (44).

d. Melphalan (FDA class D). Melphalan, or L-phenylalanine nitrogen mustard, is mainly used in the treatment of multiple myeloma. Other plasma cell dyscrasias such as scleromyxedema and the Crow-Fukase syndrome, which consists of plasma cell dyscrasia, polyneuropathy, organomegaly, endrocrinopathy, M-protein, and skin changes (POEMS), may improve after chlorambucil administration of melphalan. The drug is teratogenic, mutagenic, and carcinogenic and must be avoided in pregnancy and lactation.

2. *Antimetabolites*

a. Methotrexate (FDA class D). Methotrexate is a methylated derivative of aminopterin which exerts strong cytostatic and immunosuppressant activities by blocking the conversion of folic acid to tetrahydrofolic acid (95). Methotrexate is one of the most effective treatments for recalcitrant psoriasis, and it is used as well in the management of various inflammatory dermatoses.

Like its congener aminopterin, methotrexate exhibits potent embryotoxic and teratogenic properties (96,97). At least one-third of surviving infants will present with one or many of the congenital abnormalities listed in Table 1.

It appears therefore that methotrexate should not be administered during the first trimester of pregnancy. Its use during the second and third trimesters may cause growth retardation and bone marrow suppression.

Methotrexate crosses into breast milk in small amounts (98). However, its long tissue persistence could lead to accumulation in the neonate, and its use in breast-feeding is contraindicated (12).

b. Azathioprine (FDA class D). Azathioprine is a purine analogue antimetabolite derived from 6-mercaptopurine by the addition of an imidazole ring (99). Its immunosuppressive activity is greater than its cytostatic properties, and for years, azathioprine has been the drug of choice to prevent rejection in organ transplant recipients. In dermatology, it is successfully used as a steroid-sparing agent in a variety of autoimmune or inflammatory conditions such as pemphigus vulgaris, bullous pemphigoid, dermatomyositis, lupus erythematosus, or chronic actinic dermatosis.

Table 1 Methotrexate and Aminopterin Teratogenesis

Skull	Face	Skeleton
Oxycephaly	Wide nasal bridge	Absent digits
Absent coronal sutures	Malformed ears	Talipes equinovarus
Absent frontal bone	Low-set ears	Abnormal ribs
Absent parietal bone	Hypertelorism	Hip dislocation
Large fontanels	Micrognathia	
Hydrocephalus	Cleft palate or lip	
Anencephalus		

Azathioprine and its metabolites readily cross the placenta (100). Animal studies have shown azathioprine to be teratogenic at high doses in rabbits and mice but not in rats (101,102). In addition, decreased thymic size and suppressed hematopoiesis have been noted with azathioprine administration in late pregnancy.

In human gestation, azathioprine has been reasonably safe (103,104). Although reversible chromosomal breaks have been reported, major teratogenicity has not been encountered in association with the use of azathioprine (105). Congenital defects, reported in three children only, were pulmonary stenosis, atrial septal defects, and preaxial polydactyly (16,106). The possibility that these associations were coincidental with azathioprine use cannot be excluded.

Lymphoid tissue hypoplasia and transient depression of hematopoiesis in the newborn have been observed by some investigators to be associated with the use of azathioprine (107–109). Davison and colleagues have demonstrated that neonatal thrombocytopenia and leukopenia correlate with maternal leucocyte count at 32 weeks of gestation: halving the dosage of azathioprine when the maternal leukocyte count falls below 8.6×10^9/L affords complete protection to the newborn (109).

Despite the apparent relative short-term safety of azathioprine in pregnancy, concerns still exist about the long-term consequences of its use on the offspring of those taking the drug. 6-Mercaptopurine, the major metabolite of azathioprine, decreases the fertility of female mice exposed in utero (110). Whether fertility problems will plague the offspring of women treated in pregnancy still remains unknown. Furthermore, long-term administration of azathioprine predisposes to the emergence of secondary neoplasias, most commonly non-Hodgkin's lymphoma: children exposed to azathioprine in pregnancy could theoretically face the same risk of iatrogenic carcinogenicity and should be followed for an extended period of time.

In summary, a pregnancy which occurs during azathioprine treatment does not have to be terminated, as it will likely result in a normal child. However, it appears reasonable for women so treated to avoid pregnancy through reliable contraception. Insufficient data are available concerning the safety of azathioprine during lactation. One investigator concludes that levels found in breast milk are too small to be harmful, whereas another discourages breast-feeding (44,110).

3. *Natural Products*

a. Vinca alkaloids (FDA class D). Vincristine and vinblastine are complex dimeric alkaloids extracted from the periwinkle (*Vinca rosea*). They exert their strong cytostatic activity by disruption of the mitotic spindle, thereby arresting cellular division in metaphase. As do podophyllotoxin and colchicine, vincristine and vinblastin bind to tubulin but at a different site on the protein. Although chemically very similar, these drugs differ in their toxicity, with vincristine causing neurotoxicity and vinblastine leukopenia. Both agents are used in combination regimens for the treatment of lymphomas, leukemias, and a variety of solid tumors. In dermatology, their main indications are the classic form of Kaposi sarcoma, histiocytosis X, and mycosis fungoides.

In animal studies, vinca alkaloids administered during pregnancy have produced a high rate of fetal resorption and malformations in surviving offspring (95). Although vincristine and vinblastine have been used in pregnancy, often without evidence of fetal adverse effects, both agents should be considered teratogenic, and their use should be avoided or restricted to life-threatening conditions (16). No information is available concerning their safety during lactation.

b. Bleomycin (FDA class D). Bleomycin is a complex glycopeptide antibiotic extracted from *Streptomyces verticillus* (111). It generates superoxide radicals which cause scission and fragmentation of the DNA chain (18). Tissues poor in bleomycin hydrolase, such as the lung and the skin, are particularly sensitive to the cytotoxic effects of bleomycin.

The drug is useful by parenteral administration in the treatment of squamous cell carcinoma of the head and neck, skin, and lung, as well as in testicular tumors and mycosis fungoides. Intralesional injections are effective in the treatment of resistant warts.

Bleomycin can induce chromosomal aberrations. Although bleomycin therapy has not been linked with the production of congenital malformations, its safety during pregnancy is unknown and it should be avoided unless it is deemed absolutely necessary. Data about its transfer into breast milk are lacking, but the risk of harmful effects in the neonate appears low owing to its poor absorption from the gastrointestinal tract.

4. *Miscellaneous Drugs*

a. Hydroxyurea (FDA class D). Hydroxyurea is a cytostatic agent which selectively prevents DNA synthesis by inhibition of the ribonucleotide reductase enzyme system (112). In 1970, Leavell and Yarbro successfully used hydroxyurea in the treatment of severe plaque-type psoriasis (113). Although less effective than methotrexate or cyclosporine, it can be used when alternative therapies fail or are contraindicated.

Animal studies have demonstrated the strong teratogenic potential of hydroxyurea (114). A case report later described central axis deformities and spina bifida in a child exposed to hydroxyurea in utero (115). Pregnancy and lactation constitute absolute contraindications to the use of hydroxyurea (112).

b. Cyclosporine (FDA class C). Cyclosporine is a cyclic, 11 amino acid peptide isolated from soil fungi. The drug is endowed with strong immunosuppressive properties directed against T cells, macrophages, and antigen-presenting cells. Target cells are not destroyed, but the release of several cytokines is prevented (116). Since 1978, it has become the drug of choice for the prevention of rejection in organ transplant recipients. Cyclosporine has also found a special place in the treatment of selected dermatoses such as refractory psoriasis, pyoderma gangrenosum, epidermolysis bullosa acquisita, and lichen planus, mostly as a steroid-sparing agent with less toxicity than azathioprine or cyclophosphamide (117).

Cyclosporine is not mutagenic in the Ames test. In animal studies, chromosomal damage, carcinogenicity after long-term exposure, and teratogenic effects were not observed (118). In humans, a number of reports have documented successful pregnancies in women, mostly renal transplant recipients, treated with cyclosporine (119–121). As of 1989, information was available on 51 exposed pregnancies: The number of preterm deliveries was higher in these patients than in corresponding normal pregnancies, and fetal growth retardation was also more common. These characteristics were attributed to the health status of the mothers and not to their treatment regimens. This survey clearly showed that cyclosporine does not induce birth defects (122).

Cyclosporine crosses the placenta and levels paralleling maternal concentrations have been measured in cord blood (123). The drug is eliminated from the baby's circulation in about 1 week. No nephrotoxicity or persistent immunosuppression have been noted in exposed infants, but studies are lacking about long-term potential complications such as carcinogenicity. Thus, although cyclosporine appears relatively safe during pregnancy, common sense dictates that a woman treated with this drug for a skin condition should use effective contraception (124). A highly lipophilic substance, cyclosporine also readily diffuses into breast milk. Breast-feeding is therefore contraindicated in cyclosporine-treated women (12).

F. Anti-inflammatory and Immunomodulating Agents

1. *Acetylsalicylic Acid* (FDA classes C [first and second trimesters] and D [third trimester])

Aspirin has been synthesized in 1853 as an analgesic and antipyretic drug. Its mechanism of action involves inhibition of cyclooxygenase, an enzyme which mediates the transformation of arachidonic acid into prostaglandins, prostacyclins, and thromboxanes. Salicylates are highly lipophilic and rapidly cross the placenta. Levels attained in the neonate are higher than in the mother because of reduced liver conjugation and renal excretion (125).

Because of its wide availability, aspirin is the most commonly ingested drug in pregnancy (16). In dermatology, it is used topically for its keratolytic properties, in the treatment of acne, ichthyosis, psoriasis, and other keratodermas. Salicylates are readily absorbed from the skin, and it has been shown that repeated application of relatively small amounts may result in systemic toxicity (126).

High doses of aspirin are teratogenic in rodents, and scattered reports have described the association of various congenital abnormalities with maternal salicylate ingestion. However, a large prospective study assessed the outcome of 50,282 pregnancies and found no difference in the rate of fetal malformations between the 35,418 women who did not take aspirin during the first half of pregnancy and the 14,864 who were exposed to the drug (127). Thus, aspirin in the normal therapeutic range does not appear to be teratogenic in humans.

Maternal and fetal morbidity may be encountered, however, if aspirin ingestion occurs near term. The reported disturbances are probably related to impaired prostaglandin synthesis. Prostaglandins play a key role in the induction of labor and uterine contractility, and maternal aspirin intake has led to prolonged gestation and labor (128). Furthermore, interference with platelet adhesiveness may result in excessive hemorrhage at delivery or bleeding complications in the child, such as cephalhematoma, petechiae, hematuria, or intracranial hemorrhage. Finally, it has been shown that the administration of aspirin or other nonsteroidal anti-inflammatory agents such as indomethacin or naproxen to pregnant animals triggers premature closure of the ductus arteriosus. In human neonates, preterm aspirin exposure could be responsible for difficulties in establishing a normal pulmonary circulation and persistent pulmonary hypertension (125).

Salicylates are excreted into breast milk in small amounts. The risk of metabolic acidosis or bleeding complications from absorption during breast-feeding appears small but cannot be disregarded, as newborns are much more sensitive to salicylate intoxication than adults. The American Academy of Pediatrics urges caution in the use of salicylates during lactation (12).

2. *Acetaminophen* (FDA class B)

Acetaminophen is a widely used analgesic and antipyretic with an excellent safety profile. It causes less gastric intolerance than acetylsalicylic acid, and it can be safely taken by patients who are allergic to aspirin. Overdose has been associated with hepatotoxicity, and the fetus is exposed to this theoretical risk, as the drug crosses the placenta. Two cases of maternal acetaminophen intoxication unassociated with fetal liver damage have been reported (16).

Acetaminophen is not teratogenic, and unlike aspirin, it does not impair platelet function. Its use near term does not increase the risk of maternal or neonatal hemorrhage (125). Low levels of acetaminophen are found in breast milk but should not constitute a threat to the suckling infant.

3. *Nonsteroidal Anti-Inflammatory Drugs (NSAIDS)* (FDA class B [first and second trimesters] and D [third trimester])

Synthetic anti-inflammatory drugs such as, for example, ibuprofen, indomethacin, and naproxen, are nonteratogenic and appear to be safe until at least the last month of pregnancy. When used after the thirty-fifth week of gestation, their marked antiprostaglandin activity can lead to delayed or prolonged labor and to premature closure of the ductus arteriosus with persistent pulmonary hypertension in the newborn. The use of NSAIDS does not contraindicate breast-feeding.

4. *Colchicine* (FDA class C)

Colchicine is an alkaloid extracted from the plant *Colchicum autumnale*, which is of considerable value in the prophylaxis and treatment of gouty arthritis. Colchicine-responsive dermatoses, such as Behçet's disease, leukocytoclastic vasculitis, and dermatitis herpetiformis, are characterized by large accumulations of polymorphonuclear leukocytes. The usefulness of colchicine remains to be demonstrated in other neutrophilic disorders like the Sweet syndrome, subcorneal pustular dermatosis, erythema elevatum diutinum, and pustular psoriasis (129). Colchicine is an antimitotic agent which produces metaphase arrest through interference with microtubular proteins and failure of spindle formation (18). It crosses the placenta and, in high doses, is an abortifacient (130).

Teratogenesis has been reported from animal studies, and chromosomal damage has been observed in human lymphocyte cultures (16). In 1968, Ferreira and Buoniconti described a case of trisomy after maternal colchicine ingestion, but later studies by Cohen and collaborators have not found an increased risk of birth defects (131,132).

The safety of colchicine therapy in pregnancy, especially during the first trimester, therefore remains unestablished and the drug should be avoided. No data are available regarding its pharmacokinetics and innocuousness during breast-feeding.

5. *Gold Salts* (FDA class C)

Gold salts have been used in the treatment of rheumatoid arthritis since the pioneering works of Forestier in 1929. Their dermatological indications are restricted to psoriatic arthritis and pemphigus. Parenteral preparations include aurothioglucose and gold sodium thiomalate, both containing 50% gold by weight, and an oral compound, auranofin, which contains 29% gold (133). The mechanism of action of gold salts is complex and, so far, poorly understood. The anti-inflammatory properties of gold seem related to interference with lysosomal enzyme release, inhibition of prostaglandin synthesis, blockade of the complement cascade, chemotaxis inhibition, suppression of antibody production, and depression of cellular immunity (133).

Parenteral compounds are well absorbed and build up in tissues such as the synovium or the reticuloendothelial system from which they are slowly cleared over a period of months following cessation of therapy (18). Tissue accumulation of auranofin is less marked but blood levels persist longer. Both formulations readily penetrate the placenta and gold deposits have been shown in fetal tissues (134).

Gold sodium thiomalate and auranofin are embryotoxic and teratogenic in rats and rabbits when administered in high doses. Experience with gold salts during human pregnancy is anecdotal and based on a handful of small series (135). Most of these studies have reported a normal outcome from exposed pregnancies. Miyamoto and colleagues have examined the infants of 119 women treated with gold during pregnancy and have noted two cases of hip abnormalities, which may have been coincidental (16). The available evidence suggests the safety of chrysotherapy during pregnancy, but large prospective studies are lacking and the drugs should be reserved for the management of severe cases. In pemphigus, the safety of gold salts as steroid-sparing agents appears greater than that of other immunosuppressants.

Gold salts are excreted in breast milk and may expose the nursing infant to the risk of leukopenia, thrombocytopenia, nephrotoxicity, and drug eruptions. In spite of these theoretical risks, the American Academy of Pediatrics considers gold salts compatible with breast-feeding (12).

6. *D-Penicillamine* (FDA class D)

D-penicillamine is a sulfhydryl amino acid prepared by the hydrolytic degradation of penicillin. It is an effective chelator of heavy metals and is used in the therapy of mercury poisoning and Wilson disease. D-penicillamine inhibits enzymes which require pyridoxine and copper as cofactors (18). One such enzyme is lysyl oxidase, which is necessary for adequate cross linking of elastin and collagen. Therefore, D-penicillamine has been used to treat systemic scleroderma, a disease characterized by excessive collagen deposition.

A relatively small number of patients, mostly with Wilson disease or cystinuria, have been treated in pregnancy with D-penicillamine. Although most infants were normal at birth, at least eight displayed congenital anomalies (16,136,137). Six of these neonates exhibited signs of acquired faulty collagen or elastin synthesis, such as cutis laxa, poor wound healing, varicosities, hernias, or soft-tissue contractures (16). In one case, the anomalies were transient (138). In three other children, they were severe enough to cause death (139–141). On the basis of these data, the use of D-penicillamine to treat skin conditions in pregnancy does not appear justified. No data are available regarding use of D-penicillamine during lactation.

7. *Thalidomide* (FDA class X)

Thalidomide was first developed in 1956 by Grünenthal Laboratories in West Germany. In animal studies, it was found to be an excellent sedative with minimal toxicity. In 1958, clinical trials demonstrated that thalidomide appeared to be a perfect hypnotic and antiemetic, with a rapid onset of action, induction of a natural sleep pattern, and no residual drowsiness (142). Thereafter, the drug was mass marketed, used in adult and pediatric populations, and it was even sold as an over-the-counter drug. It was later distributed to the United Kingdom, countries of the British Commonwealth, in most European countries, as well as in Brazil and Japan.

Starting in 1959, cases of phocomelia, a previously rare congenital malformation, began to be seen with an increasing frequency that reached epidemic proportions over a short period of 2 years. The saga of epidemiological investigations that led to blame thalidomide as the cause of the syndrome has been well summarized by Taussig (142). In November of 1961, the drug was withdrawn, and exactly 9 months later, the epidemic died out, leaving in its wake thousands of crippled children who still have to cope with major handicaps to this day (143).

Retrospective and prospective studies have demonstrated the strong teratogenic potential of thalidomide. The constellation of manifestations has been varied, as shown in Table 2, but the most characteristic changes involve the limbs: The long bones are defective and the extremities, which resemble the flippers of a seal, arise directly from the shortened limb (142). The abnormalities are bilateral but asymmetrical and involve the upper limbs only in 65% of the cases, both upper and lower extremities in 10–25%, and the lower limbs only in 2–5% (144). There is no correlation between the severity of the manifestations and the total amount of ingested thalidomide: malformations have been seen after a single dose, whereas normal children were born of women who took thalidomide for many weeks. Instead, the concept of a critical window soon became apparent when it was shown that up to 50% of children exposed during gestation weeks 4–8 bore anomalies (142).

After the initial shock of the phocomelia epidemic, researchers tried again to reproduce in animals the pattern of malformations seen in humans. Early experiments failed, but some investigators eventually obtained positive results with high oral doses (150 mg/kg) in rabbits and intraperitoneal injections (500 mg) in rats (144).

In the aftermath of the tragedy, thalidomide seemed consigned to oblivion until its remarkable immunomodulatory activities were discovered. Nowadays, the drug is used extensively in the treatment of lepra reactions and has been found effective in the management of actinic prurigo, chronic lupus erythematosus, prurigo nodularis, Behçet's disease, and graft-versus-host reactions (145). Thalidomide, or α-(N-phtalimido)glutarimide, is a molecule composed of a phtalimide double ring linked to a piperidine structure. The piperidine ring is responsible for the sedative properties of the drug and is closely related to glutethimide, a nonteratogenic hypnotic. Substitutions on the phtalimide nucleus abolish the teratogenic effects of thalidomide while maintaining its sedative activity. Unfortunately, it seems that the immunomodulatory properties of the drug are mediated by an intact phtalimide structure and cannot be dissociated from teratogenicity (145).

Table 2 Thalidomide Teratogenicity

System or organ	Malformation
Musculoskeletal	Amelia
	Phocomelia
	Absent or hypoplastic ulna, radius, humerus
	Absent or hypoplastic tibia, fibula, femur
	Hip dislocation
	Loss of prehensile grasp of the hand
	Polydactyly or syndactyly of the toes
Cranium	Anencephaly, microcephaly
	Hydrocephalus, meningomyelocele
	Anophthalmia, microphtalmia
	Low-set ears, deformed pinnae, atretic ear canal
	Saddle nose, cleft palate, choanal atresia
	Midfacial nevus flammeus
Cardiovascular	Aortic hypoplasia, pulmonary stenosis
	Tetralogy of Fallot, transposition of great vessels
	Atrial and ventricular septal defects
Respiratory	Bilobed right lung
Gastrointestinal	Pyloric stenosis, duodenal atresia
	Malrotation of the gut
	Imperforate anus
Genital tract	Bicornuate uterus, vaginal atresia
	Rectovaginal fistulas
Urinary tract	Agenesis or hypoplasia of kidneys and ureters
	Horseshoe kidney

Thalidomide can safely be administered to women of childbearing potential provided that guidelines, similar to those that govern the use of synthetic retinoids, are strictly adhered to: (a) pregnancy should be excluded by a negative pregnancy test, (b) therapy is started on the last day of a normal menstrual period, and (c) the patient should use an effective contraceptive method throughout the treatment period.

The pharmacokinetics of thalidomide during lactation are unknown, but the drug has been used as a sedative in the postpartum period and administered to nursing mothers without adverse effects in their neonates (144).

G. Hormones and Antagonists

1. *Glucocorticosteroids* (FDA classes B [prednisone], C [betamethasone], C [dexamethasone], and D [hydrocortisone])

Systemic glucocorticosteroids are often administered as replacement or suppressive therapy or, in higher doses, for the treatment of various inflammatory disorders. The agents most commonly used are cortisone acetate, prednisolone or its inactive precursor prednisone, and dexamethasone. All glucocorticosteroids will enter fetal circulation to some extent, but their rate of inactivation by the placenta is variable. Prednisolone is inactivated to prednisone, so that its fetal concentration reaches only 10% of maternal blood levels. On the other hand, betamethasone and dexamethasone are freely transferred to the fetus without inactivation (9).

In mice and rabbits, cortisone administration during pregnancy leads to a high rate of abortion and cleft palate in the surviving litter (146). Impaired central nervous system maturation, decreased thymic size with long-lasting immunosuppression, and low birth weight have been highlighted by other animal studies using cortisone (147).

Few reports have documented adverse effects from glucocorticosteroids in human pregnancy. In 1968, Warrell and Taylor described the outcome of 34 prednisolone-exposed pregnancies as compared with the same number of pregnancies in women with similar medical conditions who did not receive corticosteroids. They reported an excess of stillbirths in the treated group, which they attributed to placental dysfunction (148). Reinisch and colleagues, in 1978, showed that mothers who received 10 mg of prednisone per day throughout pregnancy had a significant decrease in the birth weight of full-term infants by comparison with a control group (149). One report has linked congenital cataracts with prenatal cortisone administration (150). Cleft palate as a complication of intrauterine corticosteroid exposure was the subject of at least two publications (151). Finally, transient adrenal suppression has rarely been reported (148,152).

The results of numerous other well-conducted studies, often with a larger sample size, contradict the above-mentioned findings (16). Investigations by Bongiovanni and McPadden (260 cases), Yackel and colleagues (21 cases), Schatz and coworkers (70 cases) and Heinonen and collaborators (299 cases) have all failed to show a significant increase in maternal morbidity and fetal wastage, growth retardation, or congenital malformations (13,153–155). In their reviews, Gallant (152), Briggs (16), and Jurecka (9) agree that prednisone and prednisolone constitute a very small risk to the developing fetus.

Milk excretion of prednisolone amounts to 5–25% of maternal serum levels (16). It has been estimated that the amount ingested by a nursing infant would remain below physiological levels. Therefore, the American Academy of Pediatrics considers prednisone and prednisolone compatible with breast-feeding (12).

2. *Estrogens and Progestins*

Although rarely used by dermatologists, synthetic sex hormones hold a place in the treatment of hyperandrogenic states such as acne vulgaris and hirsutism. These agents will suppress ovarian, but not adrenal, androgen production. Inhibition of adrenal androgens requires suppressive therapy with glucocorticosteroids. Hydroxyprogesterone may be used alone in women over the age of 35, but more commonly estrogens and progestins are combined. Although the combination of estrogens and progestins usually functions as an efficient contraceptive, it is not entirely fail-safe, and it may be prescribed before pregnancy is suspected.

a. Estrogens (FDA class X). Between 1940 and 1971, it was current practice to administer diethylstilbestrol (DES) to women who experienced bleeding during pregnancy. Not only was such therapy later proven to be ineffective, it was also shown to expose the offspring to serious consequences, the most ominous being glycogen-rich, clear-cell adenocarcinoma of the vagina with a peak onset between 15 and 22 years of age (156). In animal studies, Forsberg later demonstrated that the normal fetal transformation of pseudostratified epithelium of Müllerian duct origin into squamous epithelium is prevented by maternal administration of DES and estradiol-17-β (157). At puberty, these persistent Müllerian remnants are stimulated by endogenous ovarian hormones to produce vaginal adenosis and adenocarcinoma. In addition, other reproductive tract malformations can occur, such as septate vagina, altered fornix, and uterine and Fallopian tube defects (16). In the male offspring, reported anomalies have included epididymal cysts, hypotrophic testis, microphallus, and altered semen (16). In view of these potentially catastrophic complications, all estrogenic preparations should be avoided in pregnancy, especially during the critical first trimester (158). Estrogens are compatible with breast-feeding but may decrease milk production and cause gynecomastia in the child (12).

b. Progestins (FDA class X). In 1974, studies by Nora and Nora and by Janerich and colleagues provided evidence that the administration of oral contraceptives could induce a constellation of fetal malformations. These anomalies, preferentially expressed in the male offspring, became known by the acronym VACTERL (vertebral, anal, cardiac, tracheal, esophageal, renal, and limb malformations) (159,160). Later studies, however, have produced conflicting results, some claiming, and others denying, a teratogenic potential for progestins. In 1985, Katz and coworkers published the results of a large prospective study that assessed 1608 newborns whose mothers received medroxyprogesterone as compared with a control group of 1146 unexposed children (161). Eighty-six percent of these women were treated before 14 weeks of gestation, and the mean duration of treatment was 48 days. There was no statistical difference between the two groups with respect to the incidence of malformations. Also in 1985, Resseguie and colleagues came to the same conclusions after assessing the outcome of 988 pregnancies exposed to various progestins, mainly progesterone and 17-hydroxyprogesterone, compared with a cohort of 1976 unexposed controls (162). The risk to the fetus from these progestational agents therefore appears small.

The 19-norprogestational agents (norethindrone, norethynodrel, ethynodiol diacetate, and norgestrel) possess androgenic activity. Administration of these agents in early pregnancy can cause masculinization of the urogenital tract of female fetuses and pseudohermaphroditism (158). These substances are thus contraindicated in pregnancy.

Progestins may suppress lactation but have not been associated with adverse effect in the nursing child and are compatible with breast-feeding (12).

3. *Antiandrogens*

a. Spironolactone (FDA class D). Spironolactone is a synthetic steroid with a cyclopentanophenantrene structure that inhibits aldosterone by competitive binding to cytosolic receptors. It also exhibits moderate antiandrogenic activity through a central and a peripheral mode of action: selective destruction of cytochrome P-450 in the testes and adrenal glands reduces steroidogenesis, whereas competitive blockade of dihydrotestosterone receptors occurs at the target organ level (163). These antiandrogenic properties have been put to use in the treatment of hyperandrogenic states in women; namely, hirsutism, acne, and androgenic alopecia.

Spironolactone and its metabolites cross the placenta. In pregnant rats, administration of high doses has produced distinct feminization of external genitalia in male fetuses (164). Although no report of human malformations have been published, the use of spironolactone in pregnancy is contraindicated.

Canrenone, the major metabolite of spironolactone, has been measured in breast milk (151). Such levels are not known to be harmful to the nursing child, and the American Academy of Pediatrics considers spironolactone compatible with breast-feeding (12,44). However, none of the current dermatological indications appears so critical as to justify the use of spironolactone during lactation.

b. Cyproterone Acetate. Cyproterone acetate is a progestin with strong antiandrogenic activity. It competitively blocks androgen receptors, decreases adrenal steroidogenesis, and exerts a negative feedback on luteinizing hormone secretion. In rabbits, dogs, and rats, the feminizing potential of cyproterone acetate on male fetuses is about 10 times that of spironolactone (164). High doses have caused hepatomas in rats. It is therefore contraindicated in pregnancy.

c. Flutamide (FDA class D). This "pure antiandrogen" is a nonsteroidal compound devoid of intrinsic glucocorticoid, progestational, androgenic, or estrogenic activity. It blocks androgen action at the receptor level. It is mainly used in the treatment of prostatic cancer, but in 1990, Cusan and colleagues found it effective in the management of hirsutism (165). As with cyproterone acetate and spironolactone, the use of flutamide is contraindicated in pregnancy.

4. *Anabolic Steroids*

a. Danazol (FDA class C) *and Stanozolol* (FDA class X). These synthetic derivatives of testosterone possess strong anabolic and weak androgenic activities. The dermatological indications of both agents are restricted to the prophylactic treatment of hereditary angioedema. Androgens have been shown to induce hepatic synthesis of C_1-esterase inhibitor (C_1-INH), which is the glycoprotein responsible for inactivation of the complement cascade. Stanozolol and danazol are effective in the management of hereditary angioedema type I (quantitative C_1-INH deficiency) and type II (dysfunctional C_1-INH) (166). In addition, both drugs have met with some success in the treatment of leg ulcers associated with cryoglobulinemia.

In animal studies, exposure to both danazol and stanozolol during pregnancy has caused masculinization of the female fetus. In human pregnancy, the experience with danazol is greater, since the compound is commonly used in the treatment of endometriosis and fibrocystic disease of the breast. Reports of virilization of female fetuses have appeared in the literature; in some instances associated with transient adrenal insufficiency and features of salt-losing adrenal hyperplasia (167,168). In addition, the tendency to cholestasis, common in the pregnant state, would likely increase the known hepatotoxic potential of danazol and stanozolol. Prophylactic treatment of hereditary angioedema with attenuated androgens should be stopped as soon as pregnancy is suspected and the acute attacks treated with fresh frozen plasma or, where available, with C_1-INH concentrate. Treatment can be resumed postpartum if breast-feeding is avoided.

H. Antihistamines

1. *First-Generation H_1 Blockers*

Antihistamines are the systemic agents most often prescribed by dermatologists. They are very helpful in the control of immediate hypersensitivity reactions such as urticaria, in which histamine release plays a major causal role. All first-generation antihistamines exhibit a variable degree of sedative activity, which may account for their antipruritic properties in conditions such as eczema, in which histamine is not the main mediator. On the basis of variations on their chemical structure, these traditional antihistamines are grouped in six different classes (Table 3).

a. Alkylamines

Brompheniramine (FDA class C): The Collaborative Perinatal Project reported 65 mothers who were exposed to brompheniramine during the first trimester of pregnancy. Ten infants presented with malformations, which is a statistically significant association despite the small sample size. The relative risk of malformation after first-trimester exposure was 2.34, which is much higher than the 0.81

Table 3 First-Generation H_1-Antihistamines

Class	Generic name	Trade name
Alkylamines	Brompheniramine	Dimetane
	Chlorpheniramine	Chlortrimeton
		Chlortripolon
		Histaspan
		Teldrin
	Dexbrompheniramine	Drixoral
	Dexchlorpheniramine	Polaramine
	Pheniramine	Trimeton
	Triprolidine	Actidil
Ethanolamines	Dimenhydrinate	Dramamine
		Gravol
	Diphenhydramine	Benadryl
		Benylin
	Clemastine	Tavist
Ethylenediamines	Pyrilamine	Anthisan
		Neo-Antergan
	Tripelennamine	Pyribenzamine
Piperazines	Chlorcyclizine	Di-Paralene
		Mantadil
	Cyclizine	Marezine
	Hydroxyzine	Atarax
		Vistaril
	Meclizine	Bonamine
Piperidines	Azatadine	Optimine
	Cyproheptadine	Periactin
		Vimicon
Phenothiazines	Dimethothiazine	Promaquid
	Promethazine	Phenergan
	Trimeprazine	Panectyl
		Temaril

to 1.25 range found with other antihistamines (13). Brompheniramine should therefore be avoided in pregnancy at least during the first trimester.

One report has described irritability and sleep disturbances in a nursing infant whose mother used a combination of brompheniramine and pseudoephedrine (16). As both of the drugs are excreted in breast milk, a causal relationship with brompheniramine remains unproven. Its manufacturer, A. H. Robbins Company, considers the drug contraindicated during lactation.

Chlorpheniramine (FDA class B): Heinonen and colleagues have monitored 3931 exposures to chlorpheniramine anytime during pregnancy. Although they reported scattered individual malformations, no relationship was found to large categories of major or minor defects (13). Greenberger, as well as I, believe that chlorpheniramine is safe during pregnancy (169). Unfortunately, no data exist concerning its passage into breast milk. As with all other antihistamines, there is a hypothetical risk of sedation or paradoxical excitation in the nursing child. According to the manufacturer, Schering, chlorpheniramine should be used with caution in the lactating mother.

Pheniramine (FDA class C): When pheniramine was used in the first trimester of pregnancy (831 exposures), a possible association was found with eye or ear and respiratory malformations (13). Greenberger thinks that the judicious use of this antihistamine is safe in pregnancy (169). No data are available concerning the fate of the drug during lactation.

Triprolidine (FDA class C): Tripolidine was not found to be a teratogen in animal studies and no reports associating its use with human malformations have been published (16). The Collaborative Perinatal Project monitored only 16 exposures during the first trimester of pregnancy: no malformations were encountered, but the size of the sample is too small to draw valid conclusions (13). Its manufacturer, Burroughs Wellcome, warns that triprolidine can be secreted into human milk.

b. Ethanolamines

Diphenhydramine (FDA class B): The results of a retrospective study by Saxen in 1974 linking diphenhydramine intake during the first trimester of pregnancy with an increased risk of cleft palate in the offspring were not confirmed by later investigators (170). Heinonen and coworkers surveyed 2948 exposures anytime during pregnancy (13). Scattered individual anomalies were noted, but there was no relationship with either major or minor patterns of malformation. I agree with Greenberger that diphenhydramine appears safe for use in pregnancy (169). The drug is excreted in milk but in such low amounts that it should not affect the nursing infant. The American Academy of Pediatrics considers it safe for use during lactation (11).

Clemastine (FDA class C): High doses are embryotoxic in animals. No data are available about its safety in human pregnancy and it should thus be avoided. One report described drowsiness, irritability, neck stiffness, feeding difficulties, and a high-pitched cry in one nursing infant whose mother was treated with clemastine (16). The American Academy of Pediatrics warns that clemastine should be used with caution during breast-feeding (12).

c. Ethylenediamines

Tripelennamine (FDA class B): The Collaborative Perinatal Project documented 490 in utero exposures to tripelennamine anytime during pregnancy and 100 during the first trimester. No association was found with any pattern of malformations (13). Greenberger considers tripelennamine safe for use in pregnancy (169). The drug is excreted in bovine milk, but its fate in human milk is unknown. Tripelennamine is compatible with breast-feeding (11).

d. Piperazines

Cyclizine and Meclizine (FDA class B): In amounts 50–100 times higher than the normal human dose, both drugs are teratogenic in rats (171). In human pregnancy, however, no increased rate of malformation has been detected (13,170, 172,173). There is a lack of information about the safety of these drugs during breast-feeding.

Hydroxyzine (FDA class C): High doses are teratogenic in rodents. One study showed no adverse effect when 100 mothers were treated in the first trimester of pregnancy (16). However, Heinonen and colleagues found 5 malformed children in 50 exposed pregnancies, and they infer a possible relationship, although their sample is too small for statistical significance (13). The drug manufacturer, Pfizer, contraindicates the use of hydroxyzine in early pregnancy. Here again, the safety of the drug during breast-feeding is unknown.

e. Piperidines

Cyproheptadine (FDA class B): Cyproheptadine is unique among antihistamines in that it also possesses strong antiserotonin activity. These properties have been used in the preventive treatment of habitual abortion, and no increased rate of malformation has been reported from such use (16). The rate of excretion of cyproheptadine in milk is unknown and the manufacturer, Merck Sharp & Dome, contraindicates its use in breast-feeding.

f. Phenothiazines

Promethazine (FDA class C): The Collaborative Perinatal Project found no evidence of teratogenicity in 746 promethazine-exposed pregnancies (13). One hundred and fourteen exposures occurred during the first trimester. Other studies have shown similar results (16). When used during labor, promethazine may cause respiratory depression in the newborn, as well as impairment of platelet aggregation (16). The pharmacokinetics of promethazine during breast-feeding are unknown.

Trimeprazine (FDA class C): In the cohort of pregnant women studied by Heinonen and coworkers, 140 took trimeprazine and 5 children were born with malformations (13). This possible association remains unproven owing to the small size of the sample. Trimeprazine is excreted into human milk in amounts too low to be harmful, and it is thus compatible with breast-feeding (11).

2. *Second-Generation H_1 Blockers*

The advent of the newer, nonsedating, antihistamines has been a boon to millions of urticaria or allergic rhinitis sufferers, who constantly had to choose between the annoyance of their symptoms and the drowsiness induced by their medication. Information about the safety of these agents during pregnancy is scanty or nonexistent and, generally, they should not be used during gestation and lactation until additional data become available (9).

a. Astemizole (FDA class C). In animal studies, astemizole was not teratogenic for rats and rabbits, but doses in excess of 40 mg/kg were embryotoxic in the former species. No mutagenic or carcinogenic potential was discovered with the Ames test or with chronic oral administration of high doses (174). Astemizole is, however, contraindicated in gestation, and its long half-life precludes its use in women contemplating pregnancy.

b. Terfenadine (FDA class C). Terfenadine is absorbed rapidly and has a short half-life requiring twice daily administration. Animal studies have not shown terfenadine to be teratogenic or embryotoxic, but data in human pregnancy are lacking and its manufacturer, Merrell Dow, warns against terfenadine use in this situation.

c. Loratadine. This piperidine antihistamine is closely related to azatadine and cyproheptadine, both of which are rated B by the FDA in their risk categories. The safety of loratadine has, however, not yet been established in human pregnancy.

d. Cetirizine. This substance is a metabolite of hydroxyzine and thus belongs to the piperazine family. Unique among other second-generation antihistamines, cetirizine causes mild sedation and partially inhibits the migration of eosinophils and neutrophils (175). Its safety during pregnancy and breast-feeding is unknown. Inasmuch as its chemical structure makes it very similar to hydroxyzine, its fetal toxicity is also expected to be the same.

e. Acrivastine. Not yet widely available, acrivastine is a potent H_1-inhibitor with a rapid onset of action and a quick turnover requiring thrice daily administration. No information is available concerning its safety during pregnancy and lactation.

3. *H_2 Blocker*

Cimetidine (FDA class B). Cimetidine competitively inhibits histamine-induced gastric acid secretion by binding to specific H_2 receptors. Because such receptors are also present on blood vessels, cimetidine is occasionally added to classic H_1 antihistamines in the management of refractory, chronic urticaria. Animal studies have not shown cimetidine to be embryotoxic or teratogenic, nor have there been reports describing congenital anomalies following its use in human pregnancies (16). One report of transient liver dysfunction in a neonate exposed at term was not confirmed by other studies (16).

Cimetidine is excreted into and concentrated in breast milk. Despite this concentration, no harmful effects have been reported in the nursing child, and the drug is considered compatible with breast-feeding (12).

4. *Mast Cell Stabilizers*

Mast cell stabilizers, which prevent the release of histamine from mast cells, are clinically useful in the treatment of asthma or allergic conjunctivitis. There is no confirmed dermatological indication for their use, but they have been tried with mixed results in various conditions in which the liberation of histamine or other autacoids may be involved.

a. Sodium Cromoglycate (FDA class B). Topically applied or inhaled, cromolyn sodium is a very effective prophylactic treatment for allergic conjunctivitis or asthma. Its poor gastrointestinal absorption has been held responsible for its disappointing results in the management of urticaria, mastocytosis, and atopic dermatitis. The toxicity of sodium cromoglycate, is low and no teratogenic effects have been demonstrated in animal studies. The drug has been used in 300 human pregnancies without untoward fetal effects (176). Its pharmacokinetics during lactation are unknown.

b. Ketotifen. Ketotifen is an orally active agent which prevents release of mast cell and eosinophil mediators and which also functions as an H_1 antihistamine. Although indicated for asthma prophylaxis, it has been used in the treatment of atopic dermatitis, urticaria, systemic mastocytosis, neurofibromatosis, eosinophilic fasciitis, and the Melkerson-Rosenthal syndrome. Claims of effectiveness in these disorders are mostly based on case reports or open studies (177).

The safety of ketotifen in pregnancy has not been established, but Maclay and colleagues have documented the normal outcome of 40 ketotifen-exposed pregnancies (178). No data are available concerning the safety of the drug during lactation, but inasmuch as it has been used in very young children, it is probably safe.

I. Vitamins and Derivatives

1. *Vitamin A*

a. Beta-Carotene (FDA class C). Beta-carotene is naturally present in most fruits, vegetables, and plants. Once absorbed from the digestive tract, it is cleaved in the liver and yields two molecules of vitamin A. Beta-carotene lacks the physiological properties of vitamin A, but it has found some use as a photoprotectant, particularly in erythropoietic protoporphyria. The recommended adult dose is 180 mg/day or at least three times the normal dietary intake.

The prolonged use of pharmacological amounts of beta-carotene does not cause hypervitaminosis A. Inasmuch as a teratogenic effect in animals has not been demonstrated, this provitamin appears safe during pregnancy (179). However, data in human pregnancy are lacking. Likewise, the safety of beta-carotene during lactation has not been established.

b. Vitamin A (FDA classes A [recommended daily allowance] and X [pharmacological doses]). An essential nutrient, retinol is a high molecular weight, fat-soluble alcohol obtained from various dietary sources. Retinol is necessary for the normal development of the reproductive, skeletal, and visual systems and for the differentiation of epithelial tissues.

High doses of vitamin A retard keratinocyte maturation and have traditionally been used to treat various disorders of keratinization (e.g., ichthyoses, Darier disease, pityriasis rubra pilaris, acne vulgaris). Synthetic retinoids with better cutaneous selectivity have now replaced vitamin A for these indications.

Since 1953, the teratogenicity of high doses of retinol has been well established in experimental animals (180). More than 70 types of malformations have been observed involving the central nervous system, urogenital tract, gastrointestinal system, endocrine glands, and skeleton (181).

In humans, two cases of urogenital anomalies have been reported after maternal consumption of vitamin A 40,000 IU daily for 1 month in the first case and 25,000 IU daily in the first trimester followed with 50,000 IU daily for the remainder of pregnancy in the second case (182,183). Finally, a woman treated with vitamin A for acne between days 19 and 40 of pregnancy with 150,000 IU daily was delivered of a microcephalic baby who died shortly after birth. Autopsy also revealed hypoplastic adrenals and kidney (184).

These data, coupled with the known teratogenic effect of synthetic retinoids in humans, contraindicate the use of pharmacological amounts of vitamin A in pregnancy. The risk of high doses of vitamin A to the breast-fed infant is unknown.

c. Retinoids (FDA class X). In 1982, isotretinoin was released in North America for the treatment of severe, cystic acne. The teratogenic potential of vitamin A and retinoic acid had already been demonstrated in animal studies, and isotretinoin was assigned a category X label by the FDA. Nevertheless, in the 2 years that followed its introduction, at least 154 women were exposed to isotretinoin during pregnancy (185). By 1989, the number of exposed pregnancies had increased to 396 (186). Of these, 151 proceeded to term, and 47% of the infants presented with congenital malformations. In their earlier study, Lammer and colleagues had estimated the relative risk of malformations as 25.6 (185).

As shown in Table 4, exposure to isotretinoin in pregnancy results in a characteristic spectrum of anomalies, which may occur together or singly and involve the craniofacial structures, central nervous system, heart and great vessels, thymus, and skeleton (185,187–192).

The most common craniofacial defect associated with exposure to isotretinoin is anotia or microtia: If not totally absent, the ears are severely hypoplastic, often presenting as a low-set, rudimentary pinna. The external ear canal is often atretic

Table 4 Isotretinoin Teratogenicity

System or organ	Malformation
Craniofacial	
skull	Microtia or anotia
	Atresia or agenesis of outer ear canal
	Occipital vaulting
	Prominent or sloping forehead
	Bitemporal narrowing
	Microcephaly
midface	Depressed nasal bridge
	Hypertelorism
	Small palpebral fissures
lower face	Micrognathia
	Cleft soft or hard palate
Central nervous system	
ventricular system	Obstructive hydrocephalus
	Dandy-Walker anomaly
	Brain cysts
	Nonobstructive hydrocephalus
	Meningomyelocele
cerebrum	Focal cortical agenesis
	Focal agyria
	Heterotopias
	Calcifications
posterior fossa	Cerebellar hypoplasia
	Agenesis of the vermis
	Megacisterna magna
Cardiovascular system	
conotruncal anomalies	Tetralogy of Fallot
	Transposition of the great vessels
	Atrial or ventricular septal defects
	Truncus arteriosus communis
branchial arch anomalies	Interruption/hypoplasia of the aortic arch
	Retroesophageal right subclavian artery
Thymus	Aplasia or hypoplasia
	Ectopy
Skeleton	Adactyly
	Hypoplasia of the long bones

or absent. The skull shows occipital prominence and a high or slopy forehead with bitemporal narrowing (193). The nasal bridge is severely depressed, but hypertelorism is an inconstant feature. Micrognathia is a frequent anomaly, which may be associated with cleaving of the hard or soft palate.

Among central nervous system abnormalities associated with isotretinoin exposure, various types of hydrocephalus have been reported, either communicating or obstructive because of the Dandy-Walker anomaly or other structure-distorting defect. In addition, morphogenic errors of cortical neuronal migration and posterior fossa abnormalities, including cerebellar hypoplasia and megacisterna magna have been noted (185,188,193).

Exposure to isotretinoin has been associated with congenital heart defects, and these can involve proximal, conotruncal structures, or more distal branchial arches. Anomalies in the former group include tetralogy of Fallot, transposition of the great vessels, atrial or ventricular septal defects, and truncus arteriosus communis. Reported branchial arch malformations have included interruption or hypoplasia of the aortic arch and retroesophageal subclavian right artery.

Thymic aplasia, hypoplasia, or ectopia has been noted in association with the use of isotretinoin, more commonly in patients with associated heart defects. Finally, asymmetrical reduction deformities of all four limbs were present in a child exposed to isotretinoin between gestation days 26 and 40 (194).

Similar abnormalities have since been described after exposure to etretinate in pregnancy (195). Synthetic retinoids share with pharmacological doses of vitamin A a powerful teratogenic effect. Experience has shown that there is no safe dose or duration of exposure. In fact, embryopathy has been reported after a single dose of isotretinoin (186). As with the animal model described by Shenefeldt, timing of exposure appears to be the critical factor that determines the pattern and severity of visible malformations (181,196).

Before treating a woman of childbearing age with synthetic retinoids, a baseline pregnancy test should be obtained regardless of her sexual history. Treatment should be started only at the end of a normal menstrual period. A reliable contraceptive method must be used throughout the entire treatment period. Contraception should be maintained for 1 month after termination of treatment with isotretinoin and for at least 2 years after etretinate therapy. Patients should be ready to opt for elective abortion if contraceptive measures fail.

The safety of synthetic retinoids during lactation has not been established. Skeletal toxicity is a potential hazard in an exposed infant, and Hoffmann-La Roche, the manufacturer of these agents, advises against breast-feeding during treatment with isotretinoin or etretinate.

2. *Vitamin B*

a. Nicotinamide (FDA classes A [recommended daily allowance] and C [pharmacological doses]). Niacin and its metabolite nicotinamide are water-soluble members of the vitamin B family. They act as coenzymes in numerous metabolic pathways and their deficiency causes pellagra. In dermatology, pharmacological amounts of nicotinamide have been used in the treatment of polymorphous light eruption, erythema elevatum diutinum, dermatitis herpetiformis, and bullous pemphigoid.

No reports have linked the ingestion of nicotinamide in supraphysiological doses with congenital malformations (16). Nicotinamide is concentrated in the fetus and in breast milk.

3. *Vitamin D* (FDA classes A [recommended daily allowance] and D [pharmacological doses])

In recent years, active vitamin D metabolites as well as analogues with minimal activity on calcium homeostasis have been found to be useful in the treatment of psoriasis. These compounds interact with specific nuclear receptors present in keratinocytes, macrophages, and activated lymphocytes. They inhibit proliferation and promote differentiation. Keratinocytes appear to be their primary target, but immunomodulation may also be important to the overall improvement of psoriasis (197).

Vitamin D crosses the placenta and high doses are teratogenic in animals. In humans, a peculiar syndrome associating supravalvular aortic stenosis (SAS) with infantile hypercalcemia has been linked to a derangement of vitamin D metabolism in the mother or the fetus. The full-blown syndrome, which includes a characteristic elfin facies; cranial, dental, and ocular anomalies; growth and psychomotor retardation; aortic and pulmonary stenosis; and cryptorchidism in males and precocious puberty in females; has been reproduced in rabbits with high doses of vitamin D (198). Goodenday and Gorman, however, have reported the normal outcome of 27 pregnancies in hypoparathyroid women treated with high doses of vitamin D (199). In these cases, maternal calcium levels remained normal throughout pregnancy, suggesting that hypercalcemia, and not vitamin D, is responsible for the SAS syndrome.

Calcipotriol, the vitamin D analogue now used topically in the treatment of psoriasis, is at least 100 times weaker than 1,25-dihydroxyvitamin D_3 in its calcium-mobilizing properties (200). It has not been teratogenic in experimental animals, but its safety in human pregnancy remains unknown and it should be avoided (201). Its pharmacokinetics during breast-feeding are likewise unknown.

J. Psychotropic Agents

Timely reviews by Koblenzer and Koo have emphasized the importance of emotional factors in the production and aggravation of skin disorders and the occurrence of emotional disturbances as a consequence of such disorders (202,203). Yet, most dermatologists are reluctant to use the appropriate psychotropic drugs because of a lack of familiarity with these agents. When clearly indicated, these drugs may be extremely beneficial to a subgroup of patients who will accept medication from their dermatologist but would otherwise refuse to see a psychiatrist.

1. Anxiolytics

a. Benzodiazepines (FDA class D). Diazepam and chlordiazepoxide have been most extensively studied. Several investigators have associated the maternal use of both drugs with an increased risk of malformations (16). Cleft lip or palate and inguinal hernias were reported with diazepam, whereas chlordiazepoxide was suspected to cause mental deficiency, spastic diplegia, microcephaly, duodenal atresia, and Merkel diverticulum.

Benzodiazepines are concentrated in the fetus, and their use near term may lead to hypotonia and lethargy (floppy infant syndrome) or signs of withdrawal. All benzodiazepines should therefore be avoided during pregnancy. These drugs can accumulate in breast milk and are not recommended during lactation.

b. Buspirone (FDA class B). Buspirone is a nonbenzodiazepine anxiolytic devoid of sedative or addictive properties. It has a slow onset of action and is not suited for the treatment of acute anxiety (203). Its safety in human pregnancy has not yet been established. It is excreted in rat milk, but its fate in human milk is unknown.

2. Antidepressants

a. Tricyclic (FDA class C or D). In the risk categories established by the FDA, amitriptyline, its metabolite nortriptyline, and imipramine are classified D, whereas trimipramine, clomipramine, and doxepin are rated C. Limb reduction defects have been reported with amitriptyline and imipramine, but larger studies have not confirmed these findings (16). Clomipramine, the agent of choice in the treatment of obsessive-compulsive disorders, and doxepin, often used for its strong H_1 antihistamine properties, have not been associated with birth defects. All tricyclic antidepressants may cause withdrawal reactions in the newborn when given near term. The drugs are retrieved in breast milk in low concentrations. No adverse effect has been reported in the nursing child, but the American Academy of Pediatrics expresses concern about potential side effects with long-term administration (12).

b. Fluoxetine (FDA class B). Fluoxetine is a newer, nontricyclic antidepressant with a low toxicity profile. It is effective in adults and children with obsessive-compulsive disorders (203). Teratology studies have been negative, but the drug is relatively new and, although it may prove safer than tricyclic antidepressants, studies in human pregnancy and lactation are lacking.

3. *Antipsychotics*

a. Phenothiazines (FDA class C). Promethazine and trimeprazine are commonly used for their sedative and antihistaminic properties and have been discussed earlier. Chlorpromazine has been in use since the 1950s and is commonly prescribed for emesis gravidarum. One study has documented an increased risk of malformations in phenothiazine-exposed fetuses, but other reviewers have disproved the teratogenic potential of phenothiazines (16).

Sedation, hypotonia, or extrapyramidal manifestations may be encountered in the neonate when chlorpromazine is given near term. Chlorpromazine and its congeners are excreted into breast milk in small amounts, but at least one report has described drowsiness in a breast-fed infant whose mother was receiving chlorpromazine.

b. Butylpiperidines (FDA class C). Pimozide is the representative member of this new famiy of antipsychotic drugs closely related to the butyrophenones. Pimozide has demonstrated an exceptional efficacy in the treatment of monosymptomatic psychoses, notably delusion of parasitosis. Haloperidol, a butyrophenone, has been better studied in pregnancy than its newer congener pimozide. Haloperidol has been associated with limb abnormalities in two reports, but several other studies have not shown an increased risk of malformations. The safety of pimozide in pregnancy is not established, and the drug should be avoided until more information is available. These drugs are excreted into breast milk, and the American Academy of Pediatrics expresses concern over their potential toxicity following long-term exposure in nursing children (12).

K. Anticoagulants and Hemostatics

Anticoagulants are rarely used by dermatologists, who may occasionally need these agents in the management of the hypercoagulable state sometimes associated with livedo reticularis, the Sneddon syndrome, Degos disease, and systemic lupus erythematosus. Circulating anticoagulants or anticardiolipin antibodies are usually responsible for the thrombotic events in these disorders.

1. *Warfarin* (FDA class D)

Effective after oral administration, coumarin derivatives exert their anticoagulant activity by interfering with the synthesis of vitamin K–dependent clotting factors. Warfarin crosses the placenta and its administration to pregnant women between the sixth and ninth weeks of gestation has been associated with a specific embryopathy—the fetal warfarin syndrome (FWS). The cardinal features of the syndrome are nasal hypoplasia severe enough to result in respiratory distress in 50% of the cases and stippled calcifications of the axial skeleton, the proximal femur, and the calcanei (204).

Administration of coumarin derivatives during the second and third trimesters of pregnancy can cause central nervous system defects, which are more debilitating then the FWS (16). Two patterns have emerged: dorsal midline dysplasia, manifested by corpus callosum agenesis, the Dandy-Walker anomaly and cerebellar atrophy, and ventral mid-line dysplasia, with optic atrophy as its hallmark (204).

Analysis of the outcome of 463 exposed pregnancies shows that the fetal warfarin syndrome and CNS abnormalities affect 10% of the neonates (16). The use of safer alternatives appears justified when anticoagulant therapy is needed during pregnancy. Excretion into breast milk varies with the agent used: Warfarin and bishydroxycoumarin appear safe, but other derivatives should be avoided (12).

2. *Heparin* (FDA class C)

Heparin is a heterogeneous mixture of straight-chain glycosaminoglycans with an average weight of 15,000 D (18). It is administered parenterally and achieves its anticoagulant effect primarily by enhancement of the activity of antithrombin III and by inhibition of factor Xa.

Because of its high molecular weight, heparin does not cross the placenta. It has not been associated with the production of congenital malformations, nor will it induce bleeding tendencies in the fetus. In their review of the safety of anticoagulation in pregnancy, Hall and coworkers have concluded that based on a high rate of stillbirths, prematurity, and spontaneous abortions heparin may not be safer than warfarin (204). Recent studies, however, have demonstrated the safety of heparin during pregnancy and recommended the use of this anticoagulant for the prevention and treatment of thromboembolic disorders during gestation (205).

More recently, low molecular weight heparins (4000–6500 D) have been made available, and these newer agents, which have a longer half-life and a greater safety, have been successfully used in pregnancy (206). Neither regular nor low molecular weight heparins appear in breast milk, and both types are safe during lactation.

3. *Antifibrinolytic Agents*

a. Tranexamic Acid (FDA class B). Like its parent compound ε-aminocaproic acid, tranexamic acid is a synthetic hemostatic agent which inhibits fibrinolysis by preventing the transformation of plasminogen into active plasmin. Besides its effects on clot lysis, plasmin is a strong activator of the first component of the complement cascade. Therefore, inhibition of plasmin activation by tranexamic acid has been proven useful in the treatment of hereditary angioedema (HAE), where C_1-esterase activation is unopposed by natural C_1-esterase inhibitor (166).

Tranexamic acid crosses the placenta and its safety in pregnancy has not been clearly established. Some women with fibrinolytic hemorrhagic disorders have been treated with the drug during the second and third trimesters of pregnancy without ill effects in their neonates. Until the safety profile of tranexamic acid is better known, treatment of acute attacks of HAE in pregnancy should be limited to infusions of fresh frozen plasma or C_1-INH concentrate. Breast milk levels of tranexamic acid are approximately 100 times lower than maternal serum levels and should not expose the nursing child to an increased risk of thrombotic events.

b. Aprotinin (FDA class C). Aprotinin is a naturally derived 58 amino acid polypeptide which inhibits various proteases such as trypsin, chymotrypsin, kallikrein, and plasmin. It is administered parenterally in the treatment of acute pancreatitis and various hyperfibrinolytic hemorrhagic conditions which may occur in pregnancy following abruptio placentae. It is also effective for acute attacks of HAE through inhibition of plasmin activation.

Aprotinin has been used in late pregnancy without adverse effect on the fetus (16). Data about its safety in the first half of pregnancy are lacking. It is not known whether aprotinin is excreted into breast milk. Inasmuch as it is a polypeptide, it would likely be destroyed in the nursing infant's digestive tract.

L. Vasodilators

1. Dipyridamole (FDA class C)

Dipyridamole is a vasodilator which also inhibits platelet aggregation. The drug is indicated for the prevention of thromboembolic events associated with prosthetic valvular replacement. In dermatology, dipyridamole has been used with some success in the treatment of livedo vasculitis (atrophie blanche).

The use of dipyridamole in pregnancy has not been associated with the production of congenital malformations (16). The drug is excreted in breast milk in amounts too low to cause harmful effects in the nursing child.

2. Nifedipine (FDA class C)

Nifedipine, a coronary and peripheral vasodilator, belongs to the class of calcium channel–blocking agents. Its dermatological indications include vasospastic and occlusive disorders such as the Raynaud phenomenon and atrophie blanche.

In animal studies, high doses of nifedipine have caused fetal malformations and embryotoxicity in gravid mice, rats, and rabbits. No adverse effects have been reported in the second and third trimesters of human pregnancy when the drug was used as an antihypertensive or as a tocolytic agent (16). Nifedipine should probably be avoided during the first trimester or until its safety during this period is well established. The excretion of nifedipine into breast milk is unknown.

3. Pentoxifylline (FDA class C)

Pentoxyfylline is a xanthine derivative which improves blood rheology through peripheral vasodilatation and increased erythrocyte deformability. It may be a useful adjunct in the treatment of atrophie blanche, ischemic leg ulcers, and necrobiosis lipoidica (207).

Pentoxyfylline crosses the placenta. Animal experiments have failed to produce congenital malformations, but in rats, high doses have caused some degree of embryotoxicity. The safety of the drug in human pregnancy has not been established, and its manufacturer, Hoechst, does not recommend its use during gestation. Pentoxifylline is excreted into breast milk, and either breast-feeding or the drug should be discontinued.

M. Miscellaneous Drugs

1. Psoralens (FDA class C)

Psoralens are furocoumarin compounds which are synthetically obtained or extracted from plants such as *Ammi majus*. After activation by long-wave ultraviolet light (UVA), these substances become phototoxic and induce cellular damage by forming photoadducts that intercalate in the DNA chain. Nowadays, PUVA therapy is wisely used to treat extensive psoriasis, mycosis fungoides, vitiligo, polymorphous light eruption, and numerous other skin conditions refractory to standard therapy.

Psoralens alone are mutagenic, but after UVA irradiation, the number of mutations and sister chromatid exchanges in keratinocytes and lymphocytes is even higher (208). Long-term PUVA therapy is known to induce the appearance of nonmelanoma skin cancer and may increase the risk of leukemia (209). Agents that exhibit mutagenic or carcinogenic activities are considered potential teratogens. Animal reproduction studies have not been done, and most experts consider pregnancy and lactation a contraindication to PUVA therapy (210).

However, Stern and Lange have recently reported the outcome of 326 pregnancies, including 31 in women exposed to methoxsalen and 55 in women whose partners were undergoing PUVA treatment (211). In neither group was there an increase in the frequency of stillbirths or congenital malformations compared with a nonexposed cohort. Although these investigators do not endorse the safety of PUVA during pregnancy, they conclude that, "if an increase in the risk of adverse fetal outcome does exist, it is likely to be small" (211).

2. Phenytoin (FDA class D)

Phenytoin, or diphenylhydantoin, is an anticonvulsant with low sedative activity, which is effective in all forms of epilepsy except absence seizures. In dermatology, phenytoin has found a specific niche in the management of recessive dystrophic and some cases of junctional, epidermolysis bullosa (212). Increased synthesis of collagenase by dermal fibroblasts appears to be the key factor in the pathogenesis of these disorders, and phenytoin has been shown to inhibit collagenase synthesis or secretion (213).

Phenytoin is a known teratogen in animals as well as in humans (214). The fetal hydantoin syndrome is a recognizable pattern of malformation consisting of growth retardation, mild to moderate mental deficiency, various craniofacial deformities (e.g., microcephaly, hypertelorism, coloboma, broad nasal bridge, cleft palate, low-set ears), and hypoplasia of distal phalanges with micronychia (16). These features are found in up to 11% of exposed children, and subtler changes may be present in another 31% (215).

In addition, phenytoin is a transplacental carcinogen which exposes the fetus to an increased risk of neuroblastoma, ganglioneuroblastoma, and other tumors of mesoectodermal origin (216,217). Finally, because it may produce a deficiency of vitamin K–dependent coagulation factors, phenytoin has been associated with hemorrhagic disease of the newborn (217).

In the treatment of dermatological conditions, the fetal risk clearly outweighs the potential benefit for the mother, and pregnancy therefore contraindicates the use of phenytoin. The drug is excreted into breast milk but poses little risk to the nursing infant. It is considered compatible with breast-feeding (12).

III. TOPICAL OR INTRALESIONAL THERAPY

A. Antibiotics

1. *Neomycin and Gentamicin* (FDA class C)

No reports document the production of congenital defects by either neomycin or gentamicin even after systemic use. It is unlikely that ototoxicity would result from the small amounts of percutaneously absorbed neomycin and gentamicin.

2. *Bacitracin* (FDA class C)

Bacitracin is a polypeptide antibiotic isolated from *Bacillus subtilis*, which is effective against gram-positive bacteria through inhibition of cell wall synthesis (18). Nephrotoxicity has limited the use of bacitracin to topical application. Bacitracin has never been reported to cause congenital malformations, and its use in pregnancy appears safe (16).

3. *Polymyxin B* (FDA class B)

Polymyxin B is a polypeptide with cationic detergent properties elaborated by *Bacillus polymyxa.* It disrupts the cell wall of gram-negative bacteria but also displays significant nephrotoxicity. Therefore, it is primarily used as a topical agent (18). The use of polymyxin B has never been linked to the production of congenital defects and is probably safe to use in pregnancy (16).

4. *Fusidic Acid*

Fusidic acid is a steroidlike antibiotic that interferes with protein synthesis through inhibition of the bacterial translocase enzymatic system (218). It has a limited spectrum of activity directed mostly against gram-positive bacteria, including methicillin-resistant staphylococci. Oral and parenteral formulations of fusidic acid are available, but dermatologists are more likely to use the topical preparations.

The manufacturer of fusidic acid, Leo Laboratories, warns that the safety of fusidic acid in pregnancy has not been well established. Some investigators consider topical fusidic as totally safe (219).

5. *Mupirocin* (FDA class C)

Mupirocin, or pseudomonic acid A, is a topical antibiotic with a unique chemical structure and greatest activity against gram-positive bacteria. Its mechanism of action involves inhibition of protein and RNA synthesis. Mupirocin is rapidly cleared from the body by conversion to monic acid. Systemic absorption following topical application does not exceed 0.3% (220).

There is evidence that mupirocin crosses the placental barrier and is excreted in breast milk. However, animal studies using high parenteral doses (up to 160 mg/kg/day) have failed to show teratogenic or embryotoxic effects. In addition, mupirocin is not mutagenic in the Ames test (221). Therefore, its use during pregnancy and lactation is probably safe.

6. *Sulfonamides* (FDA class B and D [near term])

The risks of systemic sulfonamides when administered late in pregnancy have already been discussed. The small amounts that can be absorbed from vaginal or ocular preparations are probably harmless for the fetus. However, the treatment of extensive burns with silver sulfadiazine can lead to near-therapeutic plasma concentrations, and care should be exercised when the drug is used in a pregnant woman near term (18).

7. *Metronidazole* (FDA class B)

Systemic absorption of metronidazole from vaginal cream and tablets averages 20% (222). Assuming a similar penetration rate from the skin, a patient applying 2 g/day of a topical preparation containing 0.75% metronidazole would absorb 3 mg of the drug daily. Even after prolonged use, such insignificant amounts are unlikely to prove mutagenic or carcinogenic.

One large study has demonstrated the lack of teratogenic effect from vaginal preparations, and it can therefore be postulated that topical metronidazole is safe during all trimesters of pregnancy and during lactation (219).

8. *Other Agents*

Topical antibiotics, most often in alcoholic vehicles, are frequently used in the treatment of acne. Tetracycline (FDA class D), clindamycin (FDA class C), and erythromycin (FDA class B) are commonly used in this situation. Percutaneous penetration of topically applied tetracycline is small, and the minimal amounts retrieved in maternal blood are unlikely to affect the fetus adversely (27). However, clindamycin and erythromycin are better choices, as they are not only safer for use in pregnancy, but because they are generally more effective than topical tetracycline. Both drugs are nonteratogenic, but clindamycin carries a small risk of inducing pseudomembranous colitis even after topical application (223). This side effect has not been described with erythromycin.

B. Antifungals

1. *Polyenes* (FDA class B)

Nystatin, like amphotericin B, is a polyene antifungal which alters cell wall permeability by binding to ergosterol. No parenteral formulation of the drug is available, and absorption following oral administration is negligible. Nystatin is used exclusively to treat cutaneous, mucosal, or intestinal candidiasis. Its use in pregnancy has not been associated with congenital malformations or fetal toxicity (16,219). The drug should not appear in breast milk, as it is poorly absorbed.

2. *Imidazoles* (FDA classes B [Clotrimazole, Oxiconazole] and C [All others])

Older imidazoles, such as clotrimazole and miconazole, have been used in pregnancy, most often to treat vaginal candidiasis, without maternal or fetal ill effect (151,224,225). The safety of newer agents such as ketoconazole, tioconazole, and sulconazole has not been established, and these antifungals are better avoided in pregnancy. Omoconazole binds strongly to stratum corneum and its systemic absorption is minimal. Its manufacturer does not contraindicate administration of omoconazole during pregnancy (219).

3. *Miscellaneous Agents*

Ciclopirox olamine (FDA class B) is a pyridone ethanolamine salt with a spectrum similar to the imidazoles and a better ability to penetrate nails. Its systemic administration in high doses has caused some degree of fetal loss in animal studies, and its manufacturer, Hoechst, does not recommend its use during pregnancy or lactation.

Undecylenic acid (FDA class C), tolnaftate (FDA class C), and haloprogin (FDA class B) have been in use for respectively 50, 30, and 20 years (226). They are generally available as over-the-counter agents and are not contraindicated during pregnancy. Naftifine and terbinafine (FDA class B) are representative members of the allylamines, a new class of antifungals which inhibit ergosterol synthesis. Although teratology studies have been negative in animals, data concerning their use in human pregnancy and lactation are lacking. Until their safety profile is well established, they are better avoided in the pregnant patient or nursing mother.

Selenium sulfide (FDA class C) has an antiyeast activity which makes it a popular agent for the treatment of dandruff and tinea versicolor. Repeated use over prolonged periods on damaged skin has led to systemic absorption and selenium poisoning. A recent study has shown no rise in selenium levels during the 2 days that followed a single overnight application of a 2.5% selenium sulfide preparation to the entire torso (227). Such treatment appears safe for the pregnant patient.

C. Antivirals

1. *Acyclovir* (FDA class C)

Percutaneous absorption of topically applied acyclovir may result in detectable, albeit low, serum levels of the drug (16). No reports of adverse fetal effects have been reported from topical maternal application. Topical application of acyclovir does not appear contraindicated during pregnancy (219).

2. *Idoxuridine* (FDA class C)

Idoxuridine is a halogenated pyrimidine which, in its triphosphorylated form, becomes incorporated into viral and mammalian DNA (18). It is available as a topical solution for the treatment of cutaneous herpesvirus infection despite minimal effectiveness for that indication. Herpetic keratitis, however, usually responds well to intraconjunctival instillation of idoxuridine. The drug was found teratogenic in rabbits after parenteral and ophthalmic use (16). No studies are available in human pregnancy, a condition which contraindicates the use of idoxuridine (219).

3. *Podophyllin*

Podophyllotoxin, a cytostatic glucoside, is the active ingredient of podophyllin, a resin extracted from the rhizomes of *Podophyllum peltatum* (mandrake root) or *P. emodi*. This substance shares with colchicine and *Vinca* alkaloids a mitostatic effect by inhibition of spindle formation. Podophyllin and podophyllotoxin are used to treat genital warts. The drug is systemically absorbed in significant amounts when liberally applied to mucous membranes or inflamed skin, and it may be responsible for severe toxicity including fever, myelosuppression, profound sensorimotor neuropathy, coma, and death (228).

Experimental studies in mice, rabbits, and rats with intraamniotic or intraperitoneal injections of podophyllotoxin have demonstrated a strong, dose-related, embryotoxic effect (130,229). The injections induced a high number of stillbirths, but no congenital malformations were noted in the surviving animals.

Maternal toxicity and death, stillbirth, and congenital malformations following the use of podophyllin in pregnancy have been reported by several investigators. Bargman has critically reviewed these publications, emphasizing that in each case compounding factors were present; for example, general anesthesia, biopsy of the lesions, application of large amounts of podophyllin, or failure to wash off the drug after 4–6 hr (230). Bargman therefore concludes that, "podophyllin must be an extremely safe drug when used properly. . . . It would seem unwarranted to say that podophyllin is contraindicated in pregnancy" (230). In reply to Sundharam, Bargman later qualified this statement by saying, "I am *not* proposing that podophyllin is safe for use in pregnancy. I am simply saying that, in my opinion, it has not been proven unsafe" (231).

Podophyllotoxin is an antimitotic agent with a toxicity profile similar to *Vinca* alkaloids. Its systemic absorption after topical application has been demonstrated. If not a teratogen, it is undoubtedly an abortifacient. Therefore, podophyllotoxin should not be used in pregnancy, especially since other effective modalities (cryotherapy, electrosurgery, trichloracetic acid, laser vaporization) are available for the treatment of condylomata acuminata.

4. *Cantharidin*

Cantharidin is a powerful vesicant secreted by *Cantharis vesicatoria*, a coleopter better known as "Spanish fly" or "blister beetle." The extract is used in concentrations of 0.5–1.0% in the treatment of warts and mollusca contagiosa. When ingested or topically applied in large amounts, it can cause severe toxicity such as gastroenteritis, nephritis, shock, and death (232).

The precise mode of action of cantharidin on epithelial tissues is not fully elucidated: Besides changes in cell membranes and acantholysis, mitochondrial poisoning has been observed (18). No studies have addressed the safety of cantharidin therapy during pregnancy and lactation. In view of this absence of data, the drug should be avoided.

D. Parasiticides

1. *Lindane* (FDA class C)

Lindane is the gamma isomer of hexachlorocyclohexane, an organochlorinated insecticide widely used in agriculture and in the treatment of scabies and pediculosis. The substance is well absorbed through skin, and multiple reports describing human toxicity have been published. Acute intoxication is usually manifested by nausea, vomiting, tremors, muscle spasms, seizures, blindness, and death, whereas chronic low-grade exposure may produce aplastic anemia (233). In a critical review of published reports of lindane toxicity, Rasmussen mentioned that most cases followed agricultural exposure, whereas ingestion or mishandling of the drug was responsible for the mishaps that occurred after medical use of the insecticide (234).

Lindane has been dubbed a carcinogen, because oral ingestion over a period of 2 years has caused a high incidence of hepatomas in mice (235). However, similar studies in other species have failed to demonstrate a carcinogenic effect, and the National Cancer Institute does not consider lindane carcinogenic (236).

High oral doses have produced an increased rate of stillbirths in animal experiments, but no teratogenic or mutagenic effects have been seen. No reports have described congenital malformations or spontaneous abortion after topical lindane application in human pregnancy (16,236). Therefore, little evidence exists to contraindicate the use of lindane during pregnancy. However, because of the potential neurotoxicity of lindane, it is advisable to choose an equally effective alternative such as permethrin when treating pregnant patients, infants, or individuals with seizure disorders.

The passage of lindane in milk has not been studied, and no adverse effect from its use during lactation has been reported. Theoretical calculations estimate the amount that a nursing infant would ingest as similar to what would occur following topical application (16).

2. *Other Agents*

a. Sulfur. Five to ten percent precipitated sulfur in petrolatum is a time-honored and effective scabicide and pediculicide. This preparation has been used for centuries without causing any ill effect other than transient cutaneous irritation. Sulfur ointment is often recommended as a safe alternative to lindane in pregnant patients and infants. Rasmussen, however, cautions that the safety of sulfur has not been thoroughly assessed, and he cites a German study in which application of 25% sulfur ointment to the abraded skin of experimental animals resulted in paralysis, convulsions, and death (234).

b. Benzyl Benzoate (FDA class C). This synthetically prepared derivative of balsam of Peru has been used as a scabicide since 1937 (237). Oral ingestion has produced incoordination and convulsions in experimental animals (232). No studies have documented the safety of benzyl benzoate in human pregnancy, but toxic effects have not been reported either. It appears to be innocuous in pregnancy and lactation when properly used.

c. Malathion. Malathion is a thiophosphate insecticide which inhibits cholinesterase. When used in a 0.5% lotion, it is as effective as lindane as a scabicide and pediculicide. It will eradicate lindane-resistant parasites, but resistance to malathion has also appeared (235). Malathion has not been reported to affect the outcome of pregnancy adversely, but its safety has not been fully assessed. According to Burns, "there is no absolute contraindication to the use of any of the currently available scabicides in pregnancy" (237).

d. Pyrethrins (FDA classes C [Pyrethrins] and D [Permethrin]). The insecticidal properties of pyrethrum, the crude extract of *Chrysanthemum cinerariaefolium*, have been exploited for more than 150 years. Synthetic pyrethroids have been available since 1949, and permethrin, the first photostable compound, was introduced in 1973 (238). Today, permethrin is used to treat scabies and pediculosis. It is used in concentrations ranging from 1 to 5%, alone or combined with piperonyl butoxide, which inhibits its enzymatic degradation by the parasite. Permethrin is one of the safest insecticides known, and less than 2% of an applied dose is percutaneously applied (238). Animal studies have demonstrated a lack of teratogenic or embryotoxic potential in mice, rats, and rabbits fed oral doses of 200–400 mg/kg/day. Transfer into breast milk is unknown, but the use of permethrin during lactation is expected to be safe.

e. Crotamiton (FDA class C). N-ethyl-o- crotonotoluidine is a yellowish oil with fungicidal, acaricidal, and antipruritic activities. Data concerning its percutaneous absorption and safety in pregnancy are lacking (234). Despite this paucity of data, crotamiton is often advocated as an alternative to lindane for pregnant women and infants (9). Treatment failures are common with crotamiton, and other agents such as permethrin and malathion appear equally safe and are more effective.

E. Antiseptics

1. Hexachlorophene

Hexachlorophene is a polychlorinated bisphenol with bacteriostatic activity against gram-positive bacteria. It is less effective than povidone-iodine or chlorhexidine. Systemic absorption occurs rapidly through damaged or immature skin and through mucous membranes. Neurotoxicity characterized by lethargy, twitchings, convulsions, and death has occurred following daily hexachlorophene baths in perinatal units. Some surviving children have been left with permanent cerebral damage (239). Hexachlorophene is embryotoxic and teratogenic in rats. One investigator has reported teratogenic effects in pregnant nurses routinely exposed to hexachlorophene (240). Thus, the use of hexachlorophene is contraindicated in pregnancy, and it appears to constitute an occupational hazard to pregnant health personnel.

2. *Povidone-Iodine*

Povidone-iodine is an effective topical germicide based on the loose association of elemental iodine with polyvinylpyrrolidone, which acts as a carrier. A 10% solution will release 1% of available iodine, which has the capacity to penetrate damaged skin, intact mucous membranes, and even burn eschars. The peripartum use of povidone-iodine solution as vaginal and perineal disinfectants has led to detectable urinary levels of iodine in the newborns and transient hypothyroidism (241). Its use in pregnancy is therefore discouraged.

3. *Chlorhexidine*

Chlorhexidine is a chlorinated biguanide with potent bactericidal activity against both gram-positive and gram-negative bacteria. It displays low toxicity and poor systemic absorption (18). Chlorhexidine has been safely used to decrease bacterial colonization of neonatal skin. Its use in pregnancy is probably safe.

4. *Quinolines*

8-Hydroxyquinolines such as iodoquinol and clioquinol (FDA class C), are halogenated compounds which are used orally for their amebicidal action. Topical formulations take advantage of the weak antibacterial and antifungal properties of the drugs. Because of their iodine content, 8-hydroxyquinolines may interfere with thyroid function. Their oral administration has been linked to a peculiar syndrome of subacute myelo-optic neuropathy (SMON) which attained epidemic proportions in Japan in the 1960s. It is not known whether systemic absorption of topically applied hydroxyquinolines occurs in significant amounts. Until this information is available, it is best to avoid the use of these compounds in pregnancy.

F. Anti-inflammatory Agents

1. *Glucocorticosteroids* (FDA class C)

Percutaneous absorption of topically applied glucocorticosteroids is extremely variable and depends on the molecular structure of the compound, its liposolubility, the nature of its vehicle, the presence or absence of occlusion, the site and area of the treated zone, and the degree of integrity of the epidermal barrier. Multiple studies have shown that application of medium- to high-potency corticosteroids to large areas may lead to transient or persistent hypothalamus-pituitary- adrenal (HPA) axis suppression with biological or clinical signs of hypercorticism (242,243). Amounts as low as 2 to 7 g/day of clobetasol-17-propionate can temporarily suppress the HPA axis when applied to diseased skin (243). Similar situations will undoubtedly arise with "optimized vehicles" and other "superpotent" corticosteroids. With regard to pregnancy, application of these drugs to large areas should be considered with the same prudent approach as the use of systemic glucocorticosteroids.

2. *Tar and Anthralin*

These messy, smelly, and often irritating agents are still widely used in the treatment of psoriasis. Coal and shale tar, from which ichthammol is extracted, are complex mixtures of aliphatic and aromatic hydrocarbons such as benzenes, anthracenes, naphthalenes, and phenols. Tars are known carcinogens, although evidence of tumor formation from their use in dermatology is scarce.

Because topically applied tars have led to the systemic absorption of measurable levels of mutagenic by-products, Jurecka and Gebhart do not recommend their use in pregnancy (9).

Anthralin and its derivatives are anthracenic compounds which inhibit DNA synthesis and mitochondrial function. Anthralin causes sebaceous gland suppression in mice and induces ornithine decarboxylase activity, two effects that indicate a carcinogenic potential (244). Anthralin causes extrachromosomal mutations in yeasts but has shown no mutagenic effect in *Salmonella* (244). In view of these findings, anthralin therapy should be avoided during pregnancy.

G. Keratolytics

1. *Benzyl Peroxide* (FDA class C)

Benzyl peroxide breaks down on the skin to release free-radical oxygen which is bacterial for *Propionibacterium acnes*. It also demonstrates keratolytic and comedolytic properties and has gained wide acceptance in the treatment of mild to moderate acne vulgaris. Benzyl peroxide is entirely metabolized to benzoic acid in the skin and excreted as benzoates in the urine.

Five percent of an applied amount of benzoyl peroxide will be systemically absorbed (245). No harmful effect has ever been reported from use in pregnancy or lactation, and the use of benzoyl peroxide in these conditions appears perfectly safe (27).

2. *Retinoids* (FDA class B)

Synthetic retinoids are among the most potent teratogens known, and it has been established that a single dose administered during the first trimester can have catastrophic repercussions. Consequently, topical tretinoin application has been discouraged in pregnancy. However, percutaneous absorption and embryotoxicity studies performed on animals with various synthetic retinoids have failed to show a teratogenic effect with tretinoin or etretinate, whereas repeated applications of the arotinoid Ro 13-6298 resulted in significant embryopathy (246).

Camera and Pregliasco have reported the case of a baby with unilateral atresia of the external ear canal coupled with a malformed, hypoplastic ear (247) born to a mother treated with tretinoin cream 0.05% during the first 11 weeks of pregnancy (247). The pattern of malformation presented by the child is identical to what has been reported following systemic exposure. It is, however, impossible to draw definitive conclusions based on a single case report.

A retrospective study recently compared 215 women exposed to topical tretinoin during the first trimester of pregnancy and 430 age-matched, nonexposed women (248). The prevalence of major defects in the offspring was slightly *lower* in the exposed group. The investigators conclude that topical tretinoin does not carry an increased risk of congenital disorders. Isotretinoin, however, is contraindicated in pregnancy (219). The risk to the breast-fed infant of maternal topical tretinoin use appears negligible.

H. Antineoplastic Drugs

1. *Nitrogen Mustard* (FDA class D)

Mechlorethamine was the first nitrogen mustard introduced in clinical practice. This very unstable alkylating agent is part of the MOPP, [nitrogen mustard, Oncovin (vincristine), procarbazine, and prednisone], chemotherapeutic protocol for the treatment of Hodgkin lymphoma. Topically applied in dilute aqueous suspensions or anhydrous ointments, mechlorethamine constitutes the mainstay of treatment for the patch and plaque stages of mycosis fungoides, and it is also effective in Langerhans cell histiocytosis.

Mechlorethamine is mutagenic, teratogenic, and carcinogenic. Because of its high reactivity, topical mechlorethamine exerts the bulk of its action at the epidermal level, which accounts for its reported absence of systemic toxicity (249). Despite this apparent safety, it should be remembered that applications must be made to the entire body surface, often to large areas of skin which has lost its normal barrier function. The potential for absorption therefore remains high, and the drug should be avoided in pregnancy or used only after completion of embryogenesis. Breast-feeding is contraindicated during mechlorethamine therapy.

2. *5-Fluorouracil* (FDA class D)

5-Fluorouracil (5-FU) is a pyrimidine antimetabolite that competes with uracil-derived nucleotides to block thymidilate synthetase, which is a key enzyme in DNA synthesis (18). Its systemic administration to pregnant mice and monkeys causes congenital malformations, fetal death, or intrauterine growth retardation. Stephens and collaborators have reported major visceral and skeletal defects in a fetus exposed to 5-FU in utero between 11 and 16 weeks of pregnancy (250).

In dermatology, the use of 5-FU is restricted to topical application or intralesional injections for the treatment of precancerous and benign tumors, warts, and selected dermatoses such as porokeratosis and acrodermatitis continua. There has been no report of fetotoxicity following the topical use of 5-FU (16). Percutaneous absorption is in the range of 10%: Application of 2 g/day of 5-FU 5% cream systemically delivers 10 mg/day, a subtoxic amount 80 times lower than the maximum intravenous daily dose (251). Intralesional injections may expose the patient to higher peak levels, as 25–50 mg is administered at each session; however, lesions are usually infiltrated on a weekly or twice weekly basis, so that the total dose remains within the same range.

In summary, topical or intralesional administration of 5-FU is unlikely to be deleterious during pregnancy and lactation. Nevertheless, sound medical judgment dictates the selection of safer alternatives in these particular situations.

3. *Masoprocol* (FDA class B)

Meso-nordihydroguaiaretic acid represents the newest addition to the chemotherapeutic armamentarium against actinic keratoses. Its cytotoxic mechanism of action probably involves the generation of free radicals. In addition, masoprocol is a potent inhibitor of 5-lipooxygenase and thus may exhibit anti-inflammatory activities.

Teratology studies in rats and rabbits have been negative, but masoprocol is mutagenic in the Ames test. After topical application, systemic absorption is in the range of 3%. Proof of toxicity in human pregnancy is lacking, but it appears wise to elect safer alternatives, such as cryotherapy or curettage, for the treatment of actinic damage in the pregnant woman. The excretion of masoprocol in breast milk is unknown.

I. Miscellaneous Agents

1. *Minoxidil* (FDA class C)

Minoxidil is a potent vasodilator used systemically for the treatment of hypertension. Because it commonly causes hypertrichosis, a topical formulation has been developed to take advantage of this side effect in the management of alopecia.

Approximately 1.5% of a topically applied dose of minoxidil is absorbed. Animal studies in rats and rabbits have shown a lack of teratogenic potential. Nevertheless, the manufacturer, Upjohn, contraindicates the use of minoxidil during pregnancy, because the safety of the drug has not been established. One woman was treated with oral minoxidil throughout pregnancy without adverse effect in the newborn (16). Another woman gave birth to a child with hypertrichosis, omphalocele, dysmorphic facies, and bilateral fifth finger clinodactyly (252). In addition to minoxidil, she had also been treated with captopril and propanolol, two drugs which have occasionally been linked to sporadic congenital malformations. In this case, minoxidil was probably responsible for the abnormal hair growth, but it is impossible conclusively to attribute the other anomalies to this particular drug. Minoxidil passes into milk, but is considered compatible with breast-feeding (12).

2. *Azelaic Acid*

Azelaic acid is a 9-carbon dicarboxylic acid with antimicrobial activity against aerobic and anaerobic bacteria, antityrosinase activity, and a specific cytotoxic effect on hyperactive melanocytes and keratinocytes (253). In a 20% cream formulation, azelaic acid is effective in the treatment of acne, melasma, and lentigo maligna.

In vitro and animal studies have failed to show embryotoxic, teratogenic, or mutagenic activities (253). Only 3–8% of a topically applied quantity is absorbed, and systemic toxicity has not occurred in experimental animals with doses up to 4000 mg/kg. Therefore, azelaic acid appears safe for use in pregnancy, but controlled studies in this setting have not been conducted. Until additional information is available, it is prudent to select therapeutic modalities with a proven record of safety during pregnancy.

REFERENCES

1. F. Howard and J. M. Hill. Drugs in pregnancy, *Obstet. Gynecol. Surv. 34*:643 (1979).
2. D. Sasseville, R. D. Wilkinson, and J. Y. Schnader. Dermatoses of pregnancy, *Int. J. Dermatol. 20*:223 (1981).
3. R. C. Holmes and M. M. Black. The specific dermatoses of pregnancy, *J. Am. Acad. Dermatol. 8*:405 (1983).
4. G. B. Winton and C. W. Lewis. Dermatoses of pregnancy, *J. Am. Acad. Dermatol. 6*:977 (1982).
5. G. B. Winton. Skin diseases aggravated by pregnancy, *J. Am. Acad. Dermatol. 20*:1 (1989).
6. M. R. Juchau and E. Faustman-Watts. Pharmacokinetic considerations in the maternal-placental-fetal unit, *Clin. Obstet. Gynecol. 26*:379 (1983).
7. G. T. Livezey and W. F. Rayburn. Principles of perinatal pharmacology, *Drug Therapy in Obstetrics and Gynecology*, 3rd ed. (W. F. Rayburn and F. P. Zuspan, eds.), Mosby-Year Book, St. Louis, 1992, p. 3.
8. G. C. Cupit and H. H. Rotmensch. Principles of drug therapy, *Principles of Medical Therapy in Pregnancy*, 2nd ed. (N. Gleicher, ed.), Appleton & Lange, Norwalk, CT, 1992, p. 68.
9. W. Jurecka and W. Gebhart. Drug prescribing during pregnancy, *Semin. Dermatol. 8*:30 (1989).
10. R. A. Lawrence. Breastfeeding and medical disease, *Med. Clin. North Am. 73*:583 (1989).
11. American Academy of Pediatrics, Committee on Drugs. The transfer of drugs and other chemicals into human breast milk, *Pediatrics 72*:375 (1983).
12. American Academy of Pediatrics, Committee on Drugs. Transfer of drugs and other chemicals into human milk, *Pediatrics 84*:924 (1989).

13. O. P. Heinonen, D. Slone, and S. Shapiro. *Birth Defects and Drugs in Pregnancy*, Publishing Sciences Group, Littleton, Mass., 1977.
14. A. W. Chow and P. J. Jewesson. Pharmacokinetics and safety of antimicrobial agents during pregnancy, *Rev. Infect. Dis. 7*:287 (1985).
15. D. V. Landers, J. R. Green, and R. L. Sweet. Antibiotic use during pregnancy and the postpartum period, *Clin. Obstet. Gynecol. 26*:391 (1983).
16. G. G. Briggs, R. K. Freeman, and S. J. Yaffe. *Drugs in Pregnancy and Lactation*, 3rd ed. Williams & Wilkins, Baltimore, 1990.
17. H. Graber and T. Magyar. Pharmacokinetics of ceftriaxone in pregnancy, *Am. J. Med. 77*:117 (1984).
18. A. G. Gilman, L. S. Goodman, and A. Gilman. *Goodman and Gilman's The Pharmacological Basis of Therapeutics,* 6th ed., Macmillan, New York, 1980.
19. A. Philipson, L. D. Sabath, and D. Charles. Erythromycin and clindamycin absorption and elimination in pregnant women, *Clin. Pharmacol. Ther. 19*:68 (1976).
20. W. M. McCormack, H. George, A. Donner, et al. Hepatotoxicity of erythromycin estolate during pregnancy, *Antimicrob. Agents Chemother. 12*:630 (1977).
21. A. J. Weinstein, R. S. Gibbs, and M. Gallagher. Placental transfer of clindamycin and gentamycin in term pregnancy, *Am. J. Obstet. Gynecol. 124*:688 (1976).
22. D. L. Tuffanelli. Successful pregnancy in a patient with dermatitis herpetiformis treated with low-dose dapsone, *Arch. Dermatol. 118*:876 (1982).
23. G. Kahn. Dapsone is safe during pregnancy, *J. Am. Acad. Dermatol. 13*:838 (1985).
24. J. F. Lucey and T. J. Driscoll, Jr. Hazard to newborn infants of administration of long-acting sulfonamides to pregnant women, *Pediatrics 24*:498 (1959).
25. S. W. Sanders, J. J. Zone, R. L. Foltz, et al. Hemolytic anemia induced by dapsone transmitted through breast milk, *Ann. Int. Med. 96*:465 (1982).
26. C. R. Lowe. Congenital defects among children born to women under supervision or treatment for pulmonary tuberculosis, *Br. J. Prev. Soc. Med. 18*:14 (1964).
27. K. F. Rothman and P. E. Pochi. Use of oral and topical agents for acne in pregnancy, *J. Am. Acad. Dermatol. 19*:431 (1988).
28. C. T. Kunelis, J. L. Peters, and H. A. Edmondson. Fatty liver of pregnancy and its relationship to tetracycline therapy, Am. J. Med. 38:359 (1965).
29. R. E. Wenk, F. C. Gebhart, B. S. Bhagavan, et al. Tetracycline-associated fatty liver of pregnancy, including possible pregnancy risk after chronic dermatologic use of tetracycline, J. Reprod. Med. 26:135 (1981).
30. M. R. Eckman. Tetracyclines and dental staining, *J. Infect. Dis. 131*:307 (1975).
31. C. J. Witkop and R. O. Wolf. Hypoplasia and intrinsic staining of enamel following tetracycline therapy, *JAMA 185*:1008 (1963).
32. M. T. Genot, H. P. Golan, P. J. Porter, et al. Effect of administration of tetracycline in pregnancy on the primary dentition of the offspring, *J. Oral Med. 25*:75 (1970).
33. S. Cohlan, G. Bevelander, and T. Tiamsic. Growth inhibition of prematures receiving tetracycline, *Am. J. Dis. Child. 105*:453 (1963).
34. J. D. Harley, J. F. Farrar, J. B. Gray, et al. Aromatic drugs and congenital cataracts, *Lancet 1*:472 (1964).
35. M. P. Carter and F. Wilson. Tetracycline and congenital limb abnormalities, *Br. Med. J. 2*:407 (1962).

36. R. Corcoran and J. M. Castles. Tetracycline for acne vulgaris and possible teratogenesis, *Br. Med. J. 2*:807 (1977).
37. G. M. Ruiz, B. F. Perez, S. C. Lopez, et al. Syndrome of hypomelia, hypotrichosis and facial hemangioma (Pseudothalidomide syndrome) (abstract), *An Esp. Pediatr. 17*:229 (1982).
38. A. C. Reboli and V. E. Del Bene. Oral antibiotic therapy of dermatologic conditions, *Dermatol. Clin. 6*:497 (1988).
39. D. M. Campoli-Richards, J. P. Monk, A. Price, et al. Ciprofloxacin. A review of its antibacterial activity, pharmacokinetic properties and therapeutic use, *Drugs 35*:373 (1988).
40. D. E. Snider, P. M. Layde, M. W. Johnson, et al. Treatment of tuberculosis during pregnancy, *Am. Rev. Respir. Dis. 122*:65 (1980).
41. J. Warkany. Antituberculous drugs, *Teratology 20*:133 (1979).
42. J. S. M. Steen and D. M. Stainton-Ellis. Rifampin in pregnancy, *Lancet 2*:604 (1977).
43. E. Eggermont, N. Logghe, W. Van de Casseye, et al. Haemorrhagic disease of the newborn in the offspring of rifampicin and isoniazid treated mothers, *Acta Paediatr. Belg. 29*:87 (1976).
44. L. Beely. Drugs and breast feeding, *Clin. Obstet. Gynaecol. 13*:247 (1986).
45. N. E. Morrison and G. M. Marley. Clofazimine binding studies with deoxyribonucleic acid, *Int. J. Lepr. 44*:475 (1976).
46. D. T. Woodley. Clofazimine and its uses in dermatology, *J. Assoc. Mil. Dermatol. 8*:41 (1982).
47. H. Farb, D. P. West and A. Pedvis-Leftick. Clofazimine in pregnancy complicated by leprosy, *Obstet. Gynecol. 59*:122 (1982).
48. M. A. Ismail and S. A. Lerner. Disseminated blastomycosis in a pregnant woman. Review of amphotericin B usage during pregnancy, *Am. Rev. Respir. Dis. 126*:350 (1982).
49. R. B. Disasio, D. E. Lakings, and J. E. Bennett. Evidence for conversion of 5-flucytosine to 5-fluorouracil in humans: Possible factor in 5-flucytosine clinical toxicity, *Antimicrob. Agents Chemother. 14*:903 (1978).
50. J. Faergemann and H. Maibach. Griseofulvin and ketoconazole: a review with special emphasis on dermatology, *Semin. Dermatol. 6*:31 (1987).
51. A. Rubin and D. Dvornik. Placental transfer of griseofulvin, *Am. J. Obstet. Gynecol.* 92:882 (1965).
52. M. F. Klein and J. R. Beall. Griseofulvin: a teratogenic study, *Science 175*:1483 (1972).
53. F. W. Scott, A. De La Hunta, R. D. Schultz, et al. Teratogenesis in cats associated with griseofulvin therapy, *Teratology 11*:79 (1974).
54. S. P. Clissold. Pharmacokinetic properties, *Ketoconazole today. A review of Clinical Experience* (H. E. Jones, ed.), Adis, Manchester, U.K., 1987, p. 24.
55. J. A. McGregor and A. Pont. Contraindications of ketoconazole in pregnancy, *Am. J. Obstet. Gynecol. 150*:793 (1984).
56. J. E. Birnbaum. Pharmacology of the allylamines, *J. Am. Acad. Dermatol. 23*:782 (1990).
57. M. Samsoen. La terbinafine (Lamisil®). La première allylamine fongistatique et fongicide per os, *Nouv. Dermatol. 11*:743 (1992).

58. J. A. Balfour and D. Faulds. Terbinafine. A review of its pharmacodynamic and pharmacokinetic properties, and therapeutic potential in superficial mycoses, *Drugs 43*:259 (1992).
59. P. S. Mehta, S. J. Mehta, and H. Vorherr. Congenital iodide goiter and hypothyroidism: a review, *Obstet. Gynecol. Surv. 38*:237 (1983).
60. D. H. King. History, pharmacokinetics, and pharmacology of acyclovir, *J. Am. Acad. Dermatol. 18*:176 (1988).
61. D. C. Lagrew, Jr., T. G. Furlow, W. D. Hager, et al. Disseminated herpes simplex virus infection in pregnancy. Successful treatment with acyclovir. *JAMA 252*:2058 (1984).
62. L. Grover, J. Kane, J. Kravity, et al. Systemic acyclovir in pregnancy: A case report, *Obstet. Gynecol. 65*:284 (1985).
63. C. L. S. Leen, B. K. Mandal, and M. E. Ellis. Acyclovir and pregnancy, *Br. Med. J. 294*:308 (1987).
64. E. B. Andrews, H. H. Tilson, B. A. L. Hurn, et al. Acyclovir in pregnancy registry: An observational epidemiologic approach, *Am. J. Med. 85*(Suppl. 2A):123 (1988).
65. V. T. De Vita, Jr., S. Hellman, and S. A. Rosenberg, eds. *AIDS. Etiology, Diagnosis, Treatment and Prevention*, 2nd ed. Lippincott, Philadelphia, 1988, p. 286.
66. H. L. Minkoff. Care of pregnant women infected with human immunodeficiency virus, *JAMA 20*:2714 (1987).
67. D. Isaacson, M. Elgart, and M. L. Turner. Antimalarials in dermatology, *Int. J. Dermatol. 21*:379 (1982).
68. W. A. Neill, G. S. Panayi, J. J. R. Duthie, et al. Action of chloroquine phosphate in rheumatoid arthritis: Chromosome damaging effect, *Ann. Rheum. Dis. 32*:547 (1973).
69. M. S. Wolfe and J. F. Cordero. Safety of chloroquine in chemosuppression of malaria during pregnancy, *Br. Med. J. 290*:1466 (1985).
70. R. Lewis, N. H. Lauersen, and S. Birnbaum. Malaria associated with pregnancy, *Obstet. Gynecol. 42*:696 (1973).
71. R. Suhonen. Hydroxychloroquine administration in pregnancy, *Arch. Dermatol. 119*:185 (1983).
72. A. Parke. Antimalarial drugs and pregnancy, *Am. J. Med. 85*(Suppl. 4A):30 (1988).
73. L. Paufique and P. Magnard. Dégénérescence rétinienne chez deux enfants consécutive à un traitement préventif anti-paludéen chez la mère pendant la grossesse, *Bull. Soc. Ophthalmol. Fr. 69*:466 (1969).
74. C. W. Hart and R. F. Naunton. The ototoxicity of chloroquine phosphate, *Arch. Otolaryngol. 80*:407 (1964).
75. G. J. Matz and R. F. Naunton. Ototoxicity of chloroquine, *Arch. Otolaryngol. 88*:370 (1968).
76. L. M. McEwen. Trimethoprim/Sulphamethoxazole mixture in pregnancy, *Br. Med. J. 4*:490 (1971).
77. A. Molavi, J. L. LeFrock, and R. A. Prince. Metronidazole, *Med. Clin. North Am. 66*:121 (1982).
78. M. O. Robbie and R. L. Sweet. Metronidazole use in obstetrics and gynecology: A review, *Am. J. Obstet. Gynecol. 145*:865 (1983).
79. T. H. Shepard and A. G. Fantel. Is metronidazole teratogenic?, *JAMA 237*:1617 (1977).

80. P. Rodin and G. Hass. Metronidazole and pregnancy, *Br. J. Vener. Dis. 42*:210 (1966).
81. A. Berget and T. Weber. Metronidazole and pregnancy, *Ugeskr. Laeger 134*:2085 (1972).
82. R. Kubba and Y. Al-Gindan. Leishmaniasis, *Dermatol. Clin. 7*:331 (1989).
83. Anonymous. Safety of antimicrobial drugs in pregnancy, *Med. Lett. Drugs. Ther. 29*:61 (1987).
84. S. K. Jones, N. J. Reynolds, S. Oliwiecki, et al. Oral albendazole for the treatment of cutaneous larva migrans, *Br. J. Dermatol. 122*:99 (1990).
85. C. J. Ellis. Antiparasitic agents in pregnancy, *Clin. Obstet. Gynaecol. 13*:269 (1986).
86. H. D. Davies, P. Sakuls, and J. S. Keystone. Creeping eruption. A review of clinical presentation and management of 60 cases presenting to a tropical disease unit, *Arch. Dermatol. 129*:588 (1993).
87. L. A. Weber and K. J. Tomecki. Drug therapy of fungal and parasitic diseases, *Dermatol. Clin. 7*:387 (1989).
88. A. R. Ahmed and S. M. Hombal. Cyclophosphamide (Cytoxan*). A review on relevant pharmacology and clinical uses, *J. Am. Acad. Dermatol. 11*:1115 (1984).
89. G. R. Mohn and T. Ellenberger. Genetic effects of cyclophosphamide, *Mutat. Res. 32*:331 (1976).
90. J. E. Lergier, E. Jimenez, N. Maldonado, et al. Normal pregnancy in multiple myeloma treated with cyclophosphamide, *Cancer 34*:1018 (1974).
91. L. H. Greenberg and K. R. Tanaka. Congenital anomalies probably induced by cyclophosphamide, *JAMA 188*:423 (1964).
92. T. M. Toledo, R. C. Harper and R. H. Moser. Fetal effects during cyclophosphamide and irradiation therapy, *Ann. Int. Med. 74*:87 (1971).
93. H. O. Nicholson. Use of cytotoxic drugs in pregnancy: review of reported cases, *J. Obstet Gynecol. B. Commonw. 75*:307 (1968).
94. D. Amato and J. S. Niblett. Neutropenia from cyclophosphamide in breast milk, *Med. J. Austral. 1*:383 (1977).
95. P. I. Dantzig. Immunosuppessive and cytotoxic drugs in dermatology, *Arch. Dermatol. 110*:393 (1974).
96. A. Milunsky, J. W. Graef and M. F. Gaynor. Methotrexate- induced congenital malformations, *J. Pediatr. 72*:790 (1968).
97. H. R. Powell and H. Eckert. Methotrexate-induced congenital malformations, *Med. J. Austr. 2*:1076 (1971).
98. D. G. Johns, L. D. Rutherford, P. C. Leighton, et al. Secretion of methotrexate into human milk, *Am. J. Obstet. Gynecol. 112*:978 (1972).
99. I. R. Younger and D. W. S. Harris. Azathioprine in dermatology, *J. Am. Acad. Dermatol. 25*:281 (1991).
100. S. Saarikoski and M. Sepala. Immunosuppression during pregnancy: Transmission of azathioprine and its metabolites from mother to the fetus, *Am. J. Obstet. Gynecol. 115*:1100 (1973).
101. J. H. Githens, J. G. Rosenkrantz and S. M. Tunnock. Teratogenic effects of azathioprine (Imuran), *J. Pediatr. 66*:959 (1965).
102. J. G. Rosenkrantz, J. H. Githens, S. M. Cox, et al. Azathioprine (Imuran) and pregnancy, *Am. J. Obstet. Gynecol. 97:387 (1967).*

103. R. M. Caplan, J. B. Dossetor and G. B. Maugham. Pregnancy following cadaver kidney homotransplantation, *Am. J. Obstet. Gynecol. 111*:1120 (1971).
104. The Registration Committee of the European Dialysis and Transplant Association. Successful pregnancies in women treated by dialysis and kidney transplantation, *Br. J. Obstet. Gynaecol. 87*:839 (1980).
105. D. W. Leb, B. Weisskopf and B. D. Kanovitz. Chromosome aberrations in the child of a kidney transplant recipient, *Arch. Intern. Med. 128*:44 (1971).
106. R. A. Williamson and L. E. Karp. Azathioprine teratogenicity: review of the literature and case report, *Obstet. Gynecol. 58*:247 (1981).
107. G. D. Lower, L. E. Stevens, J. S. Najarian, et al. Problems from immunosuppressives during pregnancy, *Am. J. Obstet. Gynecol. 111*:1120 (1971).
108. C. J. Côté, H. J. Meuwissen and R. I. Pickering. Effects on the neonate of prednisone and azathioprine administrated to the mother during pregnancy, *J. Pediatr. 85*:324 (1974).
109. J. M. Davison, H. Dellagrammatikas and J. M. Parkin. Maternal azathioprine therapy and depressed haemopoiesis in the babies of renal allograft patients, *Br. J. Obstet. Gynaecol. 92*:233 (1985).
110. J. M. Davison and M. D. Lindheimer. Pregnancy in women with renal allografts, *Semin. Nephrol. 4*:240 (1984).
111. C. J. McDonald. Cytotoxic agents for use in dermatology. I, *J. Am. Acad. Dermatol. 12*:753 (1985).
112. A. S. Boyd and K. H. Neldner. Hydroxyurea therapy, *J. Am. Acad. Dermatol. 25*:518 (1991).
113. U. W. Leavell and J. W. Yarbro. Hydroxyurea: A new treatment for psoriasis, *Arch. Dermatol. 102*:144 (1970).
114. M. L. Murphy and S. Chaube. Preliminary survey of hydroxyurea (NSC-32065) as a teratogen, *Cancer Chemother. Rep. 40*:1 (1964).
115. V. H. Ferm. Teratogenic activity of hydroxyurea, *Lancet 1*:1338 (1965).
116. A. K. Gupta, M. D. Brown, C. N. Ellis, et al. Cyclosporine in dermatology, *J. Am. Acad. Dermatol. 21*:1245 (1989).
117. V. C. Ho and D. M. Zloty. Immunosuppressive agents in dermatology, *Dermatol. Clin. 11*:73 (1993).
118. T. S. B. Zwannenburg, W. Soter and B. E. Matter. Absence of genotoxic potential for cyclosporine in experimental systems, *Transplant Proc. 20*(Suppl. 3):931 (1988).
119. G. J. Lewis, C. A. R. Lamont, H. A. Lee, et al. Successful pregnancy in a renal transplant patient taking cyclosporine A, *Br. Med. J. 286*:603 (1983).
120. H. J. Deeg, M. S. Kennedy, J. E. Sanders, et al. Successful pregnancy after marrow transplantation for severe aplastic anemia and immunosuppression with cyclosporine, *JAMA 250*:647 (1983).
121. G. Klintmalm, P. Althoff, G. Appleby, et al. Renal function in a newborn baby delivered of a renal transplant patient taking cyclosporine, *Transplantation 38*:198 (1984).
122. I. Cockburn, P. Krupp and C. Monka. Present experience of Sandimmune in pregnancy, *Transplant Proc. 21*:3730 (1989).
123. S. M. Flechner, A. R. Katz, A. J. Rogers, et al. The presence of cyclosporine in body tissues and fluids during pregnancy, *Am. J. Kidney Dis. 5*:60 (1985).

124. M. S. Fradin, C. N. Ellis and J. J. Voorhees. Management of patients and side effects during cyclosporine therapy for cutaneous disorders, *J. Am. Acad. Dermatol. 23*:1265 (1990).
125. A. M. Rudolph. Effects of aspirin and acetaminophen in pregnancy and in the newborn, *Arch. Int. Med. 141*:358 (1981).
126. B. K. Birmingham, D. S. Greene, and C. T. Rhodes. Systemic absorption of topical salicyclic acid, *Int. J. Dermatol. 18*:228 (1979).
127. D. Slone, O. P. Heinonen, D. W. Kaufman, et al. Aspirin and congenital malformations, *Lancet 1*:1373 (1976).
128. E. Collins and G. Turner. Maternal effects of regular salicylate ingestion in pregnancy, *Lancet 2*:335 (1975).
129. F. D. Malkinson. Colchicine. New uses of an old, old drug, *Arch. Dermatol. 118*:453 (1982).
130. J. Didcock, D. Jackson, and J. M. Robson. The action of some nucleotoxic substances on pregnancy, *Br. J. Pharmacol. 11*:437 (1956).
131. N. R. Ferreira and A. Buoniconti. Trisomy after colchicine therapy, *Lancet 2*:1304 (1968).
132. M. M. Cohen, M. Levy, and M. Eliakim. A cytogenetic evaluation of long-term colchicine therapy in the treatment of familial Mediterranean fever (FMF), *Am. J. Med. Sci. 274*:147 (1977).
133. I. Thomas. Gold therapy and its indications in dermatology. A review, *J. Am. Acad. Dermatol. 16*:845 (1987).
134. I. Rocker and W. J. Henderson. Transfer of gold from mother to fetus, *Lancet 2*:1246 (1976).
135. D. L. Cohen, J. Orzel, and A. Taylor. Infants of mothers receiving gold therapy, *Arthritis Rheum. 24*:104 (1981).
136. I. H. Scheinberg and I. Sternlieb. Pregnancy in penicillamine-treated patients with Wilson's disease, *N. Engl. J. Med. 293*:1300 (1975).
137. W. H. Lyle. Penicillamine in pregnancy, *Lancet 1*:606 (1978).
138. A. Linares, J. J. Zarranz, J. Rodriguez-Alarcon, et al. Reversible cutis laxa due to maternal D-penicillamine treatment (letter), *Lancet 2*:43 (1979).
139. O. K. Mjolnerod, K. Rasmussen, S. A. Dommerud, et al. Congenital connective tissue defect probably due to D-penicillamine treatment in pregnancy, *Lancet 1*:673 (1971).
140. L. Solomon, G. Abrams, M. Dinner, et al. Neonatal abnormalities associated with D-penicillamine treatment during pregnancy, *N. Engl. J. Med. 296*:54 (1977).
141. P. Gal and S. D. Ravenel. Contractures and hydrocephalus with penicillamine and maternal hypotension, *J. Clin. Dysmorphol. 2*:9 (1984).
142. H. B. Taussig. A study of the German outbreak of phocomelia, *JAMA 180*:1106 (1962).
143. G. R. Brugio. The thalidomide disaster briefly revisited, *Eur. J. Pediatr. 136*:229 (1981).
144. G. W. Mellin and M. Katzenstein. The saga of thalidomide: neuropathy to embryopathy with case reports of congenital anomalies, *N. Engl. J. Med. 267*:1184 (1962).
145. E. Grosshans and G. Illy. Thalidomide therapy for inflammatory dermatoses, *Int. J. Dermatol. 23*:598 (1984).
146. T. Fainstat. Cortisone-induced congenital cleft palate in rabbits, *Endocrinology 55*: 502 (1954).

147. H. Taeusch. Glucocorticoid prophylaxis for respiratory distress syndrome: A review of potential toxicity, *J. Pediatr. 87*:617 (1975).
148. D. Warrell and R. Taylor. Outcome of the fetus of mothers receiving prednisolone during pregnancy, *Lancet 1*:117 (1968).
149. J. M. Reinisch, N. G. Simm, W. G. Karou, et al. Prenatal exposure to prednisone in humans and animals retard intrauterine growth, *Science 202*:436 (1978).
150. A. M. Kraus. Congenital cataract and maternal steroid injection, *J. Pediatr. Ophthalmol. 12*:107 (1975).
151. D. L. Stockton and A. S. Paller. Drug administration to the pregnant or lactating woman: a reference guide for dermatologists, *J. Am. Acad. Dermatol. 23*:87 (1990).
152. C. Gallant and P. Kenny. Oral glucocorticoids and their complications: A review, *J. Am. Acad. Dermatol. 14*:161 (1986).
153. A. M. Bongiovanni and A. J. McPadden. Steroids during pregnancy and possible fetal consequences, *Fertil. Steril. 11*:181 (1960).
154. D. B. Yackel, R. D. Kempers, and W. M. McConahey. Adrenocorticosteroids in pregnancy, *Am. J. Obstet. Gynecol. 96*:985 (1966).
155. M. Schatz, R. Patterson, S. Zeitz, et al. Corticosteroid therapy for the pregnant asthmatic patient, *JAMA 233*:804 (1975).
156. A. L. Herbst, H. Ulfelder, and D. C. Poskanzer. Adenocarcinoma of the vagina: Association of maternal stilbestrol therapy with tumour appearance in young women, *N. Engl. J. Med. 284*:878 (1971).
157. J. G. Forsbeg. Estrogen, vaginal cancer, and vaginal development, *Am. J. Obstet. Gynecol. 113*:83 (1972).
158. A. C. Wentz. Assessment of estrogen and progestin therapy in gynecology and obstetrics, *Clin. Obstet. Gynecol. 20*:461 (1977).
159. J. J. Nora and A. H. Nora. Can the pill cause birth defects?, *N. Engl. J. Med. 291*:731 (1974).
160. D. T. Janerich, J. M. Piper, and D. M. Glebatis. Oral contraceptives and congenital limb reduction, *N. Engl. J. Med. 291*:697 (1974).
161. Z. Katz, M. Lancet, J. Skornik, et al. Teratogenicity of progestagens given during the first trimester of pregnancy, *Obstet. Gynecol. 65*:775 (1985).
162. L. J. Resseguie, J. F. Hick, J. A. Bruen, et al. Congenital malformations among offspring exposed in utero to progestins, Olmsted County, Minnesota, 1936–1974, *Fertil. Steril. 43*:514 (1985).
163. J. C. Shaw. Spironolactone in dermatologic therapy, *J. Am. Acad. Dermatol. 24*:236 (1991).
164. A. Hecker, S. H. Hasan, and F. Neumann. Effect of spironolactone on the sexual differentiation of rat fetuses, *Acta Endocrinol. 215*(Suppl.):32 (1978).
165. L. Cusan, A. Dupont, A. Bélanger, et al. Treatment of hirsutism with the pure antiandrogen flutamide, *J. Am. Acad. Dermatol. 23*:462 (1990).
166. M. Greaves and F. Lawlor. Angioedema: manifestations and management, *J. Am. Acad. Dermatol. 25*:155 (1991).
167. M. Castro-Magana, T. Cheruvanky, P. J. Collip, et al. Transient adrenogenital syndrome due to exposure to danazol in utero, *Am. J. Dis. Child. 135*:1032 (1981).
168. S. C. Duck and K. P. Katayama. Danazol may cause femae pseudohermaphroditism, *Fertil. Steril. 35*:230 (1981).

169. P. Greenberger and R. Patterson. Safety of therapy for allergic symptoms during pregnancy, *Ann. Int. Med. 89*:234 (1978).
170. I. Saxen. Cleft palate and maternal diphenhydramine intake, *Lancet 1*:407 (1974).
171. J. F. Sadusk and P. A. Palmisano. Teratogenic effect of meclizine, cyclizine and chlorcyclizine, *JAMA 194*:987 (1965).
172. L. Milkovich and B. J. Van Den Berg. An evaluation of the teratogenicity of certain antinauseant drugs, *Am. J. Obstet. Gynecol. 125*:244 (1976).
173. J. Yerushalmy and L. Milkovich. The evaluation of the teratogenic effect of meclizine in man, *Am. J. Obstet. Gynecol. 93*:553 (1965).
174. D. M. Richards, R. N. Brogden, R. C. Heel, et al. Astemizole. A review of its pharmacodynamic properties and therapeutic efficacy, *Drugs 28*:38 (1984).
175. N. A. Soter. Treatment of angioedema and urticaria: low-sedating H_1-type antihistamines, *J. Am. Acad. Dermatol. 24*:1084 (1991).
176. J. Wilson. Use of cromoglycate during pregnancy, *J. Pharm. Med. 8*:45 (1982).
177. C. Zip. Ketotifen review, *Can. J. Dermatol. 5*:497 (1993).
178. W. P. Maclay, D. Crowder, and S. Spiro. Postmarketing surveillance: practical experience with ketotifen, *Br. Med. J. 288*:911 (1984).
179. H. Nishimura and T. Tanimura. *Clinical Aspects of the Teratogenicity of Drugs*, American Elsevier, New York, 1978, p. 252.
180. S. G. Cohlan. Excessive intake of vitamin A as a cause of congenital anomalies in the rat, *Science 117*:535 (1953).
181. R. E. Shenefelt. Animal model: treatment of various species with a large dose of vitamin A at known stages in pregnancy, *Am. J. Pathol. 66*:589 (1972).
182. G. Pilitti and A. Scorta. Ipervitaminosi A gravidica e malformazioni neonatali dell'apparato urinario, *Minerva Ginecol. 87*:1103 (1965).
183. I. B. Bernhardt and D. J. Dorsey. Hypervitaminosis A and congenital renal anomalies in a human infant, *Obstet. Gynecol. 43*:750 (1974).
184. L. Stange, K. Carlstöm and M. Eriksson. Hypervitaminosis A in early human pregnancy and malformations of the central nervous system, *Acta. Obstet. Gynecol. Scand. 57*:289 (1978).
185. E. J. Lammer, D. T. Chen, R. M. Hoar, et al. Retinoic acid embryopathy, *N. Engl. J. Med. 313*:837 (1985).
186. W. S. Dai, J. M. LaBraico, and R. S. Stern. Epidemiology of isotretinoin exposure during pregnancy, *J. Am. Acad. Dermatol. 26*:599 (1992).
187. R. S. Stern, F. Rosa, and C. Baum. Isotretinoin and pregnancy, *J. Am. Acad. Dermatol. 10*:851 (1984).
188. P. J. Benke. The isotretinoin teratogen syndrome, *JAMA 251*:3267 (1984).
189. E. De La Cruz, S. Sun, K. Vangvanichyakorn, et al. Multiple congenital malformations associated with maternal isotretinoin therapy, *Pediatrics 74*:428 (1984).
190. P. M. Fernhoff and E. J. Lammer. Craniofacial features of isotretinoin embryopathy, *J. Pediatr. 105*:595 (1984).
191. J. T. Braun, R. A. Franciosi, A. R. Mastri, et al. Isotretinoin dysmorphic syndrome, *Lancet 1*:504 (1984).
192. R. M. Hill. Isotretinoin teratogenicity, *Lancet 1*:1465 (1984).
193. I. T. Lott, M. Bocian, H. W. Pribram, et al. Fetal hydrocephalus and ear anomalies associated with maternal use of isotretinoin, *J. Pediatr. 105*:597 (1984).

194. W. G. McBride. Limb reduction deformities in a child exposed to isotretinoin in utero on gestation days 26–40 only, *Lancet 1*:1276 (1985).
195. D. Lambert, S. Dalac, F. Escallier, et al. Malformations foetales après étrétinate, *Nouv. Dermatol. 7*:448 (1988).
196. J. H. Hersh, D. S. Danhauer, M. E. Hand, et al. Retinoic acid embryopathy: timing of exposure and effects on fetal development, *JAMA 254*:909 (1985).
197. J. Berth-Jones and P. E. Hutchinson. Vitamin D analogs and psoriasis, *Br. J. Dermatol. 127*:71 (1992).
198. W. F. Friedman and L. F. Mills. The relationship between vitamin D and the craniofacial and dental anomalies of the supravalvular aortic stenosis syndrome, *Pediatrics 43*:12 (1969).
199. L. S. Goodenday and G. S. Gordan. No risk from vitamin D in pregnancy, *Ann. Intern. Med. 75*:807 (1971).
200. K. Kragballe. Treatment of psoriasis with calcipotriol and other vitamin D analogues, *J. Am. Acad. Dermatol. 27*:1001 (1992).
201. K. Kragballe and L. Iversen. Calcipotriol. A new topical antipsoriatic, *Dermatol. Clin. 11*:137 (1993).
202. C. S. Koblenzer. Psychosomatic concepts in dermatology. A dermatologist-psychoanalyst viewpoint, *Arch. Dermatol. 119*:501 (1983).
203. J. Y. M. Koo and C. T. Pham. Psychodermatology. Practical guidelines on pharmacotherapy, *Arch. Dermatol. 128*:381 (1992).
204. J. G. Hall, R. M. Pauli, and K. M. Wilson. Maternal and fetal sequelae of anticoagulation during pregnancy, *Am. J. Med. 68*:122 (1980).
205. C. Demers and J. S. Ginsberg. Deep venous thrombosis and pulmonary embolism in pregnancy, *Clin. Chest Med. 13*:645 (1992).
206. E. Melissari, C. J. Parker, N. V. Wilson, et al. Use of low-molecular weight heparin in pregnancy, *Thromb. Haemostat. 68*:652 (1992).
207. H. Ely. Pentoxifylline therapy in dermatology. A review of localized hyperviscosity and its effects on the skin, *Dermatol. Clin. 6*:585 (1988).
208. J. K. Dunnick. *Toxicology and carcinogenesis studies of 8-methoxypsoralen in F 344/N rats*, US Dept of Health and Human Services, Public Health Service National Toxicology Program, 1989, Triangle Park, NC, National Institute of Health Publication 89-2814.
209. A. K. Gupta and T. F. Anderson. Psoralen photochemotherapy, *J. Am. Acad. Dermatol. 17*:703 (1987).
210. W. L. Morison. *Phototherapy and photochemotherapy of skin disease*, 2nd ed., Raven Press, New York, 1991, p. 67.
211. R. S. Stern and R. Lange. Outcomes of pregnancies among women and partners of men with a history of exposure to methoxsalen photochemotherapy (PUVA) for the treatment of psoriasis, *Arch. Dermatol. 127*:347 (1991).
212. J. D. Fine and L. Johnson. Efficacy of systemic phenytoin in the treatment of junctional epidermolysis bullosa, *Arch. Dermatol. 124*:1402 (1988).
213. E. A. Bauer, T. W. Cooper, D. R. Tucker, et al. Phenytoin therapy of recessive dystrophic epidermolysis bullosa, *N. Engl. J. Med. 303*:776 (1980).
214. P. M. Loughnan, H. Gold and J. C. Vance. Phenytoin teratogenicity in man, *Lancet 1*:70 (1973).

215. J. W. Hanson, N. C. Myrianthopoulos, M. A. S. Harvey, et al. Risks to the offspring of women treated with hydantoin anticonvulsants, with emphasis on the fetal hydantoin syndrome, *J. Pediatr. 89*:662 (1976).
216. R. A. Seeler, J. N. Israel, J. E. Royal, et al. Ganglioneuroblastoma and fetal hydantoin-alcohol syndrome, *Pediatrics 63*:524 (1979).
217. R. W. Allen, B. Ogden, F. L. Bentley, et al. Fetal hydantoin syndrome, neuroblastoma and hemorrhagic disease in a neonate, *JAMA 244*:1464 (1980).
218. L. Verbist. The antimicrobial activity of fusidic acid, *J. Antimicrob. Chemother. 25(Suppl. B)*:1 (1990).
219. L. Machet, L. Vaillant, and G. Lorette. Les risques des traitements topiques au cours de la grossesse, *Ann. Dermatol. Venereol. 119*:503 (1992).
220. K. A. Pappa. The clinical development of mupirocin, *J. Am. Acad. Dermatol. 22*:873 (1990).
221. J. J. Leyden. Mupirocin: A new topical antibiotic, *Semin. Dermatol. 6*:8 (1987).
222. M. M. Alper, B. N. Barwin, W. M. McLean, et al. Systemic absorption of metronidazole by the vaginal route, *Obstet. Gynecol. 65*:781 (1985).
223. E. B. Milstone, A. J. McDonald, and D. F. Scholhamer, Jr. Pseudomembranous colitis after topical application of clindamycin, *Arch. Dermatol. 117*:154 (1981).
224. C. G. Tan, C. S. Good, L. J. R. Milne, et al. A comparative trial of six-day therapy with clotrimazole and nystatin in pregnant patients with vaginal candidiasis, *Postgrad. Med. J. 50*(Suppl. 1):102 (1974).
225. C. Culbertson. Monistat—A new fungicide for treatment of vulvovaginal candidiasis, *Am. J. Obstet. Gynecol. 120*:973 (1974).
226. E. B. Smith. Topical antifungal agents, *Dermatol. Clin. 2*:109 (1984).
227. J. Kalivas. Lack of serum selenium rise after overnight application of selenium sulfide, *Arch. Dermatol. 129*:646 (1993).
228. P. D. Silva, J. P. Micha, and D. G. Silva. Management of condyloma acuminatum, *J. Am. Acad. Dermatol. 13*:457 (1985).
229. J. B. Thiersch. Effect of podophyllin (P) and podophyllotoxin (PT) on the rat litter in utero, *Proc. Soc. Exp. Biol. Med. 113*:124 (1963).
230. H. Bargman. Is podophyllin a safe drug to use and can it be used during pregnancy?, *Arch. Dermatol. 124*:1718 (1988).
231. J. A. Sundharam. Is podophyllin safe for use in pregnancy?, *Arch. Dermatol. 125*:1000 (1989).
232. R. E. Gosselin, H. C. Hodge, R. P. Smith, et al., *Clinical Toxicology of Commercial Products*, 4th ed., Williams & Wilkins, Baltimore, 1976.
233. L. M. Solomon, L. Fahrner, and D. P. West. Gamma benzene hexachloride toxicity: A review, *Arch. Dermatol. 113*:353 (1977).
234. J. E. Rasmussen. The problem of lindane, *J. Am. Acad. Dermatol. 5*:507 (1981).
235. B. Schacter. Treatment of scabies and pediculosis with lindane preparations: An evaluation, *J. Am. Acad. Dermatol. 5*:517 (1981).
236. J. E. Rasmussen. Lindane. A prudent approach, *Arch. Dermatol. 123*:1008 (1987).
237. D. A. Burns. The treatment of human ectoparasite infection, *Br. J. Dermatol. 125*:89 (1991).
238. D. Taplin and T. L. Meinking. Pyrethrins and pyrethroids in dermatology, *Arch. Dermatol. 126*:213 (1990).

239. H. Powell, O. Swarner, L. Gluck, et al. Hexachlorophene myelinopathy in premature infants, *J. Pediatr. 82*:976 (1973).
240. W. Check. New study shows hexachlorophene is teratogenic in humans (editorial), *JAMA 240*:513 (1978).
241. D. L'Allemand, A. Grüthers, P. Heidemann, et al. Iodine-induced alterations of thyroid function in newborn infants after prenatal and perinatal exposure to povidone iodine, *J. Pediatr. 102*:935 (1983).
242. J. M. Garden and R. K. Freinkel. Systemic absorption of topical steroids. Metabolic effects as an index of mild hypercortisolism, *Arch. Dermatol. 122*:1007 (1986).
243. E. A. Olsen and R. C. Cornell. Topical clobetasol-17-propionate: Review of its clinical efficacy and safety, *J. Am. Acad. Dermatol. 15*:246 (1986).
244. R. E. Ashton, P. André, N. J. Lowe, et al. Anthralin: historical and current perspectives, *J. Am. Acad. Dermatol. 9*:173 (1983).
245. S. Nacht, D. Young, J. N. Beasley, et al. Benzoyl peroxide percutaneous penetration and metabolic disposition, *J. Am. Acad. Dermatol. 4*:31 (1981).
246. C. C. Willhite, R. P. Sharma, P. V. Allen, et al. Percutaneous retinoid absorption and embryotoxicity, *J. Invest. Dermatol. 95*:523 (1990).
247. G. Camera and P. Pregliasco. Ear malformation in baby born to mother using tretinoin cream, *Lancet 339*:687 (1992).
248. S. S. Jick, B. Z. Terris, and J. Hick. First trimester topical tretinoin and congenital disorders, *Lancet 341*:1181 (1993).
249. E. C. Vonderheid. Topical mechlorethamine chemotherapy. Considerations on its use in mycosis fungoides, *Int. J. Dermatol. 23*:180 (1984).
250. J. D. Stephens, M. S. Golbus, T. R. Miller, et al. Multiple congenital anomalies in a fetus exposed to 5-fluorouracil during the first trimester, *Am. J. Obstet. Gynecol. 137*:747 (1980).
251. D. K. Goette. Topical chemotherapy with 5-fluorouracil, a review, *J. Am. Acad. Dermatol. 4*:633 (1981).
252. S. F. Kaler, M. E. Patrinos, G. H. Lambert, et al. Hypertrichosis and congenital anomalies associated with maternal use of minoxidil, *Pediatrics 79*:434 (1987).
253. M. Nazzaro-Porro. Azelaic acid, *J. Am. Acad. Dermatol. 17*:1033 (1987).

10

Dermatological Surgery During Pregnancy

Marwali Harahap
University of North Sumatra Medical School, Medan, Indonesia

I. INTRODUCTION

Pregnancy is a situation in which special considerations are necessary when dermatological surgery is required. The primary concern when providing care for a pregnant patient is that a fine balance should be maintained. No harm should be allowed to befall the fetus because of drug administration, but equally no harm must come to the mother because a disease is being inadequately treated.

II. FETAL RISK

An area of dermatological surgical management with a potential for creating fetal damage is drug administration. Since it is virtually impossible to perform a dermatological surgical procedure properly without the administration of medication, one option is to defer any elective dermatological surgery until after delivery to avoid fetal risk.

The critical period of organogenesis in humans is from the third to the eleventh week of pregnancy, and only essential surgery should be carried out in this period. During this period of organogenesis, drugs can produce fetal malformation (teratogenicity) or spontaneous abortion. During the second and third trimesters, drugs can affect the growth and functional development of the fetus, in particular the central nervous system (CNS) (1). Drugs may be employed in the second trimester if necessary, but caution should be used, especially when administering CNS depressants (2). Anesthesia and surgery in late pregnancy are also undesirable. Considerable respiratory and cardiovascular changes occur as a result of pregnancy, and there is a risk also of precipitating premature labor (3). As the patient nears term in late pregnancy, it might be prudent to postpone any nonemergency treatment. Thus, where possible without increased maternal morbidity, dermatological surgery should be performed under local anesthesia, preferably in the middle trimester of pregnancy. Although local anesthetics are in no way contraindicated in a pregnant patient, it is prudent to be conservative in the administration of all drugs at this time.

In general, elective surgery should be delayed until after the termination of pregnancy and at least 6 weeks postpartum (4). However, urgent dermatological surgery should be done.

III. INDICATIONS FOR SURGERY

The primary indications for urgent dermatological surgery during pregnancy are the diagnosis and/or treatment of skin malignancies and removal of benign lesions that are inflamed or infected and/or associated with pain or bleeding (5).

IV. PREOPERATIVE AND INTRAOPERATIVE MANAGEMENT

As drugs may cross the placental barrier and produce adverse effects on the fetus, it is wise to limit medication in pregnant women as far as is practicable. The amount of local anesthesia used for dermatological surgery is probably small enough to be destroyed in the liver before reaching the fetal circulation. For purposes of dermatological surgery, local anesthetics, that is, lidocaine and bupivacaine, are considered safe when used in moderate amounts.

From the initiation of any dermatological surgery plan for the pregnant woman, communication between dermatologist, obstetrician, and patient is essential. Consultation with the patient's obstetrician outlining the degree of urgency of the proposed surgery, its duration, and the anesthetic planned is always in order (Table 1).

The dermatologist may or may not be aware that the patient is pregnant at the time of surgery. At some point in the future, the patient may allege or blame a miscarriage or the birth of a retarded or deformed child on the surgery experience. It goes without saying that women of childbearing age should be carefully queried about possible pregnancy and tested for pregnancy if necessary to avoid administering anesthetic and medication to a patient with early first-trimester pregnancy for routine elective surgery. If the patient is pregnant or suspects that she is

Table 1 Management of the Pregnant Patient

1. Defer surgery until after delivery if possible.
2. The primary indication for urgent dermatological surgery is the diagnosis and/or treatment of skin malignances and removal of benign lesions that are inflamed or infected and/or associated with pain or bleeding.
3. Consult the patient's obstetrician or general physician if surgery cannot be delayed.
4. Urgent dermatological surgery should be delayed until after the first trimester if possible without increased maternal morbidity. Where possible, urgent dermatological surgery should be performed preferably in the middle trimester of pregnancy.
5. Allay the patient's apprehension by personal assurance.
6. Avoid the use of drugs with teratogenic potential. Use local anesthetics when anesthesia is necessary. The teratogenicity of local anesthetics has not been reported in animals or humans.
7. Avoid keeping the patient in the supine position during the second and third trimesters. The enlarged uterus may compress the vena cava and thus impede venous return, leading to decreased cardiac output and hypotension.
8. Monitoring of the fetal heart rate before, during, and after surgery is advisable in the late second and third trimesters.
9. Allow the patient to take frequent breaks to the restroom, because of fetal pressure on the patient's urinary bladder.

pregnant, have a forthright and informative discussion with her about the potential hazards to the fetus. Do not hesitate to cancel the procedure if there is any reluctance on the part of the patient to go ahead, particularly if the surgery could be postponed without any difficulty. If the patient elects to proceed with the surgery, prior consultation with her obstetrician is advisable, and suspected teratogenic drugs which can produce spontaneous abortion or the development of fetal malformation should be avoided. All this information should be carefully documented on the patient's chart.

Preoperative contact with the patient must be professional, thorough, reassuring, and confident. Pregnancy can be emotionally as well as physiologically stressful and an urgent surgery causes anxiety. Psychological preparation for surgery is the best premedication. Verbal reassurance is essential to control anxiety. Premedication is usually not necessary. The patient's vital signs should be obtained, with particular attention being paid to any elevation in blood pressure (a possible sign of preeclampsia).

Fetal cardiac rhythm can be monitored electronically or by auscultation. In late second- and third-trimester patients, fetal heart tones should be monitored before, during, and after the operation if possible.

V. SUPINE HYPOTENSIVE SYNDROME

A woman in late pregnancy should not be placed in the supine position, because her enlarged gravid uterus will compress the soft-walled inferior vena cava and to a lesser extent the aorta. Caval obstruction leads to reduced venous return to the heart. The cardiac output falls and except in a minority of patients, despite a compensatory rise in the peripheral resistance, the blood pressure also falls. This can lead to a loss of up to 30% of the effective circulating blood volume (6). This manifests in the signs and symptoms of supine hypotensive syndrome, such as fainting, sweating, nausea, pallor, and often bradycardia (7,8). The aorta is compressed subrenally, which leads to reduced uterine blood flow and decreased femoral pulses with consequent detriment to the fetus. Owing to poor placental perfusion, fetal hypoxia occurs, usually associated with bradycardia or other signs of fetal distress. The treatment for supine hypotensive syndrome consists of relieving the compression on the inferior vena cava by turning the patient to the left lateral position or by displacing the uterus to the left (9). Tilting the patient from the supine to the lateral position increases cardiac output by 20–100% (10). In 97% of patients, a tilt to the left is more satisfactory than to the right (11). The symptoms and signs rapidly disappear if these procedures are effective in relieving the compression, but the blood pressure may take a few minutes to return to its previous level. Vena caval compression can begin to develop during the second trimester and become maximal at 36–38 weeks. The supine hypotensive syndrome has been reported in approximately 10% of pregnant women during the third trimester (12).

For this reason, the supine position in late pregnancy must be scrupulously avoided at all times. Whenever possible, the patient should be laid on her left side. If this is inappropriate, a wedge or rolled-up towel must be inserted under the right buttock or the operating table tilted to the left. Displacing the uterus manually to the left is a useful additional precaution.

VI. LOCAL ANESTHETICS

There is no evidence that local anesthetics are teratogenic. In general, local anesthesia in pregnancy creates no problems. Although local anesthetics rapidly cross the placenta, the blood concentrations in the fetus and neonate are usually low. Local anesthetic toxicity can occur, however, when large doses are used. Careful attention must be paid to the maximum recommended doses of local anesthetics to beware of inadvertent intravenous administration and to have resuscitative facilities available. Clearly, a toxic reaction with its associated derangement of maternal circulation could result in secondary fetal teratogenesis due to fetal hypoxia. The rare convulsive reaction to local anesthetics could give rise to fetal anoxia if prompt attention was not paid to the patient's airway. Anoxic episodes in the first trimester might interfere with fetal development (13). The doses of local anesthetics used for dermatological surgery are very unlikely to cause serious toxic effects unless they accidentally injected into a vein. Gormley (5) and Schneider and Webster (14) reported no increase in complications in pregnant women who received surgical treatment using local anesthetic.

Most of the local anesthetics have a certain basic formulation: an aromatic nucleus which is joined to the active amino groups by either an amide or ester linkage. Based on this linkage, the anesthetics are separated into two groups: the amide group and the ester group. Those most useful for injection are nearly all in the amide group, whereas the ester group contains some valuable topical agents.

Amide anesthetics	*Ester anesthetics*
Lignocaine	Cocaine
Mepivacaine	Procaine
Prilocaine	Benzocaine
Bupivacaine	Amethocaine
Etidocaine	Chloroprocaine

Drugs which cross the placenta may cause harmful effects to the fetus in many ways. The time of fetal exposure to the drug may be an important factor determining unwanted effects on the fetus and newborn. Placental transfer occurs principally by passive diffusion. The rate and degree is proportional to the total anesthetic dose administered to the mother but is dependent on the extent of the maternal plasma protein binding. It has been postulated that the higher the maternal plasma protein binding, the less toxic the drug may be for the fetus. The ratio between the concentration in the umbilical vein blood and that in the maternal venous blood is lower in the case of bupivacaine and etidocaine when compared with lignocaine and mepivacaine. In other words, the placental transfer rate is lower for bupivacaine and etidocaine. For this reason, bupivacaine and etidocaine should be considered as drugs of first choice (15). Bupivacaine is the most commonly used agent in obstetrical analgesia. Its principal advantage is a longer duration of action (2 hr) than other agents, relatively low incidence of fetal adverse effects, and clinical efficacy with low doses (16). Bupivacaine is safer than mepivacaine or lignocaine, because it is more highly protein bound, requires less frequent administration, and is more rapidly eliminated by the neonate (17).

Prilocaine has free placental transfer and was reported to have caused fetal methemoglobinemia, and it therefore should be avoided during any stage of pregnancy (18). Lignocaine, prilocaine, and mepivacaine are poorly bound to serum proteins and are therefore more toxic, have more extensive placental transfer, and are relatively unsuited to use in obstetrics.

Lidocaine (Xylocaine) is considered safe but easily crosses the placental barrier and in high doses causes decreased muscle tone in the neonate and abnormal neurobehavioral scores (19,20) as does mepivacaine.

Chloroprocaine, with its rapid metabolism and inactive metabolites, offers distinct theoretical advantages for pregnant women who have normal cholinesterase levels, although its brief duration and abrupt offset of action may be less than ideal (21).

Ropivacaine is the most recent amide-type local anesthetic which appears promising for obstetrical use. Its toxicity appears to be less than that of bupivacaine (22) and is not increased by pregnancy (23).

Epinephrine added to either lidocaine 1.5% (24,25) or bupivacaine 0.5% (26) to provide a concentration of 1:300,0000 has no significant adverse effects in pregnant women. The addition of epinephrine to the aforementioned drugs is considered to provide the following advantages: prolongation of duration of anesthesia and diminished placental transfer of the anesthetic agent from the mother to the fetus.

Fortunately, in the volumes and concentration used in dermatological surgery, local anesthetics are safe (5,27). Nevertheless, the dermatologist must be careful to use solutions with minimal amounts of vasoconstrictor injected slowly and after careful aspiration. With these safeguards, local anesthesia offers little risk to the pregnant patient.

VII. DRUG SELECTION IN THE PREGNANT PATIENT

Before, during, and after dermatological surgery, the dermatologist will often prescribe an analgesic, some form of antibiotic, or both in order to control pain and infection.

The U.S. Food and Drug Administration (FDA) has established a classification of the potential fetal risk of drugs (28) (see Chap. 9, p. 253).

There are very few drugs in FDA class A. Of approximately 600 compounds reviewed in a standard reference source (29), only 5% were placed in class A. This highlights the paucity of human data regarding the potential teratogenicity of the vast majority of therapeutic agents currently used.

Most drugs are classified in category C, which includes a statement that the drug should be given only if potential benefits justify potential risks to the fetus. Clinicians may overutilize drugs in class C, interpreting this designation as evidence of safety. The clinician should be cautioned not to view drugs in class C as safe. Such a classification should be interpreted as a warning that unknown adverse fetal effects may occur. Rely on those few drugs with a well-documented history of efficacy and safety and avoid administration of newer, inadequately investigated drugs. Only a few agents have been studied sufficiently to consider their usage as safe in the pregnant woman. Unnecessary or excessive medication of the pregnant patient should be stringently avoided.

Most drugs will pass the placental barrier. The agent ingested by the mother may directly affect the fetus (or its metabolites may be toxic) according to its distribution to or affinity for fetal tissue, or it may exert an indirect effect by interfering with metabolic processes in the mother. This results in the transmission of potentially toxic metabolites from mother to the fetus or embryo.

A. Antibiotics

Virtually all antibiotics cross the placenta to some degree (30,31). No antibiotic has been certified as safe for use in pregnancy by FDA, nor are adequate data available from comparative studies. Therefore, recommendations for antibiotic usage in pregnancy tend to be based on a long history of safe usage in pregnant women.

1. Penicillins (FDA class B)

Penicillins are among the most widely employed antibiotics for the treatment of common infections of the pregnant woman. Penicillin or its derivatives is safe and has exhibited no teratogenic effects when administered in the first trimester of pregnancy (32). No adverse effects on fetal development have been reported. Because these substances are quite safe, they are often the agent of choice in a variety of bacterial infections.

2. Cephalosporins (FDA class B)

Cephalosporins are widely used agents in obstetrics. They have a similar mode of action to that of the penicillins, and they do not appear to be teratogenic (33).

3. Erythromycin (FDA class B)

The estolate ester of erythromycin is specifically contraindicated in pregnancy (34). This drug is associated with hepatotoxicity (35). Erythromycin base, however, is relatively safe and without known teratogenic effect on the fetus.

4. Tetracyclines (FDA class D)

Tetracyclines are contraindicated in pregnancy, because they stain the deciduous teeth of infants by binding with calcium orthophosphates (36–38). Also, they deposited in long bones, producing temporary inhibition of long bone growth (39,40). Calcification of the deciduous teeth begins in the twelfth week of gestation, but the adverse effects of the tetracyclines are most prominent in late pregnancy. Fetal hepatic necrosis has been reported in association with azotemia and lactic acidosis in women given tetracycline in the last trimester (41).

5. *Sulfonamides* (FDA class B)

Sulfonamides should be withheld in the late stages of pregnancy. The drug crosses the placenta extremely well, competes with bilirubin for albumin binding sites, and thus raises serum-free bilirubin and increases the risk of kernicterus in the newborn (42,43). Sulfonamides may occasionally precipitate hemolytic anemia in the newborn owing to glucose-6-phosphate dehydrogenase (G6PD) deficiency.

6. *Clindamycin* (FDA class B)

Clindamycin is effective in the treatment of many aerobic and other anaerobic organisms. No adverse maternal or fetal reactions have been documented, but clindamycin does not enjoy the wealth of clinical experience that has been garnered with penicillins and erythromycin. The major contraindication to its use is an associated pseudomembraneous enterocolitis which could be fatal.

7. *Chloramphenicol* (FDA class C)

Chloramphenicol should not be used during pregnancy because it readily crosses the placenta and induces toxic effects on the fetus. In the neonate, especially the premature infant, normal doses of chloramphenicol may manifest a disease process known as the gray baby syndrome (44) with a resultant 40% mortality due to cardiovascular collapse (45).

8. *Aminoglycosides* (FDA classes C and D)

Gentamicin (C), kanamycin (D), and tobramycin (D) have not been associated with any teratological effects in humans. These drugs should be avoided, if possible, when the risk of ototoxicity is greatest. Hence, when necessary in the therapy of life-threatening infections, aminoglycosides should be administered in the lowest effective doses and for the shortest possible period of time.

B. Analgesics

1. *Aspirin* (FDA class C)

Aspirin is freely transferable across the placenta and is excreted by the newborn infant at a slower rate than in adults owing to immaturity of the excretory pathways (46).

Massive doses of aspirin given to pregnant rats cause congenital skeletal and eye defects (47). Many of the studies which claimed an association of the use of aspirin with congenital abnormalities in humans have been retrospective case-control studies. A prospective cohort study of more than 41,000 women found no evidence that the drug was a cause of fetal abnormality (48). Evidence linking ingestion of aspirin to fetal malformations is suggestive but inconclusive. However, in high doses in late pregnancy, aspirin may displace bilirubin in the fetal circulation from plasma proteins, and the free bilirubin is deposited in the basal ganglia causing the condition known as kernicterus (49).

Of more significance is the suggestion that aspirin may impair hemostatic mechanisms in newborn infants and predispose to intracranial hemorrhage in premature babies (50). Because of the possible teratogenic effect of aspirin, together with its well-documented adverse effects on hemostatic mechanisms when taken in late pregnancy, aspirin and other salicylates are probably best avoided in pregnancy.

2. *Paracetamol (Acetaminophen)* (FDA class B)

Paracetamol is much more widely used in pregnancy than aspirin and it seems to be generally safe. Studies in animals have shown no adverse effects on fetal or placental growth (51). This drug does not impair hemostatic mechanisms as does aspirin, and for this reason alone it is preferable for use in pregnancy. Paracetamol in normal dosage is recommended as the mild analgesic of choice (52).

C. Narcotics (FDA class B)

Some 70% of mothers receive intramuscular narcotics in labor, probably because of their simplicity of administration (53). The neonatal respiratory depression that can be the result of large doses of narcotic analgesics administered to relieve the pain of labor are well known.

Pethidine (mepiridine) is probably the most widely used narcotic in obstetrics, and it crosses the placenta rapidly and affects the neonate as well. Neonatal depression is most likely to occur when delivery is between 1 and 3 hr after an intramuscular dose of meperidine (54). It causes respiratory depression (54) and neurobehavioral changes in the neonate for 2–3 days (54,55) if given in too high a dose. Neonatal respiratory depression due to pethidine can be reversed by naloxone.

REFERENCES

1. L. Beeley. Adverse effects of drugs in the first trimester of pregnancy, *Clin. Obstet. Gynecol. 13*:177 (1986).
2. S. F. Malamed. *Sedation. A Guide to Patient Management*, 2nd ed. Mosby, St. Louis, 1989, p. 176.
3. T. H. L. Bryson. Anesthesia during pregnancy, *Preparation for Anesthesia* (A. J. Stevens, ed.), Pitman Medical, Kent, UK, 1980, p. 26.
4. A. G. Delaney. Anesthesia in the pregnant woman, *Clin. Obstet. Gynecol. 26*:795 (1983).

5. D. E. Gormley. Cutaneous surgery and the pregnant patient, *J. Am. Acad. Dermatol. 23*:269 (1990).
6. N. S. Assail. *Pathophysiology of Gestation*, Vol. 1 Academic Press, New York, 1972.
7. D. B. Scott. Inferior vena caval occlusion in late pregnancy and its importance in anesthesia. *Br. J. Anesth. 40*:120 (1968).
8. B. Howard, J. Goodson, and W. Mengert. Supine hypotensive syndrome in late pregnancy, *Obstet. Gynecol. 1*:371 (1953).
9. G. B. Drummond, S. E. M. Scott, M. M. Lees, and D. B. Scott. Effects of posture on limb blood flow in late pregnancy, *Br. Med. J. 2*:587 (1974).
10. M. M. Lees, D. B. Scott, M. G. Kerr, and S. H. Taylor. The circulatory effects of recumbant postural change in late pregnancy, *Clin. Sci. 32*:453 (1967).
11. B. W. Perriss. Analgesia and anesthesia, Prescribing in pregnancy (S. M. Wood and L. Beeley, eds.), *Clin. Obstet. Gynecol. 8*:475 (1981).
12. J. Sexton, K. Edelin, D. F. Booth et al. Surgery in the gravid patient, *J. Oral Surg. 36*:878 (1978).
13. J. M. Robson, E. Poulson, and F. M. Sullivan. Pharmacological principles of teratogenesis, *Embryopathic Activity of Drugs* (J. M. Robson, F. M. Sullivan, and R. L. V. Smith, eds.), Churchill Livingstone, London, 1965, pp. 21–35.
14. S. Shneider and G. Webster. Maternal and fetal hazards of surgery during pregnancy, *Am. J. Obstet. Gynecol. 92*:891 (1965).
15. L. Stern. *Drug Use in Pregnancy*, Adis Health Science Press, Sydney, 1984, p. 49.
16. F. Reynold. *Effects on the Baby of Maternal Analgesia and Anaesthesia*, Saunders, London. 1993, p. 58.
17. D. H. Ralston and S. M. Shnider. The fetal and neonatal effects of regional anesthesia in obstetrics, *Anesthesiology 48*:34 (1978).
18. D. F. Hawkins. Drug treatment of medical disorders in pregnancy, *Drugs and Pregnancy* (D. F. Hawkins, ed.), Churchill Livingstone, Edenburgh, 1983, p. 76.
19. L. F. Redick. Epidural analgesia, *Clin. Perinatol. 9*:63 (1982).
20. S. M. Shnider and G. Levinson. *Anesthesia for Obstetrics*. Williams & Wilkins, Baltimore, 1979.
21. F. Reynolds. *Effects on the Baby of Maternal Analgesia and Anaesthesia*. Saunders, London. 1993, p. 56.
22. D. B. Scott, A. Lee, D. Fagan, et al. Acute toxicity of ropivacaine compared with that of bupivacaine, *Anesth. Analg. 69*:563 (1989).
23. H. Pedersen, A. Santos, H. O. Morishima, et al. Systemic toxicity of ropivacaine in pregnant and non-pregnant ewes, *Anesthesiology 69*:A344 (1988).
24. J. J. Bonica. *Principles and Practice of Obstetric Analgesia and Anesthesia*, Davis, Philadelphia, 1967.
25. T. K. Abbound, S. David, S. Nagappala, et al. Maternal, fetal and neonatal effects of lidocaine with and without epinephrine for epidural anesthesia in obstetrics, *Anesth. Analg. 63*:973 (1984).
26. T. K. Abbound, A. Sheik-al-Eslam, T. Tanagi, et al. Safety and efficacy of epinephrine added to bupivacaine for lumbar epidural analgesia in obstetrics. *Anesth. Analg. 64*:585 (1985).
27. G. B. Winton. Local Anesthesia and Regional Anesthesia, *Complications of Derma-*

tologic Surgery. Prevention and Treatment (M. Harahap, ed.), Springer-Verlag, Berlin, 1993, p. 2.
28. American Medical Association, Dept. of Drugs, Division of Drugs and Technology. *Drug Evaluations*, 6th ed. *American Medical Association*, Chicago, 1986, pp. 41–52.
29. G. G. Briggs, R. K. Freeman, and S. J. Yaffe. *Drugs in Pregnancy and Lactation*, 4th ed. Williams & Wilkins, Baltimore, 1994.
30. D. Charles. Dynamics of antibiotic transfer from mother to fetus, *Semin. Perinatol.* *1*:89 (1977).
31. D. Charles and M. Mac Aulay. Use of antibiotics in obstetric practice, *Clin. Obstet. Gynecol. 13*:255 (1970).
32. O. P. Heinonen, D. Sloan, and S. Shapiro. *Birth Defects and Drugs in Pregnancy*, Publishing Sciences Group, Littleton, MA, 1977, p. 8.
33. G. Greenberg, W. H. W. Inman, J. A. C. Weatherall, et al., Maternal drug histories and congenital abnormalities, *Br. Med. J. ii*:853 (1977).
34. R. H. K. Barber. Symposium on drugs in pregnancy, *Obstet. Gynecol. 58*:42S (1981).
35. W. M. Mc Cormack, H. George, A. Doinner, et al. Hepatotoxicity of erythromycin estolate during pregnancy, *Antimicrob. Agents Chemother. 12*:630 (1977).
36. A. H. Kline, R. J. Blattner, and M. Lunin. Transplacental effects of tetracyclines on teeth, *JAMA 118*:178 (1964).
37. J. C. MacAulay and J. A. Leistyna. Preliminary observations on the prenatal administration of demethychlortetracycline HCl, *Pediatrics 34*:423 (1964).
38. T. J. Rendel-Short. Tetracycline in teeth and bone, *Lancet 1*:1188 (1962).
39. S. Q. Cohlan, G. Bevelander, and T. Tiamsic. Growth inhibition of prematures receiving tetracycline, *Am. J. Dis. Child. 105*:453 (1963).
40. M. Erikkson, C. S. Catz, and S. J. Yaffe. Drugs and pregnancy, *Clin. Obstet. Gynecol. 16*:199 (1973).
41. P. J. Whalley, R. H. Adams, and B. Combes. Tetracycline toxicity in pregnancy, *JAMA 189*:357 (1964).
42. P. M. Dunn. The possible relationship between the maternal administration of sulphamethoxypyridazine and hyperbilirubinemia in the newborn, *J. Obstet. Gynecol. Br. Commonw. 71*:129 (1964).
43. J. M. Dupuy, D. Frommel, and D. Alagille. Severe viral hepatitis type B in infancy, *Lancet 1*:191 (1975).
44. J. M. Sutherland. Fatal cardiovascular collapse of infants receiving large amounts of chloramphenicol, *J. Dis. Child. 97*:761 (1959).
45. C. F. Weiss, A. J. Glazko, and J. K. Weston. Chloramphenicol in the newborn infant: A physiologic explanation of its toxicity when given in excessive doses, *N. Engl. J. Med. 262*:787 (1960).
46. L. K. Garretson, J. A. Procknal, and G. Levy. Fetal acquisition and neonatal elimination of a large amount of salicylate. Study of a neonate whose mother regularly took therapeutic doses of aspirin during pregnancy, *Clin. Pharmacol. Ther. 17*:98 (1975).
47. J. Warkamy and E. Takacs. Experimental production of congenital malformation in rats by salicylate poisoning, *Am. J. Pathol. 35*:315 (1959).
48. G. Greenberg, W. H. W. Inman, J. A. C. Weatherall, et al. Maternal drug histories and congenital abnormalities, *Br. Med. J. 2*:853 (1977).

49. D. G. Grahame-Smith and J. K. Aronson. *Oxford Textbook of Clinical Pharmacology and Drug Therapy*, 2nd ed., Oxford University Press, New York, 1922, p. 154.
50. C. M. Rumac, M. A. Guggenheim, B. H. Rumack, et al. Neonatal intracranial hemorrhage and maternal use of aspirin, *Obstet. Gynecol. 58*:52 (1981).
51. D. K. Bloomfield. Fetal deaths and malformations associated with the use of coumarin derivatives in pregnancy, *Am. J. Obstet. Gynecol. 107*:883 (1980).
52. M. de Swiet. *Medical Disorders in Obstetric Practice.* Oxford, UK, Blackwell Scientific, 1984.
53. B. W. Perris. Analgesia and anesthesia, *Clin. Obstet. Gynecol. 8*:476 (1981).
54. S. M. Shnider and G. Levinson. *Anesthesia for Obstetrics*, Williams & Wilkins, Baltimore, 1979.
55. R. Hodgkinson and F. J. Husain. The duration of effect of maternally administered meperidine on neonatal neurobehavior, *Anesthesiology 56*:51 (1982).

11

Prenatal Diagnosis of Genodermatoses

Ingrun Anton-Lamprecht
Institute for Ultrastructure Research of the Skin, Ruprecht-Karls University Heidelberg, Heidelberg, Germany

I. INTRODUCTION

In this chapter, we discuss the prenatal diagnosis (PD) of severe, genetically determined disorders of the skin, or *genodermatoses*. In the context of the dermatological aspects of pregnancy. Our knowledge has been gained from 15 years of experience with prenatal diagnostic procedures performed in close cooperation between the gynecologist and dermatologist and based on fetal skin biopsy and morphological evaluation of fetal skin samples. In 1980 and 1981, when the first reports on PD of genodermatoses were published (3,19,35,41,68), fetoscopy had already been established for about 10 years (64,65), and intrauterine fetal biopsy had been proposed by Valenti in 1972 (82) as a means to obtain fetal tissue for analysis. Nevertheless, years were required before the innovative purposes of these techniques for genodermatoses were realized. This delay was caused, as usual, mainly by the lack of efficient transmittal of mutual interdisciplinary information and by the fact that dermatologists had not been aware of Valenti's report and gynecologists did not know about the needs for PD because of the severity of many genodermatoses.

Many risk pregnancies have been terminated in the past, solely based on high recurrence risks (25% for recessive disorders, 50% for dominant disorders in case one of the parents is affected), and many healthy unaffected fetuses have been aborted unnecessarily. Still, in 1978, "dermatological indications for interruption" (without previous PD) were the main topic of a dermatological congress in Germany (24).

At that time, only in some few genodermatoses were basic biochemical defects unsolved so far as to permit PD and identification of affected fetuses from the amniotic fluid. Examples are the alpha-galactosidase deficiency in Fabry disease (angiokeratoma corporis diffusum) or steroid sulfatase deficiency in X-linked ichthyosis. The great majority of genodermatoses, however, had not been gene mapped, and the underlying biochemical abnormalities were unknown.

On the other hand, the pathomorphogenesis of most of these severe genodermatoses is well known (4,7,9,11). Ultrastructural studies of large series of patients suffering from the various types of genodermatoses have led to the identification of distinctive morphological markers that are constantly expressed independent of biopsy site, age of the patient, or treatment. These ultrastructural markers are used routinely since many years for an early postnatal diagnosis, identification, and classification even in the neonate (2,9).

Finally, with the work of Holbrook (49,51,52,77), all the important aspects of the process and timing of normal fetal skin development and sequential differentiation has become similarly well known.

Thus, at present, fetoscopy as a safe means of obtaining fetal skin samples for analysis; the knowledge of normal fetal skin development, timing, and maturation; and an understanding of the specific pathomorphogenetic markers and basic defects of the genodermatoses serve as the pillars on which a reliable prenatal diagnosis is based. Currently only some few specialized international centers are performing this type of PD of genodermatoses.

In the past few years, tremendous progress has been achieved in the identification of the molecular biochemical defects underlying genetic diseases, and a steadily increasing number of disorders are being mapped in the human genome. In spite of this progress, only some few genodermatoses have been fully clarified with regard to their gene mutations on the DNA level, to structural and functional abnormalities of their gene products on the protein level, and to the subsequent phenotypic expression of the disease on the cellular (ultrastructural), tissue (histopathological), and organ levels. Some types of epidermolysis bullosa and some few dominant ichthyosis types are examples genodermatoses in which this progress has been made (1,30,31,37,40,57,62,63,69,71,80,81).

Even in those types of genodermatoses in which the kind of mutation has been identified, there is increasing evidence that each individual patient or family has its own specific mutation, that has to be determined separately for each case. Therefore, the application of molecular genetics in the prenatal diagnosis of genodermatoses is still restricted to some few disorders and here to some few selected cases. In the future, molecular genetics will permit to shift PD of genodermatoses more and more to early pregnancy (first trimester) and to use extraembryonic tissue instead of fetal skin.

II. PREREQUISITES OF PRENATAL DIAGNOSIS

1. PD of genodermatoses is no screening method. It requires a clearly defined genetic risk and the exact diagnosis and classification of the disorder (index cases!).
2. Fetal skin sampling is an invasive technique. Therefore, PD should only be performed if the severity of the disorder justifies termination of the pregnancy in case of an affected fetus. Mild disorders with a good response to therapy are no indication for PD, even if there is a high risk of recurrence (e.g., autosomal dominant ichthyosis vulgaris—50% risk; X-linked ichthyosis—50% risk for male pregnancies).
3. The underlying basic defects should be identifiable by morphological means as long as no biochemical or molecular genetic defects have been defined.
4. The basic defects should be expressed before the end of the time limit for legal interruption of the pregnancy to permit timely PD. In Germany and many other countries, this time limit is the end of week 22 of fetal life (normally corresponding to the twenty-fourth week of the pregnancy).
5. Personal experience of the investigator with the normal fetal skin development and ultrastructure as well as with the diagnostic criteria and specific markers of the genodermatosis at risk is indispensably required.
6. The fetal skin samples need to be of excellent quality to allow investigation at high electron microscopic magnifications, as most specific markers are only evaluable at the ultrastructural level and high resolution (see Section IV). The sampling procedure should, therefore, be restricted to the experienced fetoscopy specialist among gynecologists.
7. The at-risk family has to be informed extensively on the risks and reliability of PD in their specific case, in view of the severity and prognosis of the disorder at risk, to be able to decide early enough whether they can accept termination of the pregnancy in case that their baby is found to be affected. At present, prenatal or intrauterine therapy is not available for any of the disorders to be discussed in the following sections (42).

III. INDICATIONS AND TIMING OF PRENATAL DIAGNOSIS

Over the last 15 years, the main indications for PD have been for severe types of epidermolysis bullosa, various types of congenital ichthyosis, and ectodermal dysplasias. In addition, a series of other genetic skin disorders has been the reason for PD, but mostly only some few cases have been investigated (to be discussed later on).

As for obtaining fetal skin samples for analysis in PD, fetal skin biopsy has to be done in the second trimester; the exact timing within this period depends on the genodermatosis at risk and on the earliest and the optimal times of expression of the respective marker (see below).

With the development of modern molecular genetic techniques, such as the increasing mapping of the human genome, the establishment of large DNA libraries, the cloning of cDNA, the polymerase chain reaction for amplification of gene/DNA sequences, and the availability of highly specific polyclonal and monoclonal antibodies directed against specific structural constituents or synthesis products of cells, increasing numbers of gene mutations have been identified that underlie the genodermatoses of individual patients from each of the three major groups of disorders mentioned above.

Therefore, it has become more and more important to check carefully in each individual case whether PD is already possible with molecular genetic means and thus can be performed in the first trimester using chorionic villus samples, or whether morphological evaluation of fetal skin samples is required, in which case PD has to be performed in the second trimester. These alternatives are discussed in detail later in the context of the respective genodermatoses.

IV. METHODOLOGY OF PRENATAL DIAGNOSIS OF GENODERMATOSES

If molecular genetic data are already available for PD, chorionic villus (CV) samples serve as material for analysis. The specific methods of CV sampling and of molecular biology are not discussed further, as they are not the subject of this chapter. It will only be mentioned that depending on the disorder at risk and the protein in question, different specialists and laboratories have to be contacted; keratin specialists do not normally work with collagen specialists and vice versa.

A. Fetal Skin Biopsy

If analysis from the amniotic fluid or from isolated and/or cultured amniotic fluid cells is possible, fetal skin samples can serve as material for prenatal diagnosis by morphological means. Gynecological intrauterine sampling techniques (fetal blood, fetal skin, muscle or liver biopsy) have been available for many years (38,61,64,65). In brief, a trocar is introduced transabdominally into the amniotic cavity after local anesthesia of the skin, passing the abdominal and uterine walls and the fetal membranes, chorion, and amnion; here, the trocar itself is either exchanged against an endoscope, the fetoscope, or directly against the forceps (or needle) for tissue sampling. The fetoscope permits direct visualization of parts of the fetal body and skin. The diameter of the forceps determines the size of the skin samples. Forceps of too small diameter have proved to be unstable and therefore to be a high risk; forceps with a diameter of 1.7 mm have been found to be optimal

(38,55,61,64–66). In general, several skin samples per fetus are required for a safe PD.

The whole sampling procedure is performed under real-time ultrasound guidance. Modern ultrasound scanners with their excellent resolution allow omission of the fetoscope entirely. Amniotic fluid is collected in conjunction with fetal skin (tissue) and used for chromosome analysis, screening tests, such as AFP, ACHE, and others, and controls for microbial infection.

B. Handling and Preparation of Fetal Skin Samples for Light and Electron Microscopy

Fetal skin samples of the second trimester, even if obtained between weeks 20 and 23, are extremely sensitive to desiccation and any kind of mechanical stress and damage. It is therefore essential that they be removed from the tips of the forceps without squeezing. To maintain sterility of the instruments, samples are cleared from the tip of the forceps by floating them off into a sterile physiological sodium chloride solution, from where they have to be transferred immediately into fixation solution.

Fixation (3% glutaraldehyde in cacodylate buffer solution pH 7.4, 1% osmic acid in the same buffer), dehydration in graded ethanols, and embedding in epoxy resins are principally the same as for postnatal skin samples and have been discussed in detail elsewhere (9,14). Before final embedding and polymerization, the samples are subdivided into about three to four tissue blocks each to ensure their optimal utilization. Normally, the undivided skin sample is more or less round to ovoid, and well-oriented parallel blocks may be obtained after embedding in flat silicon molds.

Light microscopic investigations are performed on semithin sections and electron microscopic analysis on ultrathin sections of selected areas from these tissue blocks. In general, about 10–15 tissue blocks from a fetus at risk are investigated for PD. Sufficient experience is required for the evaluation and correct interpretation of fetal skin sections; pitfalls that might occur have been collected and discussed previously (12,14; see also Ref. 53).

C. Time Required for Prenatal Diagnosis from Fetal Skin

Preparation and embedding after receipt of the fetal skin samples require 2 days. Semithin and ultrathin sectioning can be performed after curing of the resin on the morning of the third day. Light microscopic examination (e.g., for ectodermal dysplasias) can be completed the same morning (about 51 hr). The electron microscopic investigation of ultrathin sections of course requires much more time. This depends on the difficulty of the diagnosis and on the number of sections to be examined. Generally, PD of epidermolysis bullosa can be completed on the same day (about 58 hr), whereas a risk for keratinization disorders such as congenital ichthyosis may require several days at the electron microscope, as in certain cases all areas with beginning keratinization have to be checked (20,21). Normally, PD is completed in the same week fetal skin biopsy has been performed (e.g., Monday to Friday).

V. DEVELOPMENT OF NORMAL FETAL SKIN IN THE SECOND TRIMESTER AS A BASIS FOR PRENATAL DIAGNOSIS

The detailed understanding of the normal fetal skin development that occurs in the second trimester of pregnancy, the most important time for PD, goes back to the pioneer investigations of Holbrook (49,51,52). At this period between weeks 12 and 24, all important structures, proteins, and markers—with some few exceptions—are principally organized in fetal skin. Later in the third trimester, these structures are mainly increased in number and gradually mature to reach the perinatal state.

Sections of well-oriented fetal skin samples obtained intrauterinely look like little mushrooms, more or less round, with a small "rootlet" where the sample has been pinched off by the forceps from the surrounding skin (Fig. 1a,b). The fetal epithelium, increasing from two to about five cell layers between weeks 12 and 20 or 21, covers a loose connective tissue with scattered fibroblasts, some indeterminate cells (lymphocytes, macrophage, and mast cell precursors), ingrowing small blood vessels, and accompanying unmyelinated nerve bundles (Fig. 1c,d). Small fat droplets appear at the subcutaneous borderline.

About week 20, fetal skin is still unkeratinized and covered by periderm cells that separate the basal cell layer and two to three layers of glyocogen-filled intermediate cells from the surrounding amniotic fluid (Figs. 1d and 2). *Keratinization*—the most important "invention" in evolution of vertebrates and thus also in the evolution of humans, permitted the passage of organisms from the aquatic to the arid, dry, terrestrial life at their transition from amphibia to reptilia—is not yet necessary for the 20-week fetus in its aquatic intrauterine environment. At the end of the second trimester, keratinization gradually begins to develop with first stages of cornified cells becoming visible around the orifices of the pilosebaceous follicles within the fetal epidermis and in the just developing hair roots (Fig. 1b,d). Between the twentieth and twenty-second week, the number of keratinized cells around the intraepidermal openings of the follicles increases, but the interfollicular epidermis is not completely keratinized before the twenty-fourth week in the beginning of the last trimester, when skin is no longer covered by periderm and principally corresponds to the skin of the neonate. Thus, this important step in pregnancy between the second and third trimesters is marked by the same transition

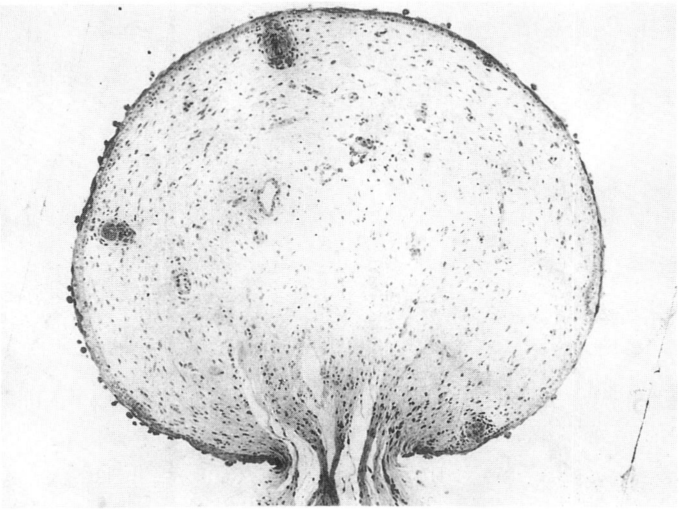

(a)

Figure 1 Normal fetal skin development in the second trimenon. Semithin sections of biopsy samples at weeks 16 + 1 (a), 17 + 6 (c), 20 (d,f), 21 (b), and 21/22 (e) show the increasing differential development of skin and appendages. Follicle primordia gradually grow down into the loose connective tissue (a,c) and keratinization is still lacking even in week 18 (c); large, well-developed hair follicles with keratinized root sheaths (b), distal hair canals (b,d–f), and hair shafts (e), sebaceous glands with sebum lipid synthesis (b,e,f), and sweat gland primordium (e) are revealed in samples from weeks 20 and 21. Interfollicular epithelium covered by periderm up to the end of the second trimenon (b,d,f) except focal areas with patchy onset of keratinization (e), where a granular layer and one to two horny cells are present in the interfollicular epidermis in part of the samples of an otherwise unkeratinized series. Unintended intrauterine sampling of amnion (f, top) together with fetal skin (f, bottom) permits comparative investigation of both types of epithelia and their junctions. Fetuses at risk of EB dystrophica (a,c), junctional EB with pyloric obstruction (f), restrictive dermopathy (b), autosomal recessive anhidrotic ectodermal dysplasia (d), and ichthyosis congenita (e), all born healthy. (b and d from Ref. 18.)

between unkeratinized epithelium and keratinized epidermis that marked the acquatic-terrestrial transition in the evolution of vertebrates.

The late appearance of keratinization-specific markers is the major problem in the prenatal diagnosis of heritable keratinization disorders or inborn errors of keratinization. Therefore, it is important to emphasize that only part of the severe keratinization disorders, such as congenital ichthyoses, may be identifiable prena-

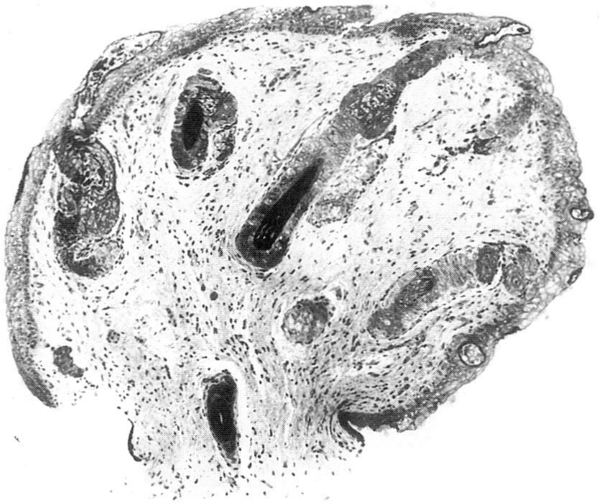

(b)

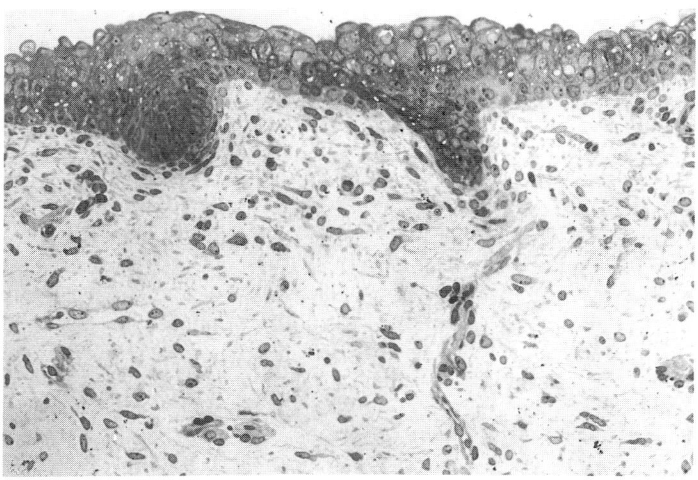

(c)

Figure 1 *(continued)*

tally. Other such disorders are not manifest before complete keratinization in the early third trimester, and false-negative diagnosis might result. Details are discussed below.

Another problem that might be responsible for false-negative and false-positive PDs is the fact that keratinization of the interfollicular epidermis starts in a patchy,

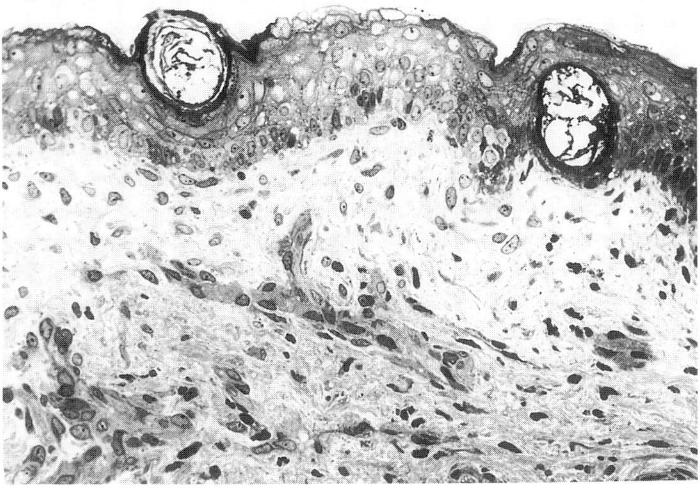

(d)

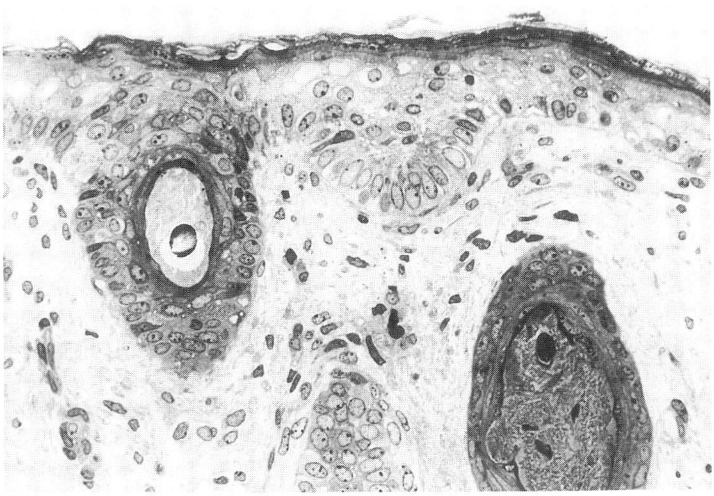

(e)

irregular distribution (Fig. 1e) that is independent from the well-established craniocaudal gradient of fetal development and maturation (12,13,18,20,21).

Finally, the keratinized portions of the distal hair canal and follicular openings may be running more or less horizontally or slightly tangential within the epidermis until reaching the surface of the fetal skin (Fig. 1b), as hairs normally grow

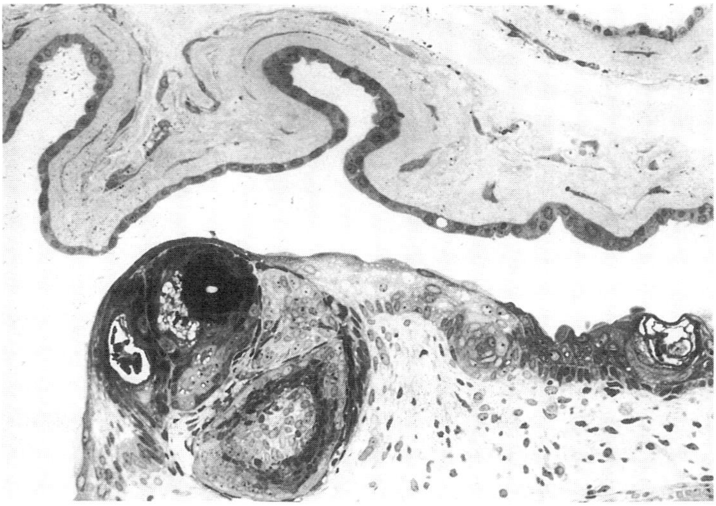

(f)

Figure 1 *(continued)*

downward from the epidermis in angles of up to 140 degrees (Fig. 1c) to enter tangentially into the epidermis (6,10,12,14). These horizontal, superficial keratinized portions of the hair canal may not be mistaken for an indication of a keratinization disorder (35).

In contrast, the borderline between the epidermis and superficial connective tissue, the *dermoepidermal junction*, develops at the transition between the first and second trimester and is complete about the twentieth week (Fig. 3), differing only quantitatively from the neonatal stage. It is this region where blister formation occurs in the various genetic types of epidermolysis bullosa (EB). Therefore, the severe genetic types of EB are identifiable from fetal skin samples with absolute reliability about week 20 or earlier (see below). Analogous junctions are already present in chorionic villi; the specific markers of EB, however, are not yet expressed in this early developmental stage, and therefore PD using morphological markers is not yet possible in the first trimester (44).

The *pigmentary system of the skin*, melanocytes and melanin synthesis, is again a late-appearing and a late-maturating part of fetal skin development. The ethnic background and the respective family-specific degree of pigmentation of skin, hair, and eyes significantly influence the time to which melanin synthesis and melanin transfer is first demonstrable in fetal epidermal melanocytes (Fig. 4) and hair bulbs. Prenatal diagnosis of *oculocutaneous albinism* (33) is therefore possible at an earlier fetal age in at-risk pregnancies from dark-tanning ethnic groups and popu-

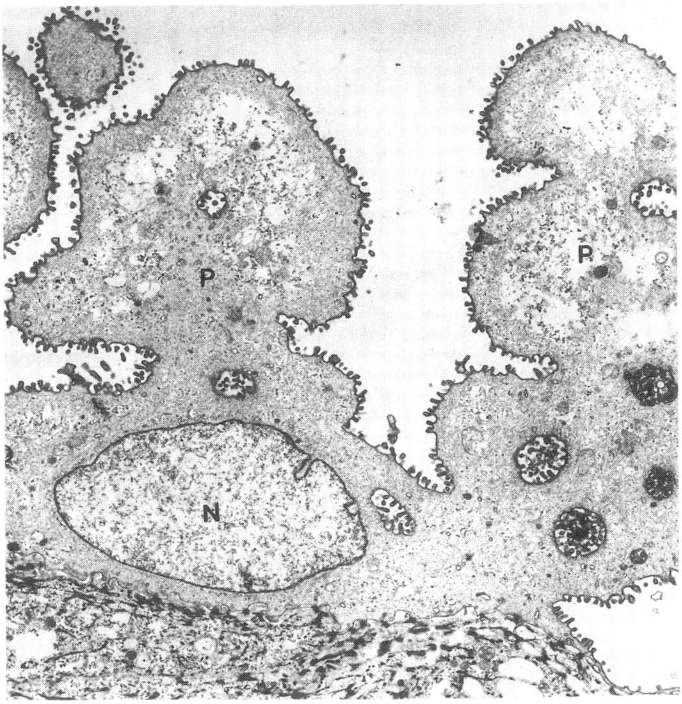

Figure 2 Periderm cell (P) covering the interfollicular epidermis of a fetus at week 20 + 4 (risk of EB Herlitz, born healthy) contains a nucleus (N) and is budding off into the amniotic fluid; microvilli on the cell surface covered with surface coat.

lations (African black, Japanese, Turks, and other Mediterranean groups) than in fetuses from fair (blond) northern European populations or families (see Fig. 7a, b in Ref. 13) using skin morphology (13). Application of the DOPA technique on the ultrastructural level to demonstrate the presence or absence of tyrosinase activity in fetal epidermal melanocytes was shown to facilitate PD of tyrosinase-negative oculocutaneous albinism (75). Meanwhile, PD may also be performed on the DNA level in selected cases by analysis of the fetal tyrosinase gene (76).

The *skin appendages*, especially hair follicles, sebaceous glands, eccrine sweat glands, and apocrine glands, develop gradually and consecutively at different times over a long period of fetal life. It is this special aspect of fetal skin development at which the craniocaudal gradient is most obviously pronounced (51,52).

Hair follicles with hair shafts and sebaceous glands are normally demonstrable in the fifth month (Fig. 1b,e). The degree of keratinization, however, is still low at about week 18. About the twentieth week, the intraepidermal portions of the hair

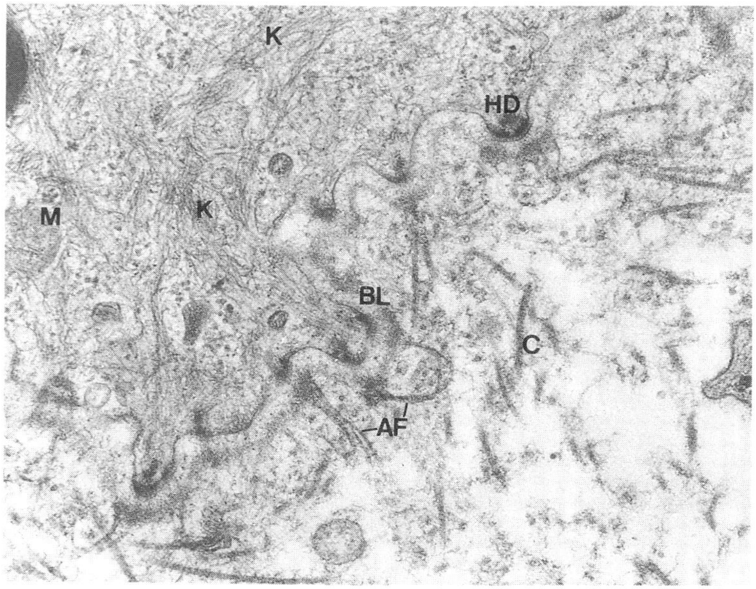

(a)

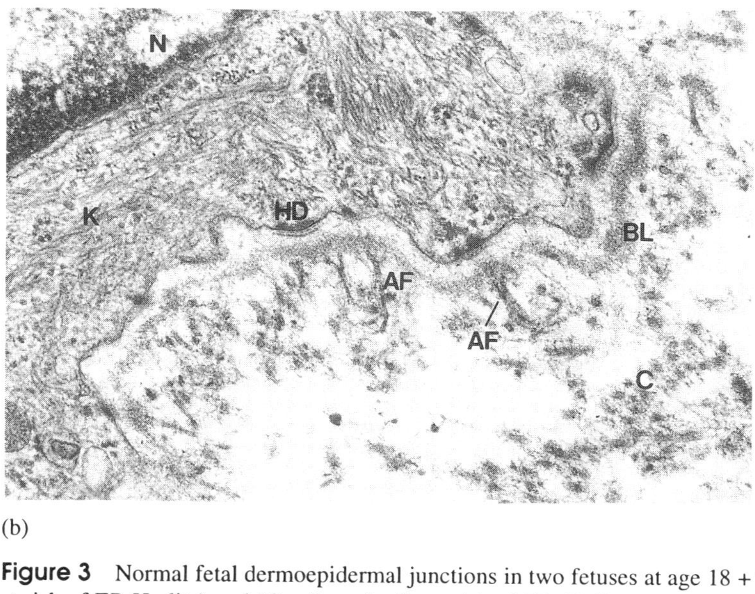

(b)

Figure 3 Normal fetal dermoepidermal junctions in two fetuses at age 18 + 7 weeks (a, at risk of EB Herlitz) and 19 + 7 weeks (b, at risk of EB, Hallopeau-Siemens type), both born healthy. The junction consists of hemidesmosomes (HD) with cytoplasmic attachment plates and clearly identifiable extracellular subbasal dense plates, the basal lamina (BL), and anchoring fibrils (AF) with specific crossbanding, interwoven with collagen fibrils (C). K, keratin filaments in basal cell cytoplasm; M, mitochondria; N, part of nucleus.

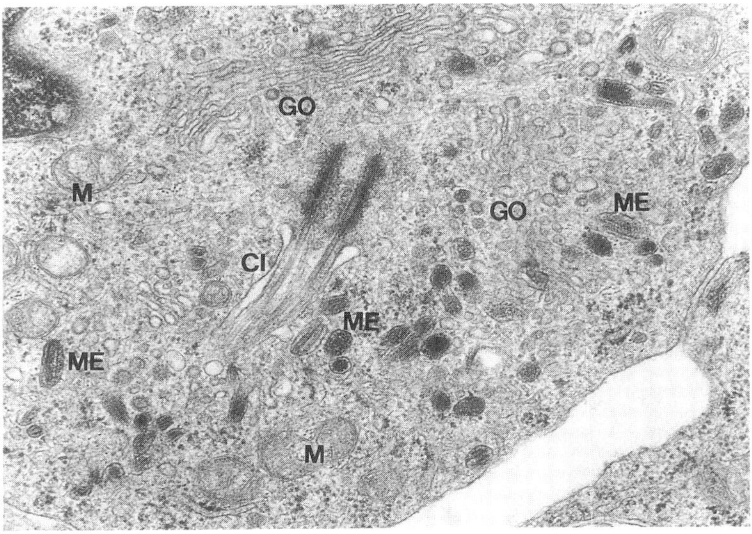

Figure 4 Fetal epidermal melanocyte at week 19 with intracellular cilium (IC) projecting downward from the centriol surrounded by Golgi bodies (GO) and many melanosomes (ME), some with beginning melanin synthesis (stages I–III). (Child well tanning with light-brown hair and green-brown eyes after birth, of German origin.) M, mitochondrion.

canal are keratinized as are the hair shafts and parts of the growing bulbs, and the sebaceous glands are already active in sebum synthesis with central cells filled with large droplets of sebum lipids (Figs. 1b,e,f and 5b). At the same time, primordia of the eccrine sweat glands just start to develop (Fig. 1e), whereas apocrine glands are not formed before the sixth month. Only on the palms and soles—locations that are out of the question for prenatal fetal skin sampling—are sweat gland primordia already developing at the end of the first trimester, 2 months earlier than in all other locations of fetal skin. This gradual consecutive development of the skin appendages has to be kept in mind in cases of PD for risk of ectodermal dysplasias (15,22,23). Lack of sweat glands in a fetal skin sample, for instance at week 18, may not be taken as indicating an ectodermal dysplasia in the fetus.

The differential development and maturation of fetal skin increases gradually and continuously from week to week in its complexity and may serve as an especially sensitive morphological marker of fetal age based on the many different component parts of fetal skin. Skin samples of weeks 17 and 21 demonstrate these significant developmental differences (Fig. 1a,b) that are, however, influenced additionally by factors of localization.

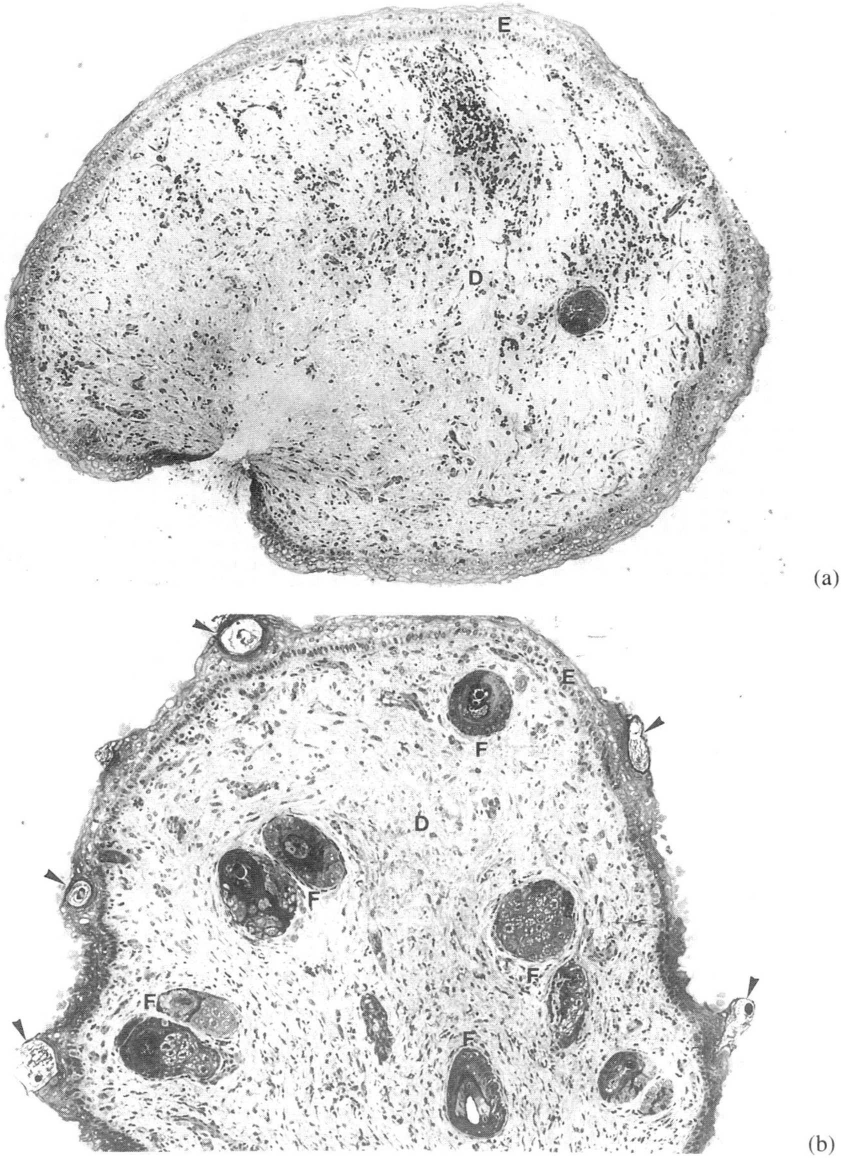

Figure 5 PD of anhidrotic ectodermal dysplasias. Skin sample of affected fetus lacks normal skin appendages and only shows one small follicular bud (a, X-AED, week 21). Safe prenatal exclusion is possible by demonstration of age-matched development of hair follicles with sebaceous glands (F) and of sweat gland primordia (b, R-AED, week 20). E, epidermis; arrowheads indicate keratinized follicular openings. (From Ref. 7.)

VI. PRENATAL DIAGNOSIS OF ECTODERMAL DYSPLASIA SYNDROMES

At present, experiences in the use of PD of ectodermal dysplasia syndromes have only been reported with the group of anhidrotic ectodermal dysplasias (AED) (10,12,13,15,18,22,23). Both, the X-linked recessive type (X-AED, in male pregnancies) and the autosomal recessive types (R-AED, in both sexes) can be identified or excluded prenatally from fetal skin. Affected fetuses are characterized by a more or less complete lack of hair follicles, sebaceous glands, and sweat gland primordia (Fig. 5a). Some few hair follicles, often of low developmental degree, may occasionally be revealed in fetal skin specimens (23). In risk pregnancies for AED, it is therefore necessary that a series of biopsies from various sites on the fetal skin be performed. The (light microscopic) evaluation of the whole series of biopsy samples normally permits a safe prenatal diagnosis or exclusion of AED in the fetus (Fig. 5), which might be impossible if only one or two biopsy samples are available. As patients with AED generally are not completely devoid of hair, fetal scalp biopsy might have the risk of a false-negative PD and therefore should be avoided.

Skin of affected fetuses often reacts to the biopsy trauma with formation of suprabasal clefts between the basal and the first intermediate cell layer in the central portions of the specimen (see Fig. 3b in Ref. 23). These clefts are artefactual but may be induced because of the lack of the normal strengthening of the fetal skin sample by the downgrowing hair follicles.

The gene for the X-linked form of AED, the Christ-Siemens-Touraine syndrome, is located on Xq11-21.1 close to the centromer (83). As far as possible, PD of X-AED is now performed in the first trimenon from chorionic villus samples on the DNA level by linkage analysis of closely adjacent X chromosomal markers. This requires informative marker combinations in the family of the at-risk fetus (84). In cases of remaining doubts, PD from fetal skin samples (about week 21) can be performed as an additional second step.

The autosomal recessive form of AED seems to be heterogeneous and to comprise several distinctive genotypes. The localization of the gene(s) for these autosomal recessive types on the chromosomal and DNA levels is still unknown. PD in at-risk pregnancies is restricted to the analysis of fetal skin samples in the second trimester (about week 21; Fig. 5b).

VII. PRENATAL DIAGNOSIS OF EPIDERMOLYSIS BULLOSA

Presently, the severest forms of epidermolysis bullosa (EB) account for the great majority of cases of PD since the very beginning because of their peculiar problems, early death in the lethal Herlitz type, and progressive handicap and multifold nondermatological complications in the severe but nonlethal mutilating Hallopeau-Siemens type.

Depending on the specific plane of blister formation, three large and heterogeneous groups of EB with more than 20 genetic types are to be distinguished: the EB simplex group with intraepidermal cleavage, the EB atrophicans group with junctional cleavage, and the EB dystrophica group with subepidermal, dermolytic cleavage (39). Electron microscopy and more recent results of molecular genetics have shown that the respective subtypes of the three groups of EB share common target structures subject to their gene mutations and basic defects that finally are responsible for the specific type of skin cleavage.

A. EB Simplex Group

Disturbances in the cytoskeleton of basal epidermal cells, the keratin filaments (tonofilaments), lead to an intraepidermal blister formation. These disturbances are caused by mutations in the basal cell–specific keratin genes K5 and K14 (on chromosomes 12 and 17, respectively). The position of the individual mutation within the keratin gene (K5 or K14) decides the resulting kind of protein abnormality. Point mutations (mostly single base exchanges) in the highly conserved N- and C-terminal portions of the rod domain induce clumping of basal cell keratins (37), which is the distinctive and unique feature of EB herpetiformis Dowling-Meara (4,7,9,11). Mutations situated outside these terminal portions (e.g., in the central part of the rod domain) induce other EB simplex types, such as the Koebner type (37), and cause instability of the keratin cytoskeleton (4,9,11,43).

These intraepidermal EB simplex types, the generalized Koebner type and the localized Weber-Cockayne type, are dominant traits. Exceptional Koebner-type patients with an autosomal recessive inheritance exist, in whom basal cells lack keratins entirely. This lack of cytoskeleton strengthening is responsible for blister formation in the cytoplasm of basal cells (7,9,11). In two such patients, the gene mutation and its structural and functional consequences have recently been solved independently at the same time (30,71). In our patient, born to consanguineous parents and suffering from EB and osteogenesis imperfecta (30), a homozygous point mutation (T to A transition) in helix 1B of the K14 gene leads to a premature termination codon and induces lack of measurable K14 protein (30). In normal basal cells, keratins 5 and 14 join to form heterodimers, the alignment of which leads to the final keratin filaments of the cytoskeleton (37). Although K5 is normal in our patient, lack of its natural partner explains the instability of K5 and lack of basal cell keratin filament networks and cytoskeleton function. In our Heidelberg material, 3 of 45 patients with the Koebner type of EB belong to this rare recessive subtype (11).

As yet, no experience with PD of EB simplex (Koebner and Weber-Cockayne) exist. Both types are mostly mild EB types with a good prognosis, and in such instances PD seems not to be indicated. As in most of the dominant Koebner types, no ultrastructural abnormalities have been identified before the onset of blister formation. It seems questionable whether such cases of EBS Koebner might be identifiable ultrastructurally in an affected fetus. In contrast, fetuses at risk of a recessive Koebner type such as discussed above should be identifiable with reliability from their lack of keratin networks in basal cells.

The Dowling-Meara type, EB herpetiformis, generally is much more severe than the dominant Koebner type and may be an indication for PD (4,5,7,9,11). One positive PD of the Dowling-Meara type has been reported by Holbrook in an at-risk fetus that clearly revealed the typical clumping of basal cell keratins (34,53). The Dowling-Meara type is much more frequently seen than the Koebner type and most other types of EB (5,9). In our Heidelberg material, it accounts for 13% of all EB cases identified by electron microscopy (EM) (76 of 616, December 1994).

B. Junctional EB or EB Atrophicans Group

The Herlitz type (EB atrophicans generalisata gravis) with its grave prognosis, and most rapidly lethal course is the most frequent genetic type of EB, at least among newborns with EB (5,7,9,10). Between 40 and 50% of all newborns suffering from EB may be Herlitz cases. In our Heidelberg material of a total of now 616 postnatal EB cases (December 1994), 110 have been analyzed to be Herlitz cases. With its severity, the lethal course and early death of affected babies, the Herlitz type is the most frequent at-risk diagnosis for which PD is requested (Table 1).

Various defects of hemidesmosomes and their constituents at the dermoepidermal junction (DEJ) have been identified in the group of junctional EB, inducing cleavage within the space of the lamina rara above the epidermal basal lamina (9).

Hemidesmosomes are important contact structures of basal cells facing the epidermal basal lamina of the DEJ (Fig. 3a,b). They have a complex organization. Ultrastructurally they are composed of the attachment plates on the cytoplasmic aspect of the basal plasma membrane, which are related to but not identical with the desmosomal plaques in which keratin filaments insert, and of filamentous extracellular constituents, the anchoring filaments and a specific interdigitation zone subjacent the attachment plates, the so-called subbasal dense plate. Anchoring filaments are also found outside of hemidesmosomes; they traverse the space of the lamina rara and insert into the basal lamina.

Biochemically various extracellular and intracellular proteins and glycoproteins were recently identified as contributing to the complex hemidesmosomal attachment device. Kalinin (nicein, laminin-5, or epiligrin) and K-laminin (laminin-6), members of the laminin family, are extracellular glycoproteins that are major components of the anchoring filaments, Kalinin, a heterotriplex, consists of three different subunits, the alpha3, beta3 and gamma2 polypeptide chains encoded by the genes LAMA3 on chromosome 18q, LAMB3 on chromosome 1q32, and

Table 1 Prenatal Diagnosis of Genodermatoses in Heidelberg

	Total	Affected
Cases of fetal skin biopsy, total (Dec. 1994)	209	
Risk for epidermolysis bullosa	111	35
EB atrophicans group	86	30
Herlitz type[a]	83	30
Herlitz type with pyloric obstruction	7	2
EB dystrophica group	21	5
EB dystrophica recessiva Hallopeau-Siemens	20	4
EB dystrophica dominans Cockayne-Touraine	1	1
EB, unclassified	4	—
Risk for keratinization disorders	37	14
Harlequin ichthyosis	11	2
Bullous congenital ichthyosiform erythroderma	5	3
Autosomal recessive ichthyosis congenita group	18	7
Type I	4	1
Type II	5	4
Type III	1	—
Type IV	1	1
Unclassified	7	1
Sjögren-Larsson syndrome	1	—
Chondrodysplasia punctata, rhizomelic type	1	1
Netherton syndrome	1	1
Risk for ectodermal dysplasias	15	3
X-chromosomal anhidrotic ED	10	3
Autosomal recessive anhidrotic ED	5	—
Risk for other genodermatoses	13	2(3?)
Restrictive dermopathy	2	1
Incontinentia pigmenti Bloch-Sulzberger	3	1(2?)
Chédiak-Higashi syndrome	1	—
Goltz-Gorlin syndrome	1	—
Ehlers-Danlos syndrome/cutis laxa	2	—
Leprechaunism	1	—
Ceroid lipofuscinosis, juvenile type	1	—
Infantile neuroaxonal dystrophy	2	—

[a]Including two twin pregnancies with two healthy fetuses each.

LAMC2 on chromosome 1q25-31 (57,80). Further hemidesmosome constituents are partly transmembranous, partly intracellular proteins such as the integrins (alpha6/beta4), and the two components of the bullous pemphigoid antigen. All their encoding genes may be candidate genes for the Herlitz type and other, nonlethal types of junctional EB. Application of monoclonal and polyclonal antibodies showed a lack of binding of antikalinin and of 19-DEJ-1, directed against another hemidesmosome-related epitope, in Herlitz cases (36,47,57,59). Recently, first mutations in the kalinin subunit genes LAMB3 and LAMC2 on chromosome 1q25-32 have been identified (1,40,62,63,80,81). Evidence is also increasing that integrins may be defective in junctional EB (40). Ultrastructurally, the Herlitz type is characterized by a mostly pronounced hypoplasia of hemidesmosomes, a lack of the specific subbasal dense plates within the lamina rare (Fig. 6a), and a lack of binding of antikalinin antibodies by immunofluorescence and immunoelectron microscopy (2,9,59).

Each of these criteria may be used for PD (5,6,10,12,13,36,47,53,67,80,81) provided that the respective marker proves to be valid in the index case. PD in early pregnancy demands a safe identification of the individual mutation in the at-risk family; this may often be difficult because of the early death of the affected infants. Molecular genetic analysis of closely linked or even intragenic markers bears some risk of false-positive or false-negative PD, as long as only indirect tests can be applied. A further difficulty is the larger number of candidate genes in junctional EB.

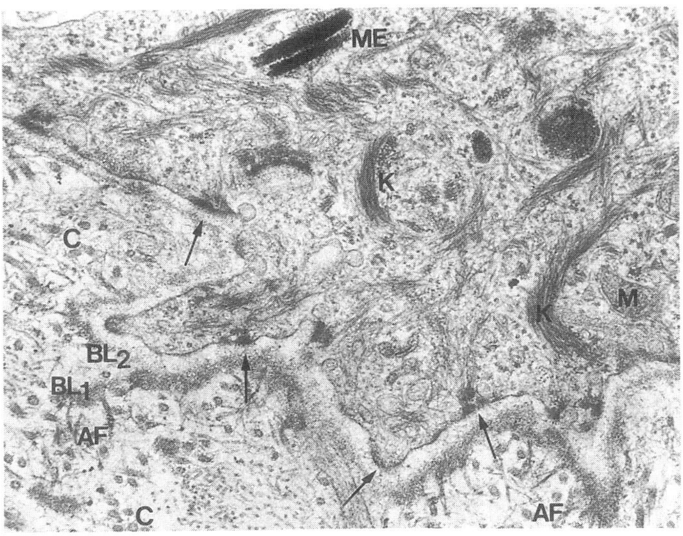

(a)

Figure 6 (a) Basic abnormality of junctional EB, Herlitz type. Basal cell and dermoepidermal junction of postnatal skin sample at 21 days of age with pronounced hypoplasia of hemidesmosomes (arrows) that entirely lack subbasal dense plates; focal detachment of old basal lamina (BL1) and subsequent repair (BL2) indicate repeated subclinical junctional split formation. AF, normal anchoring fibrils; C, collagen fibrils; K, keratin filament bundles; M, mitochondria; ME, melanin granule.

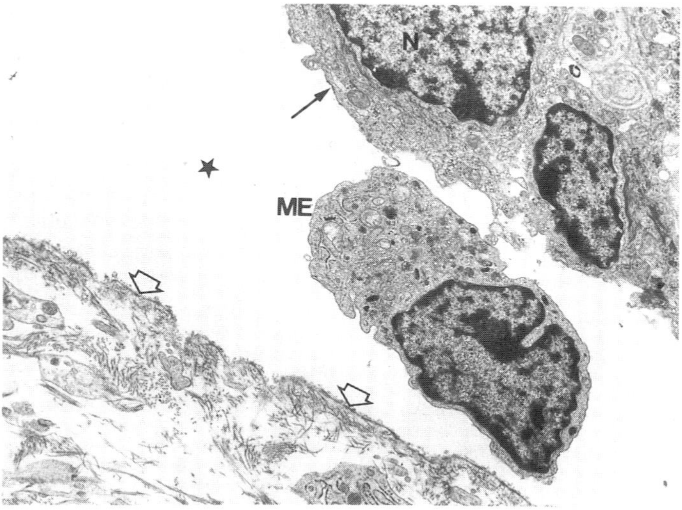

(b)

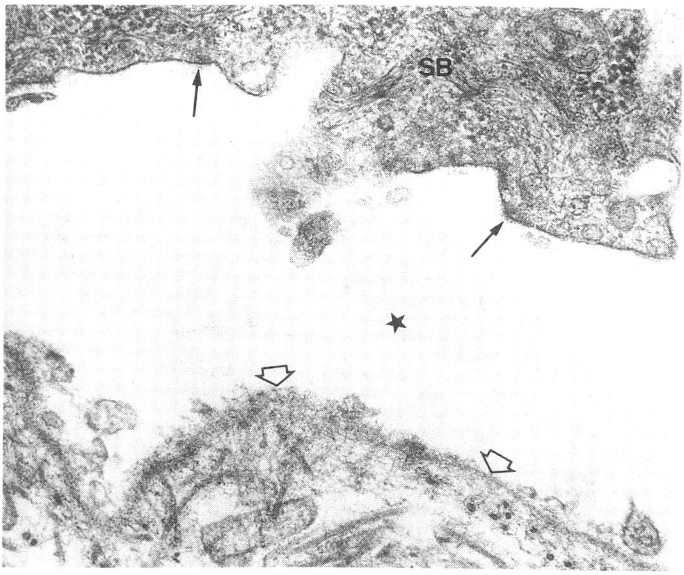

(c)

Figure 6 (b,c) Prenatal diagnosis of junctional EB, Herlitz type. Junctional split formation in affected fetus at age 18 + 0 weeks is the same as in postnatal skin with basal lamina and anchoring fibrils covering the blister floor (open arrows) and remnants of hypoplastic hemidesmosomes (arrows) at the undersurface of the blister roof. Melanocyte (ME) dropped out from basal cell layer (a) and floating in the blister cavity (*). N, nucleus; SB, basal cell.

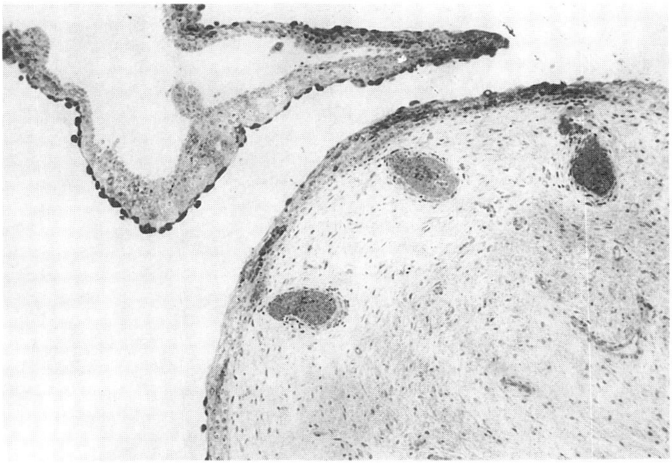

(d)

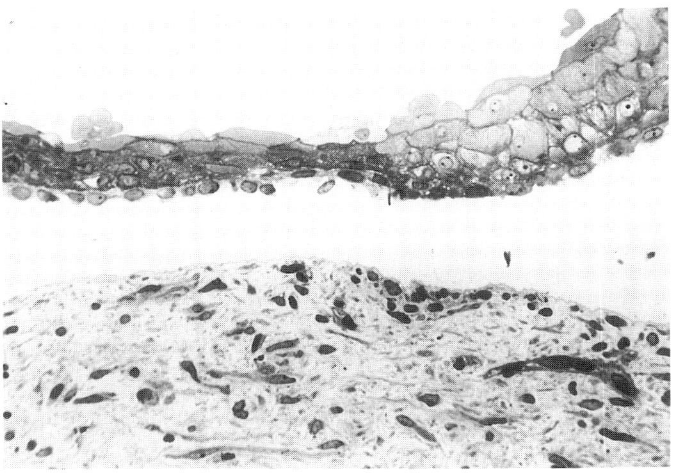

(e)

Figure 6 (d,e) Fetal expression of junctional EB, Herlitz type. Junctional detachment of fetal epithelium is induced by the pressure of the forceps and is more frequent in later stages (e, affected, week 20) than in earlier stages (d, affected, week 16 + 6, same fetus as in Figs. 6f and g); unsplit skin sample (d) at lower right and detached epithelium at upper left (d). Note low developmental degree of follicles in (d).

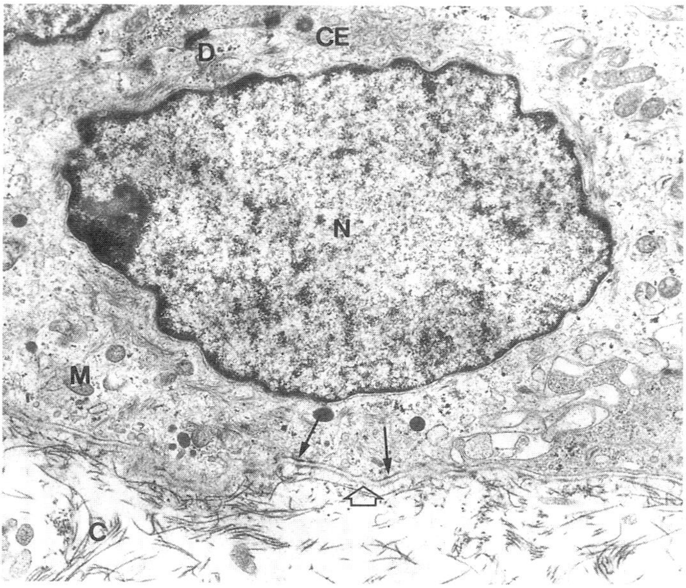

(f)

Figure 6 (f) Fetal expression of junctional EB, Herlitz type. Basal cell in unsplit skin sample of affected fetus at week 16 + 6 (same as in Figs. 6d and g) with normal general cell morphology and intact dermoepidermal junction (open arrows) with only some few hypoplastic hemidesmosomes (arrows). C, collagen; CE, centriol; D, desmosome; M, mitochondria; N, nucleus.

In contrast, the electron microscopic investigation of fetal skin samples permits us to identify the gene *action* on hemidesmosome ultrastructure and EB-specific blister formation immediately and directly even when the gene mutation itself is not known. Fetuses suffering from junctional EB react to the pressure of the forceps at biopsy with specific junctional cleavage (Fig. 6b,c) of more or less pronounced degree; this specific separation increases with age but may still be lacking—at least in part of the fetal skin samples—in fetuses at earlier gestational ages (e.g., weeks 17 to 20 or 21; Fig. 6d,e). It is therefore inevitably necessary to investigate the specific DEJ and hemidesmosome ultrastructure at high EM magnifications instead of relying on the presence or absence of blister formation alone. Affected fetuses show the same degree of hemidesmosome hypoplasia and lack of subbasal dense plates (Fig. 6f,g) as found in the index cases postnatally (5,7,9,10,12,13,18,27,66, 68). With the normal ultrastructure of the hemidesmosomes (Fig. 6h), the Herlitz type, and each other type of junctional EB, can be excluded with absolute reliability (3,5,7,9,10,12,13,27,56,74). Immunologically, antibodies that normally recognize

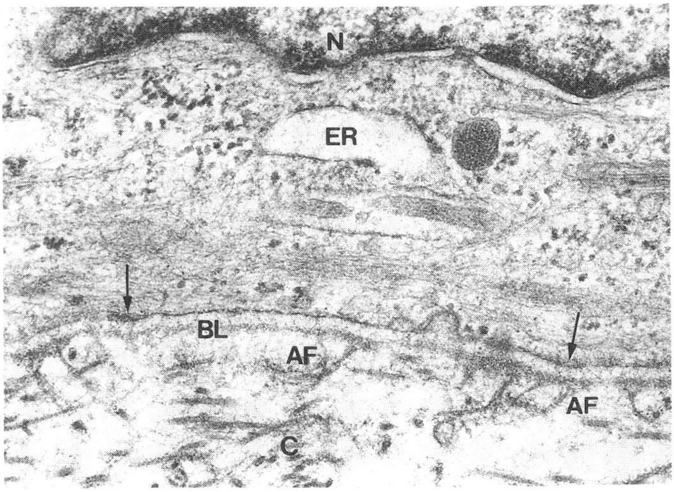

(g)

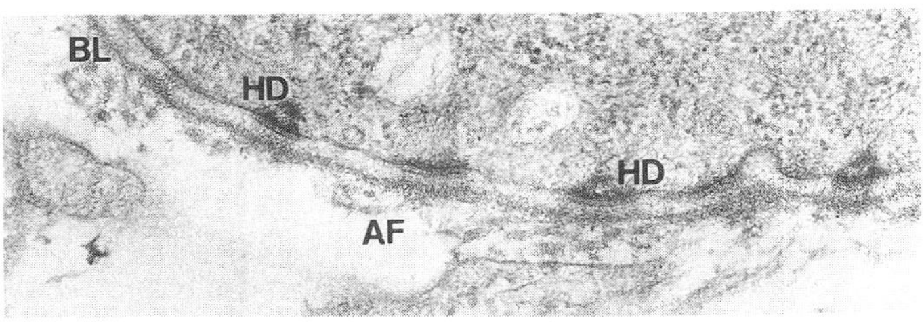

(h)

Figure 6 (g,h) Dermoepidermal junctions in fetuses at risk of the Herlitz type. Affected fetus (g, week 16 + 6, same as in Figs. 6d and f) with severe hypoplasia of hemidesmosomes (arrows). Normal ultrastructure of hemidesmosomes (HD) with prominent subbasal dense plates permits prenatal exclusion of the Herlitz type (h, unaffected, week 21). AF, anchoring fibrils; BL, basal lamina; C, collagen fibrils; ER, granular endoplasmic reticulum; K, keratin filaments; N, nucleus.

antigenes of the dermoepidermal junction (GB3, 19-DEJ-1) fail to bind to fetal or postnatal skin of junctional EB. They are used in parallel with electron microscopy for prenatal diagnosis (36,47,59).

The specific basic abnormality of hemidesmosomes is not only expressed in the skin, but also in the mucous membranes of various internal organs, which explains the wide spectrum of clinical complications. It has also been shown to be expressed in the same way at the epithelial-mesothelial junctions in the growing tooth buds of Herlitz fetuses resulting in attachment impairment of the enamel epithelium and focal junctional separation at the outer epithelium of the enamel organ, and thus inducing the pronounced enamel defects that are characteristic teeth of junctional EB (73). The "pleiotropic gene action" of the past can thus now be attributed to one single gene action on one specific gene product and structural component with essential function in many different organs.

In exceptional cases, PD of the Herlitz type can also be performed by EM analysis of amniotic membranes (Fig. 1f) where the gene(s) for junctional EB is(are) expressed analogously if no fetal skin and only fetal membranes are available (45,46). In the previously reported cases of PD from amniotic membranes (46), the failure to obtain fetal skin samples in two consecutive pregnancies (weeks 20 and 19) of the same family was mainly due to technical problems because of the obesity of the mother. In another case, the younger age (week 17 + 0) and higher mobility of the fetus together with an unsuited intrauterine position were the main reasons for failure. It should be noted, however, that epithelial detachment may occur in the amniotic membranes of healthy fetuses and that affected fetuses may not have any clefting in their amniotic membrane samples (46). The investigation at high EM magnifications is therefore also inevitable in cases of PD from amniotic membranes.

As mentioned above, the specific morphological markers of EB are not yet expressed in the first trimester in chorionic villi, and therefore PD is not yet possible by morphological means.

The first DNA-based prenatal exclusion of the Herlitz type of EB in an at-risk pregnancy was recently reported by Vailly et al. (81) using chorionic villus samples obtained in the tenth week of pregnancy.

Another biochemical approach to PD of junctional EB is demonstration of kalinin (laminin-5) in the amniotic fluid by Western blot analysis using a monoclonal antikalinin antibody (K140). Kalinin was demonstrable in the second-trimester amniotic fluids of 44 normal control pregnancies and was found to be biologically active in strongly supporting keratinocyte attachment. In contrast, kalinin was undetectable in second-trimester amniotic fluid samples from four pregnancies with Herlitz fetuses. In one additional pregnancy with a fetus affected with severe junctional EB (with pyloric obstruction, see below) and with positive binding of antikalinin antibodies to fetal skin, kalinin was normally demonstrable in the amniotic fluid (58).

C. Junctional EB with Pyloric Obstruction

Children with the Herlitz type of EB and the milder, nonlethal types of junctional EB (39) normally are born at term and often with normal-appearing skin. They start to get blisters only after they are handled and at first clinical examinations some hours after birth. Severer cases may be born with blisters and epithelial defects, often especially on the lower legs.

One subtype of junctional EB, however, is characterized by premature birth (about week 34/35), large and long-standing epithelial defects, mostly mistaken as aplasia cutis congenita, and obstruction of the pylorus, often also of the duodenal and/or esophagial tract. All carefully investigated cases revealed junctional blister formation and an exceptionally pronounced hypoplasia of hemidesmosomes (6,9, 27,36,74). However, anchoring filaments are normally expressed in the lamina rara and the DEJ, and immunologically kalinin antibodies bind normally to the junction zone (59). This type of junctional EB may be due to mutations in one of the other candidate genes, integrins, or bullous pemphigoid antigenes. Prenatal diagnosis and prenatal exclusion have been performed using EM and immunofluorescence data (6,9,10,27,36,74). In our Heidelberg material, prenatal diagnosis was performed in seven pregnancies at risk of EB of the Herlitz type with pyloric obstruction with two fetuses found to be affected (Table 1). One of these fetuses was later investigated by immunological means and found to lack binding of 19-DEJ-1 (36).

D. EB Dystrophica Group, Scarring EB

Autosomal recessive and dominant types of scarring EB are classified in the dystrophic EB group. The most important and also most frequent type in this group is the recessive Hallopeau-Siemens type, which has a broad range of severities from mild localized to generalized but nonmutilating to severe mutilating subtypes. Normally nonlethal, the mutilating Hallopeau-Siemens type represents the severest form of EB because of its many complications: With synechiae (bridge-scarring) and mutilations, leading to "mitten" hands and feet; esophageal stenosis; anemia; kidney involvement (glomerulonephritis); and risk for amyloidosis and scar carcinoma, affected individuals are increasingly handicapped, and early invalidity is the rule (39). The survival of patients (in contrast to the lethal Herlitz type) and the necessity for intensive, demanding care of affected children may explain why parents hesitate to face another pregnancy. Although with nearly 30% of all newborns with EB, one of the most frequent types of EB, the Hallopeau-Siemens type nonetheless ranges far behind the Herlitz type in PD not only in our Heidelberg series (3,5,10,18; Table 1), but also internationally (27,34,53; Dr. C. W. Chow, Melbourne, Australia, personal communication). No doubt exists regarding the indication for PD, and the Hallopeau-Siemens type of EB therefore belongs to the first cases of a proven PD from fetal skin samples (19).

Similarly, PD may be justified for the recessive inversa type of dystrophic EB (39); no experience has been reported as yet. Apart from these severe recessive types of dystrophic EB, some dominant types (39) may be so severe that PD is indicated as well. This may especially apply to the Pasini type (17).

All these types of dystrophic EB are characterized by defects of the anchoring fibrils of different degrees. Anchoring fibrils are important bandlike contact structures of the DEJ connecting the epidermal basal lamina with the papillary connective tissue (Fig. 3a,b). They consist of triple helices of three identical (alpha1) protein chains of collagen VII that form dimers by means of a C-terminal overlap. Dimers then aggregate laterally to form the ultrastructurally visible anchoring fibrils. With their N-terminal they insert in the epidermal basal lamina (57).

Defects of the anchoring fibrils are responsible for the specific cleavage plane below the basal lamina (9,17,26,57), which in turn causes scarring after wound healing and leads to dystrophic EB (39). The gene for collagen VII, COL7A1, located on chromosome 3p21.1, therefore is the candidate gene for all types of dystrophic EB. Linkage analysis of families with recessive and dominant types (54,72) and recent DNA-based mutation analyses (80) have confirmed this relationship, which was first demonstrated on the ultrastructural level (17,26). Point mutations have been identified in most of the cases analyzed so far (80; Christiano 1994, personal communication). In cases of the severe recessive forms, they mostly lead to premature termination codons, to early termination of collagen VII synthesis, and thus to a lack of anchoring fibrils. In dominant types, amino acid substitutions, mostly of glycine, were found that possibly lead to an instable protein structure and rapid destruction of preformed anchoring fibrils under mechanical stress and trauma (80).

In the fetal skin, anchoring fibrils are synthesized before the twelfth week, although at first in very low amounts (49,51,52). With the end of the fourth month, the amount and ultrastructure of anchoring fibrils (Figs. 3 and 7a,b) allow clear and reliable statements on whether or not a fetus in an at-risk pregnancy is affected (3). Fetuses suffering from dystrophic EB present with the same ultrastructural abnormality of anchoring fibrils (Fig. 7a) and back of binding of anticollagen VII antibodies as found postnatally in the respective index case. Owing to the pressure of the forceps at biopsy, cleavage in the specific subepidermal plane is induced (Fig. 7c,d) and increasing with age between weeks 16 and 20 (3,5,10,12,13,19). Good EB skin samples obtained about weeks 16–17 may lack such specific cleavage entirely (cf. Figs. 1a and 6d). Careful ultrastructural analysis of the DEJ at high EM magnifications is inevitably required to avoid a false-negative diagnosis (Fig. 7b) (18). In healthy fetuses, unspecific splitting may be induced in fetal skin samples at biopsy as well; therefore cleavage also has to be controlled at high EM magnifications for the specific cleavage plane of EB (Fig. 7c,d) to avoid a false-positive PD (14).

DNA-based PD in early pregnancy (first trimester) is becoming increasingly available and possible in all those families in whom the underlying gene mutation has already been identified (55,78). Recent experiences have, however, shown that PD by DNA-based linkage analysis, even with the use of intragenic markers, should be controlled in case of a positive result in a second step by EM analysis of fetal skin samples to check for direct gene action as long as the mutation itself has not yet been identified. In such a case of PD by means of DNA-based linkage analysis, the fetus at risk of the Hallopeau-Siemens type of EB had the same intragenic marker combination as found in the affected sibling, indicating the fetus to be affected. Unexpectedly, control of the fetal skin before planned termination of the pregnancy

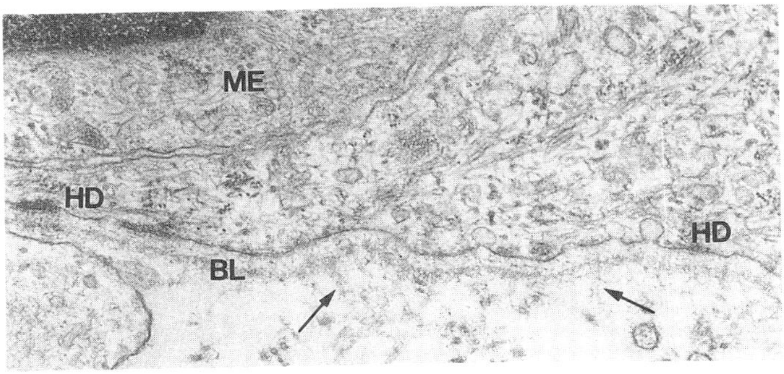

(a)

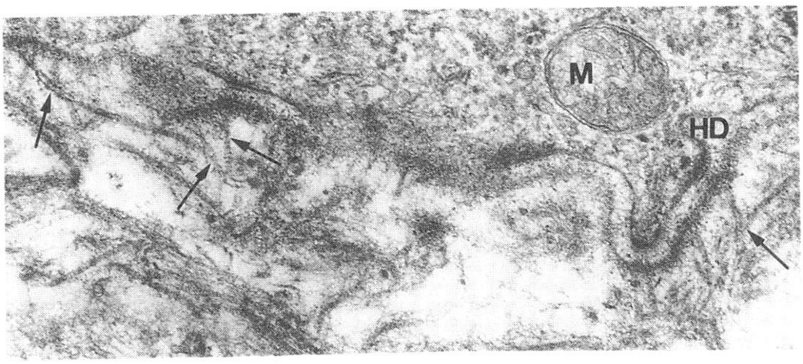

(b)

Figure 7 (a,b) Prenatal diagnosis of dystrophic EB, Hallopeau-Siemens type. Affected fetuses (a, week 21, same fetus as in Figs. 7c and d) show the same degree of defective anchoring fibrils (arrows) as found in the respective index case. Demonstration of normal amount and ultrastructure of anchoring fibrils (arrows in b) permits safe prenatal exclusion of dystrophic EB (b, week 16 + 1, same fetus as in Fig. 1a; DNA-based linkage analysis had indicated EB in this fetus, but subsequent EM of fetal skin samples revealed the fetus to be unaffected; born healthy at term; see text). BL, basal lamina; HD, hemidesmosomes; M, mitochondria; ME, melanocyte.

revealed a completely normal ultrastructure of the fetal DEJ and anchoring fibrils in week 16 + 1 (Figs. 1a and 7b) and demonstrated that the fetus was healthy and not affected with EB (Anton-Lamprecht et al. and Christiano et al., in prep.).

VIII. PRENATAL DIAGNOSIS OF KERATINIZATION DISORDERS

The main indications for PD predominantly concern congenital ichthyoses with generalized, severe disturbances of keratinization and dominant or recessive inheritance.

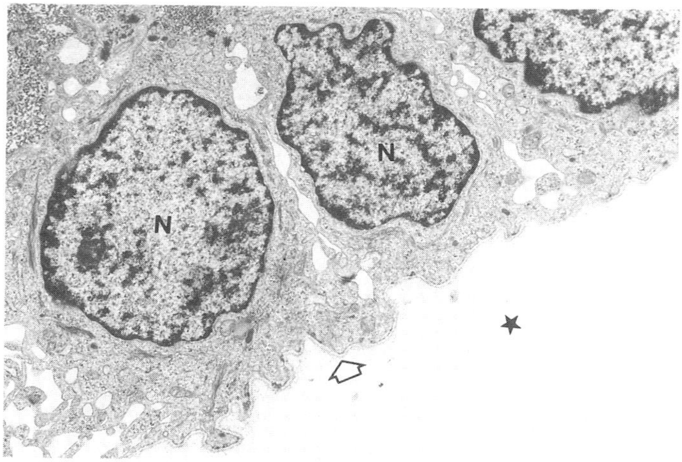

(c)

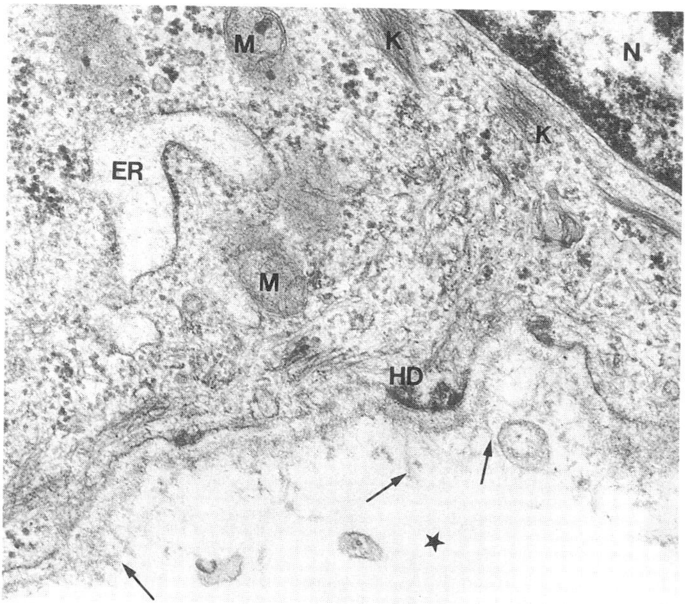

(d)

Figure 7 (c,d) Fetal expression of dystrophic EB, Hallopeau-Siemens type. Specific split formation below the basal lamina that remains at the undersurface of the blister roof (c, open arrow). This split occurs exactly in the plane of the defective anchoring fibrils (d, arrows) underneath the basal lamina (fetus affected, same as in Fig. 7a, week 21). ER, granular endoplasmic reticulum; HD, hemidesmosomes; K, keratin filaments; M, mitochondria; N, nuclei of basal cells; asterisk, blister cavity.

As discussed earlier in this chapter, keratinization is one of the fetal developmental processes with the latest onset and is complete only at the end of the second trimester (weeks 24–26), which is after the time limit for legal abortion (about week 24). Therefore, only those types of congenital ichthyosis can be diagnosed or safely excluded prenatally that are characterized by the expression of specific morphological markers at a sufficiently early stage of fetal development. This is the case for some of the dominant congenital ichthyosis types, such as bullous congenital ichthyosiform erythroderma of Brocq (or epidermolytic hyperkeratosis), as well as for some, but by far not for all, of the recessive types (nonbullous congenital ichthyosis) (3,8,10,20). Moreover, the timing of fetal skin sampling depends on the respective type of ichthyosis. The exact diagnosis and classification of index cases is therefore an essential and significant prerequisite in cases of pregnancies at risk for congenital ichthyosis.

A. Bullous Congenital Ichthyosiform Erythroderma (Brocq Ichthyosis or Epidermolytic Hyperkeratosis)

Patients suffering from this dominant ichthyosis type have a 50% recurrence risk for their offspring. The mostly pronounced severity justifies PD in at-risk pregnancies. The genes responsible have an especially high mutation rate (see below): Many of the patients represent spontaneous dominant new mutations. Healthy parents of an infant affected with this ichthyosis type do not have an increased risk of recurrence for their further children. Therefore, PD is only indicated if one of the parents is affected.

Bullous congenital ichthyosiform erythroderma of Brocq (bullous CIE) is characterized by an aggregation and clumping of suprabasal keratins, which is completely comparable to that of EB of the Dowling-Meara type: In the EB type, the low molecular weight keratins of basal cells (K5, K14) are involved; in bullous CIE, higher molecular weight keratins of suprabasal cells (K1, K10) undergo clumping (4,9,11). In the newborn such bullous CIE cytolysis and suprabasal blister formation predominate. Vulnerability and blister formation decrease gradually in parallel with the compensatory formation of hyperkeratoses with increasing age. The main differences between both dominant disorders are the groups of keratins and cell layers involved: The result of basal keratin clumping is an epidermolysis bullosa, whereas suprabasal keratin clumping induces a congenital type of ichthyosis (11).

Affected fetuses (three of five in our Heidelberg series, all from one family; Table 1) present with the typical suprabasal cytolysis between weeks 18 and 22 (Fig. 8a), whereas the specific keratin clumping only becomes evident with the onset of keratinization. It may therefore still be missing in diagnostic fetal skin samples from the trunk (3). At the same time, massive hyperkeratoses begin to develop on the palms and soles (Fig. 8b) with their much earlier developmental

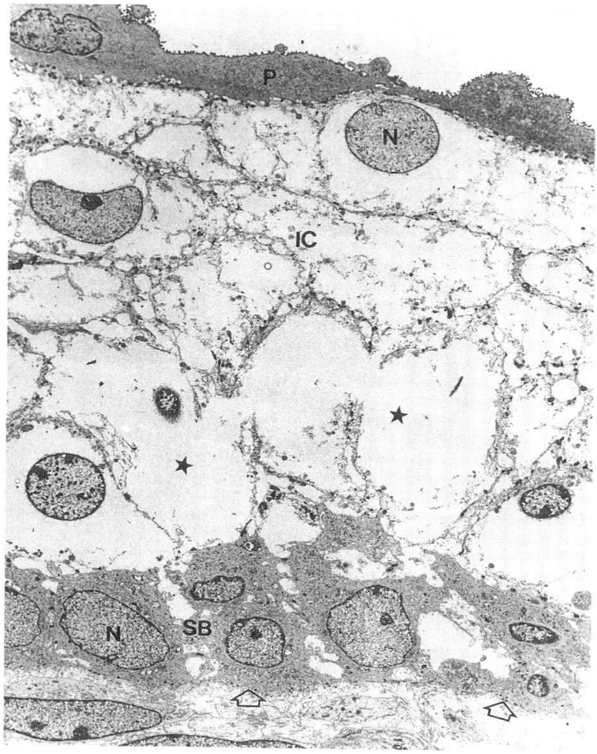

(a)

Figure 8 Fetal expression of bullous CIE. Normal basal cells (SB) and pronounced cytolysis (*) of suprabasal intermediate cells (IC) characterize affected fetuses (a and b). Fetal back skin (a, week 19) is yet unkeratinized and covered by periderm cells (P) and still lacks the specific keratin clumping, while plantar (b) and palmar skin (c) is keratinized, has already developed significant hyperkeratosis of the horny layer (SC) and a prominent granular layer (SG) with large keratohyalin granules (KH) at about the same time, and reveals the specific clumping of suprabasal keratins (arrows). b and c, fetus at 22 weeks, after termination, sibling of (a). D, desmosomes; N, nuclei.

timing (see Section V). Such samples reveal the specific aggregation of suprabasal keratins (Fig. 8c) (8,10[Fig. 7a–d],12,13,18). In fetal skin samples, PD of this severe dominant ichthyosis form is possible from about the eighteenth week (3,4,8–10,12,13,18,21,41,48,53,66).

In some, but not all, pregnancies with affected fetuses, amniotic fluid cells originating from the fetal epidermis express the specific keratin clumping (48,53).

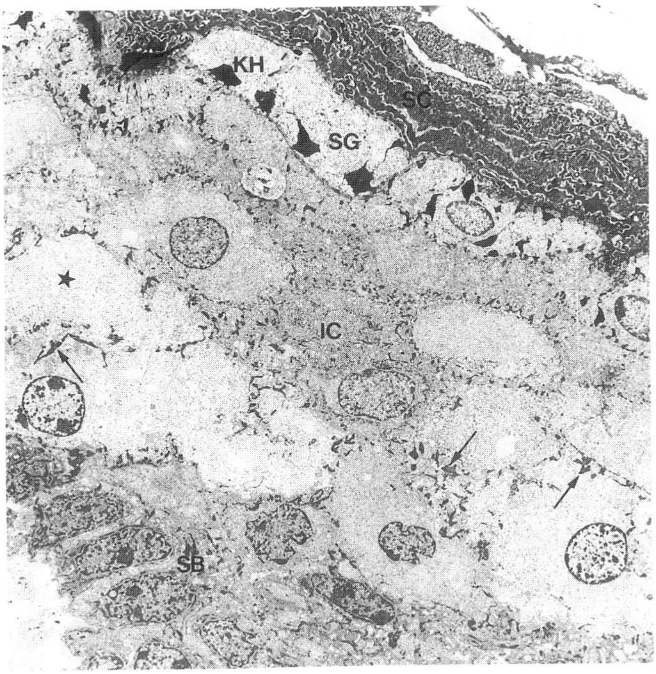

(b)

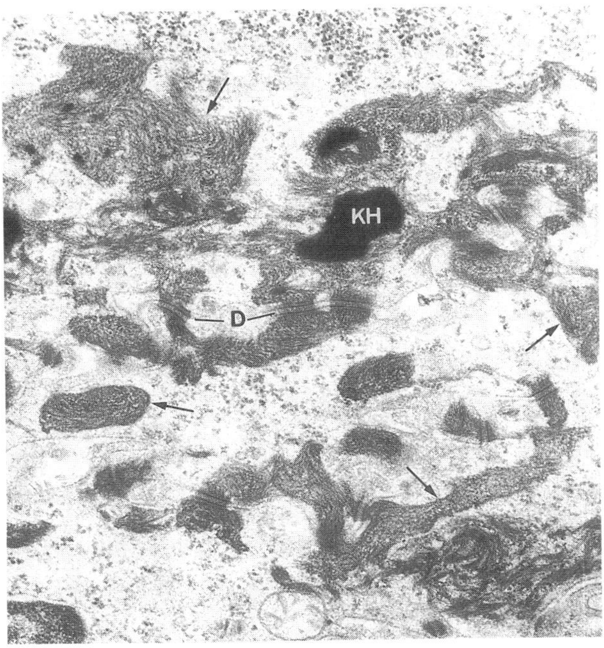

(c)

As this is not the case in every amniotic fluid cell sample of affected fetuses (4), lack of clumping in cells obtained by amniocentesis may not be taken as a guarantee for safe exclusion of bullous CIE, and amniocentesis alone is not suited for a safe and always reliable PD. Amniotic fluid samples obtained in conjunction with fetal skin sampling may, however, serve as a valuable supplemental diagnostic aid.

By molecular genetic analysis of patients with bullous CIE, mutations in the genes for keratin 1 and keratin 10 have been identified that constantly are localized in so-called hot spots in the highly conserved N- and C-terminal segments of the rod domain (triple helical region) (31,37,69). In the same hot spots of the genes for keratin 5 and 14, the mutations underlying EB herpetiformis Dowling-Meara are localized (37). In the future, in all those cases where the underlying mutation has been clearly identified, a prenatal diagnosis will be possible in early pregnancy (first trimester); as yet, no studies exist.

B. Ichthyosis Congenita Gravis, Harlequin Ichthyosis

This autosomal recessive keratinization disorder is the severest, almost always lethal form of congenital ichthyosis. Affected children are born prematurely at about weeks 32–34 with armourlike hyperkeratoses and deep fissures covering the entire skin. Severe ectropion and eclabium, grossly abnormal facial appearance, lack of helix development of the outer ear, dermatogenic contractures of large and small joints of the limbs, and edema of the hands and feet develop in consequence of the increasing thickness of the hyperkeratoses. Most of the affected infants die within a few hours or days, mostly because of respiratory distress. Spontaneous survival has been observed in some exceptional cases. Such children develop a severely scaling erythrodermic ichthyosis after shedding of the horn masses present at birth. In view of the severity of this disorder, no doubt exists regarding an indication for PD (8–10,25).

The underlying basic defects of the form of ichthyosis are unknown on the biochemical as well as on the molecular genetic and DNA levels. In contrast, the ultrastructural expression is well defined and permits an unequivocal diagnosis not only postnatally, but prenatally in risk pregnancies as well. The target structures of this basic defect are the keratinosomes (Odland bodies, or lamellar granules), which in the upper epidermal layers accumulate the epidermal barrier lipids (Fig. 9c [inset]) that are then discharged into the intercellular spaces of the horny layer. After transformation into nonpolar lipid sheets, these barrier lipids form the intercellular "mortar" between the "bricks" of horn cells that together act as a highly effective barrier against transepidermal water loss and penetration of water-soluble substances from the environment into the skin. In children with harlequin ichthyosis, keratinosomes display the primary defect of the disorder: Although many vesicular keratinosomes are formed in the uppermost living epidermal cells, no barrier lipids are synthesized; instead these defective vesicular keratinosomes are

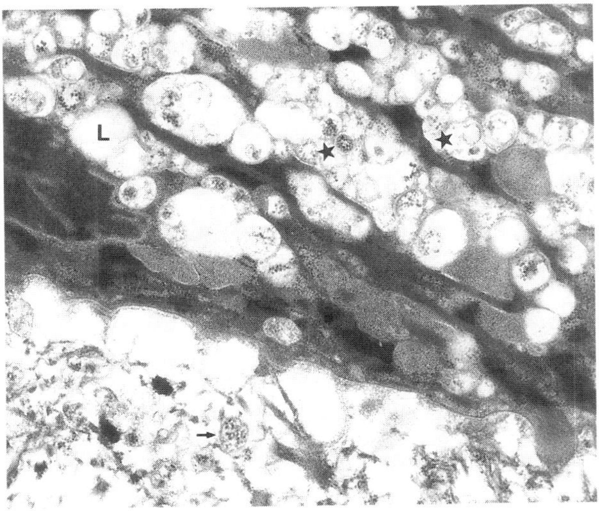

(a)

Figure 9 (a) Ichthyosis congenita gravis or harlequin ichthyosis. The basic defect concerns the keratinosomes which lack the normal epidermal barrier lipid lamellae (see inset in Fig. 9c). Vesicular keratinosomes (arrow) of the uppermost living cells containing some glycogenlike granules accumulate in the first horn cell layers in large amounts (*) together with lipid droplets (L) and remainders of keratohyalin and cell organelles. Postnatal trunk skin.

more or less empty or contain small amounts of glycogenlike granules (8–10). Glycogen is known to serve as a precursor of lipid synthesis. It is therefore to be expected that an enzyme deficiency causes an early block in the synthesis of barrier lipids from glycogen and other precursors. The defective keratinosomes are not discharged to the intercellular spaces as normally occurs but accumulate within the lowermost cells of the compact horny layer (Fig. 9a); they are especially evident in the deep follicular plugs.

With the ultrastructural demonstration of these defective keratinosomes, a safe and distinctive diagnosis of harlequin ichthyosis is possible (8–10). The same defect of keratinosomes is already revealed in skin samples of affected fetuses at week 23 (Fig. 9b,c) together with massive follicular and interfollicular hyperkeratoses (Fig. 9d,e) and the characteristic facial involvement (25). In contrast to statements in the literature, PD for risk of harlequin ichthyosis is, however, possible already about 4 weeks earlier than week 23. With the onset of keratinization in the intraepidermal follicular openings and with the first appearance of keratohyalin granules and keratinized cells at about weeks 18–19, the first keratinosomes appear

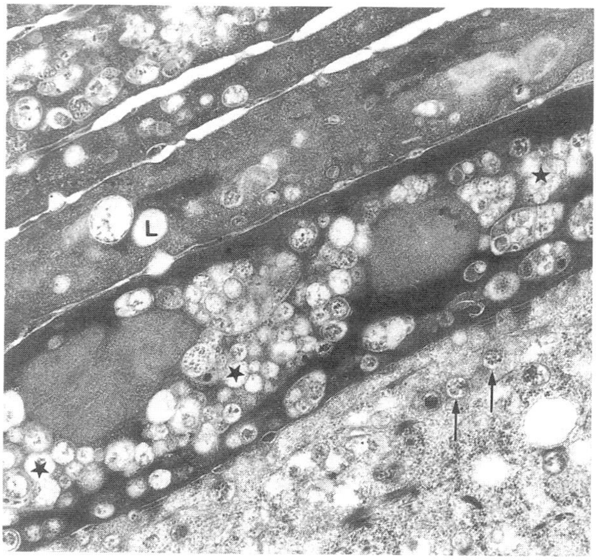

(b)

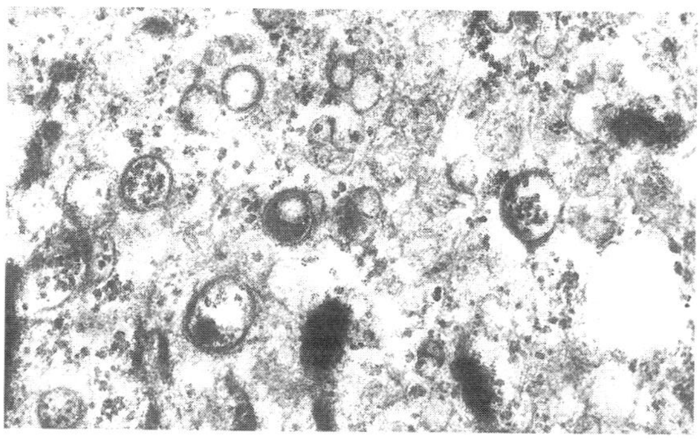

(c)

Figure 9 (b,c) Fetal expression of harlequin ichthyosis: Basic defect. Affected fetuses show the same keratinosome abnormality as in postnatal skin (see Fig. 9a). Keratinosomes lack the normal barrier lipid lamellae, are vesicular (arrows) and contain glycogen-like granules. They accumulate in large numbers (*) in the lower horny layer wherever keratinization has started, together with lipid droplets (L) and remainders of cell organelles (b). The peculiar ultrastructure of defective keratinosomes (c) is pathognomonic of harlequin ichthyosis and the crucial distinctive diagnostic marker, as compared to normal fetal keratinosomes (c inset). (b) affected fetus at week 23 + 3, after termination, back skin; (c) same fetus at week 22 + 4, diagnostic skin sample from lateral trunk; (c inset) normal keratinosomes of a fetus at 20 weeks affected with bullous CIE, another sibling of the fetuses in Fig. 8.

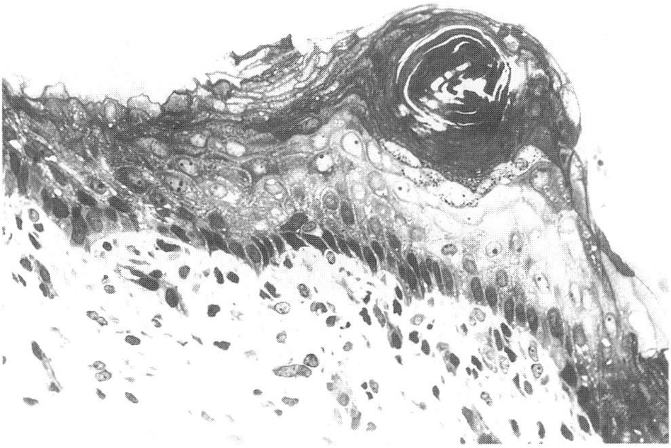

(d)

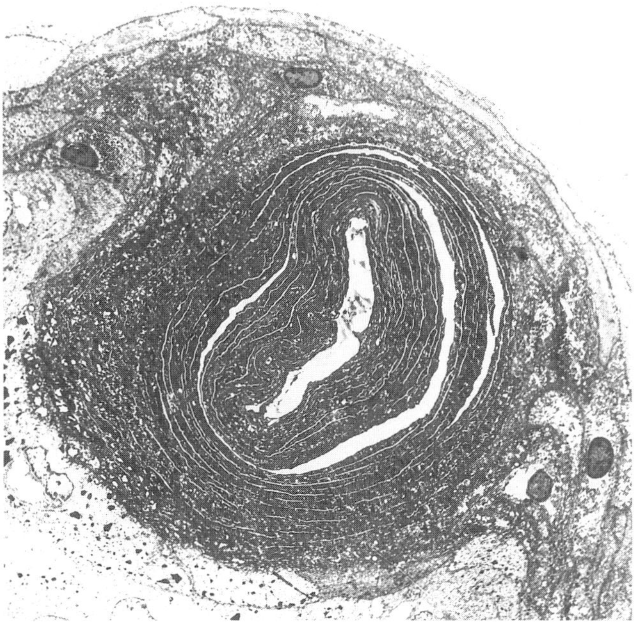

(e)

Figure 9 (d,e) Fetal expression of harlequin ichthyosis: Follicular plugging. Pronounced follicular plugging is already present in samples with yet unkeratinized interfollicular epithelium (compare Fig. 1d, normal fetal skin, and Figs. 10a and 11b, ichthyosis congenita types IV and II). Diagnostic skin sample from lateral trunk at week 22 + 4, same affected fetus and sample as in Fig. 9c. Back skin samples taken after termination 6 days later (see Fig. 9b) were already keratinized continuously also in the interfollicular epidermis. (d) semithin section; (e) ultrathin section of the same plugged follicle (see Fig. 9d, upper right).

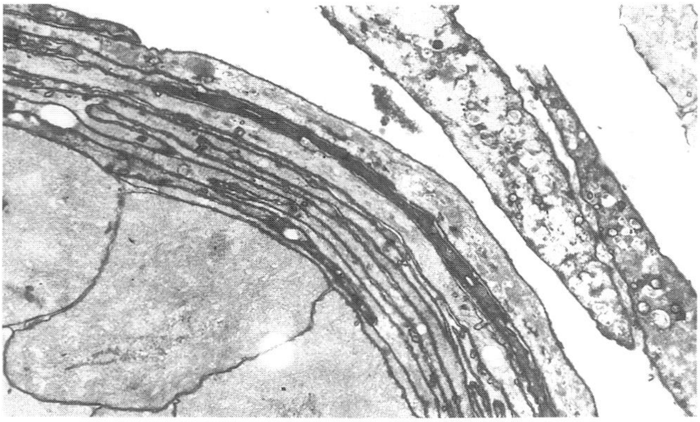

(f)

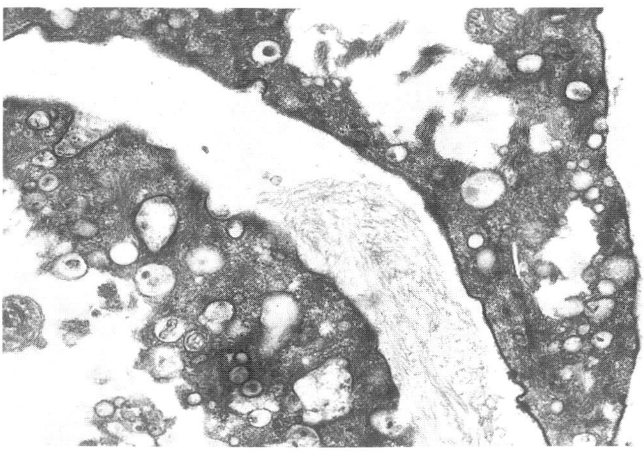

(g)

Figure 9 (f,g) Harlequin ichthyosis, amniotic fluid cells. Amniotic fluid samples of affected fetuses contain stacks of keratinized cells that originate from the plugged follicles (f) and at high magnifications reveal the remainders of accumulated defective keratinosomes (g) together with lipid droplets. Same fetus as in Figs. 9b–e at week 23 + 3.

in these areas; in harlequin fetuses, they reveal the specific defect and lack of barrier lipids, whereas in healthy fetuses, the normal lamellar stacks of the barrier lipids are formed within the keratinosomes (Fig. 9c[inset]). At present, PD is not possible before the onset of keratinization in the outer hair canal at about week 18.

Pellets of amniotic fluid cells of affected fetuses reveal striking stacks and ringlike aggregations of flat, partly keratinized cells that correspond to the horn cells of follicular plugs and intercellular epidermis. The transformed remainders of the defective keratinosomes together with lipid droplets are demonstrable in these cells (Fig. 9f,g).

The first PD for risk of harlequin ichthyosis (false-positive) was attempted in 1980 (35); this was mainly based on the erroneous interpretation of horn cells in the hair follicle openings on the epidermal surface. The first proven prenatal diagnosis of a true fetal harlequin ichthyosis (25; see also Refs. 8,9,12,13, and 21) already showed the pronounced clinical expression of the affected fetus at the end of the second trimester (25). Two additional cases of harlequin fetuses at PD have been reported from Japan (34).

Dale and coworkers (32) have proposed classification of harlequin ichthyosis into three distinct genetic types based on the amount of keratohyalin and profilaggrin/filaggrin synthesis and on the expression of keratins in the epidermis of their cases. They showed that the morphological features were also maintained in culture. Only little attention was paid to the abnormality of the keratinosomes. As to our experience now with a total of 12 postnatal and 2 prenatal cases (Table 1), it is this abnormality of keratinosomes which is the constant defect that may serve as an absolutely safe diagnostic criterion. Changes in the expression of keratins and keratohyalin proteins are probably of secondary nature.

In 1988, Holbrook et al. reported on "the expression of congenital ichthyosiform erythroderma in second trimester fetuses of the same family" (50). In this family, the index case had been diagnosed clinically and by histopathology elsewhere and was not investigated by EM and was not seen by the investigators themselves. In four consecutive pregnancies, PD was attempted (50,53). In the first and fourth pregnancies PD (fetuses 1 and 4), the disorder was excluded and both children were born healthy at term (week 40). In the second PD (fetus 2), one of two fetal skin samples proved to be abnormal, and extensive postinvestigation after abortion confirmed that the fetus had been affected. Fetus 3 in the next pregnancy was concluded to be normal, although part of the hair canals were hyperkeratotic (50[Fig. 7b]) and stacks of cells, although less numerous than in case of fetus 2, were present in the amniotic fluid. This child was born prematurely at week 33 with a strikingly abnormal facial appearance described by the neonatologists as "harlequin ichthyosis–like" (50,53). The lack of normal keratinosomes is mentioned only for fetus 2, and no detailed description of the ultrastructure of the prenatal and postnatal skin samples of fetus 3 is given (50). Only in the later review (53) is it mentioned that the postnatal biopsy "revealed histologic characteristics of lamellar ichthyosis and ultrastructural features . . . strikingly similar to harlequin ichthyosis."

Taking all information in these two reports (50,53) together, it is evident that the investigators were not dealing with a type of congenital ichthyosis as diagnosed by them (50) but with harlequin ichthyosis. The clinical description seems to be consistent with a milder expression of harlequin ichthyosis as occasionally found in spontaneously surviving cases. The same peculiar facial appearance, much less pronounced than in the case of Blanchet-Bardon (25), was seen by us in a fetus after abortion at week 23. Thus, variation in the clinical expression of affected fetuses has to be taken into account similarly as for postnatal cases. Stacks and rings of partly keratinized cells (50[Fig. 3]) are typical of the amniotic fluid of harlequin fetuses. The lack of acanthosis, piling up of very flat, only partly keratinized cells (50[Fig. 2b]), compact follicular plugging and interfollicular hyperkeratosis (50[Fig. 4a–c]), and the ultrastructural appearance of the upper epidermis and horny layer as well as prematurity are all characteristic of harlequin ichthyosis. Although at too low magnification, the illustrations in the review done by Holbrook and coworkers (50) indicate the specific defective keratinosomes (Figs. 2a and 4b) and the accumulation of defective keratinosomes in the lowermost horny cells, their transformation, and remnants in the following layers (Figs. 2f and 4d). Also in this review, illustrations of fetus 2 (Fig. 4a–c) and fetus 3 (Figs. 7b and 8a–d) are very typical of harlequin ichthyosis. The false-negative diagnosis in fetus 3 was explained (50,53) with the pronounced regional differences because of the patchy onset of keratinization (see Section V). Control of the keratinizing portions of fetal and postnatal skin samples at high EM magnification for the normal or abnormal ultrastructure of keratinosomes as presented earlier in this paragraph would not only have helped to avoid the false-negative evaluation at PD in fetus 3, but would have permitted to the correct diagnosis of harlequin ichthyosis—and not of ichthyosis congenita—to be made in this family.

C. Autosomal Recessive Ichthyosis Congenita Group

This group is considerably heterogeneous and comprises various genetic types of nonlethal congenital ichthyoses that were regarded as being one entity until about 10 years ago. Their heterogeneity was revealed by systematic ultrastructural analysis of large series of patients. At present, at least four distinctive types are to be distinguished (8,9,20). In none of these congenital ichthyosis types are the underlying biochemical and molecular genetic basic defects known. However, specific deviations from the normal differentiation are demonstrable in the uppermost living epidermis and in the horny layer by EM, which all point to different disturbances of the epidermal lipid metabolism (see 8 and 9):

Ichthyosis congenita type I: storage of nonpolar lipids in lipid droplets in the horn lamellae occur. This is the classic type of hyperproliferation hyperkeratosis and is often combined with pronounced erythroderma.

Ichthyosis congenita type II: storage of islands of cholesterol clefts in the horny layer, especially pronounced in the massive follicular plugs. Pronounced or mild polygonal scaling, with or without erythroderma, is seen.

Ichthyosis congenita type III: distended perinuclear membranes, probably consisting of polar lipids, vesicular keratinosome complexes, and membrane-bound vacuoles in the granular and horny layer occur. These patients present with a very characteristic reticular scaling pattern, normally without erythroderma.

Ichthyosis congenita type IV: lentiform blown-up paranuclear cell regions of granular cells filled with dense aggregations of shorter membrane profiles probably also of polar lipids, which are retained in the horn cells are observed. Affected infants are usually born prematurely at about weeks 32–34. They are at risk of perinatal death because of considerable shedding of horn cells into the amniotic cavity and the risk of asphyxia. Surviving cases develop a mild keratinization disorder.

Babies of all four types may be born with a collodion skin, which is most pronounced in type II and differs in appearance among the four types. The degree of severity also varies in each of the four types from very mild to very severe. As erythroderma is a variable feature and even may vary within families and within one and the same patient from time to time, it may no longer serve as a diagnostic criterion for classifying autosomal recessive congenital ichthyosis (8). The pathological patterns of the four types also remain constant under clinically successful therapy and seem to be a direct consequence of the respective underlying metabolic abnormality (8). A first hint comes from the correlation of congenital ichthyosis (unclassified) to the gene for the enzyme transaminidase and the identification of first mutations in three unrelated families (D. Hohl, personal communication, to be published).

A safe prenatal diagnosis is possible in the meanwhile for types II and IV (Figs. 10 and 11), in which the postnatal ultrastructural markers are already expressed in fetal skin, although only in relation to beginning keratinization. Type IV can be diagnosed by the demonstration of the membrane aggregations in paranuclear regions as soon as cells enter into keratinization; in the second-trimester fetus, this ichthyosis type is therefore restricted to the hair follicle openings. In view of the very mild postnatal course of the disease and in spite of the perinatal risk of asphyxia, it is questionable whether PD is really justified. In our first (and only) fetal case (Table 1), PD was requested because of the severe clinical appearance at birth and perinatal death of the index case, of which only reembedded paraffin material had been available for EM investigation (6). The significance of the morphological pattern of the index case and of the affected fetus (Fig. 10a–c) was later confirmed by the identification and follow-up of further, surviving cases (8,9).

In spite of the initial problems with PD of the ichthyosis congenita group (20,21), type II can now safely and reliably be diagnosed from fetal skin samples (8–10). The typical cholesterol clefts in the horn cells of postnatal skin (Fig. 11a) are not yet expressed in the second-trimester fetus; this and the lack of interfollicular precocious keratinization (Fig. 11b), expected at that early time internationally for

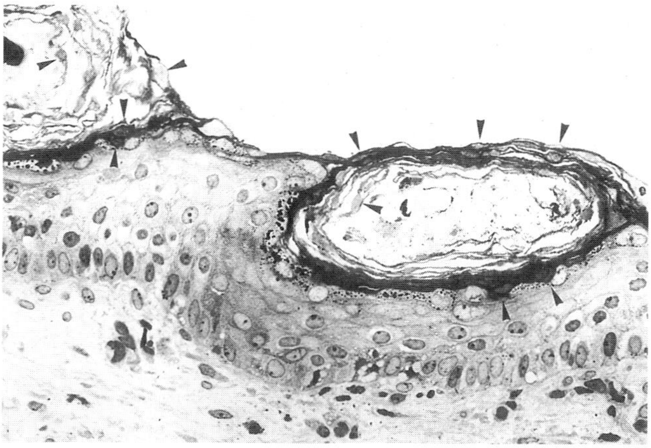

(a)

Figure 10 (a) Fetal expression of ichthyosis congenita type IV. The specific marker is expressed in the keratinized distal portions of the fetal hair canal where the surrounding horn lamellae show the typical lentiform swelling already by light microscopy in semithin sections (arrowheads, Fig. 1a, normal skin, Fig. 9d, harlequin ichthyosis, and Fig. 11b, ichthyosis congenita type II). (Micrograph courtesy of Dr. M.-L. Arnold; from Ref. 18.)

congenital ichthyoses, were the reasons for the initial problems and false-negative diagnosis in the first affected type II fetus (20). Progressive plugging of the distal hair canals occurs in fetuses affected with type II (Fig. 11b,c); the specific patterns of membrane proliferation and lipid deposition in these plugging follicles are diagnostically distinctive and may be retained in the outermost layers of the collodion skin of the newborn infant (Fig. 11d,e) (8–10,12,13,20,21). In our Heidelberg material, four of five at-risk fetuses were affected (Table 1).

No proven positive PD of type III has been reported as yet; preliminary experiences point to a possible expression in the fetal skin already at about the end of the second trimester (unpublished).

In contrast, a safe and reliable exclusion of type I congenital ichthyosis is at present not possible in at-risk fetuses. Because of the irregular and patchy onset of keratinization between weeks 20 and 23 (see Section V), samples of risk fetuses may be completely inconspicuous before week 24 in spite of involvement of the fetus. This problem has led to repeated false-negative PDs in most international centers (16,20,34).

One positive PD of a fetus affected with an unclassified type of congenital ichthyosis has been reported from Adelaide, Australia (78).

As discussed earlier in this chapter, the ichthyosis family investigated by

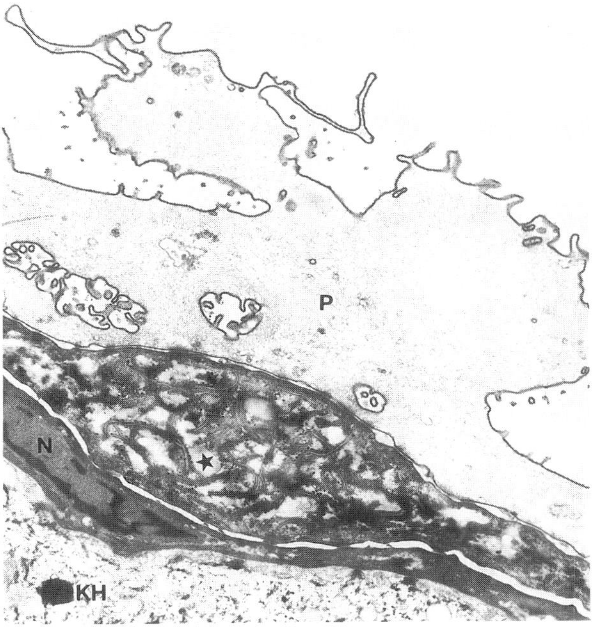

(b)

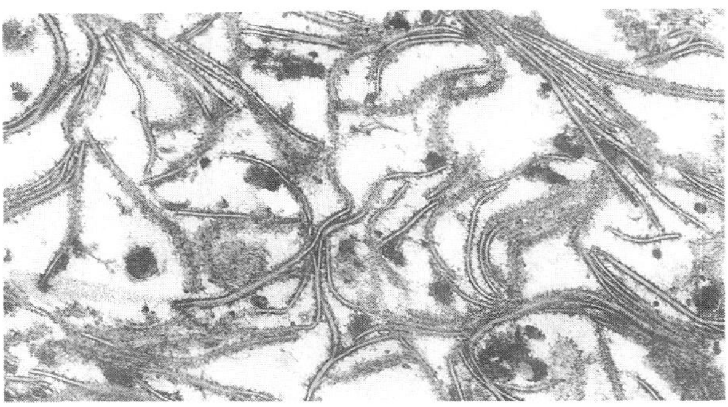

(c)

Figure 10 (b,c) Fetal expression of ichthyosis congenita type IV. Interfollicular epidermis with beginning keratinization in week 22 + 4 with lentiform swelling of one of two horn lamellae (*) where lipid membranes are accumulated (b). Detail of these lipid membranes in another horn cell is shown in (c). KH, keratohyalin granules in the granular layer; N, nucleus of 2nd horn cell in (b); P, periderm cell at skin surface.

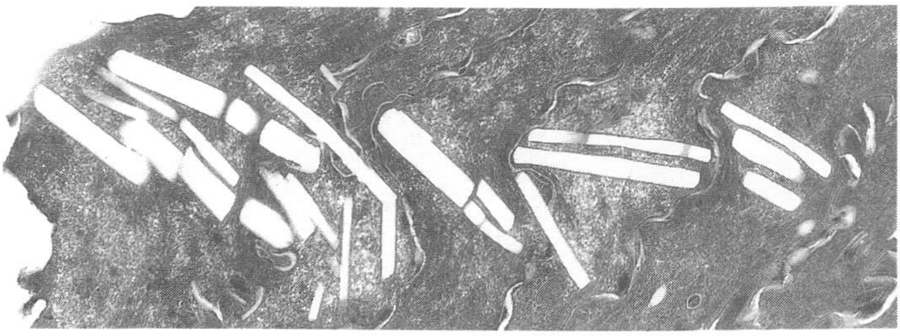

(a)

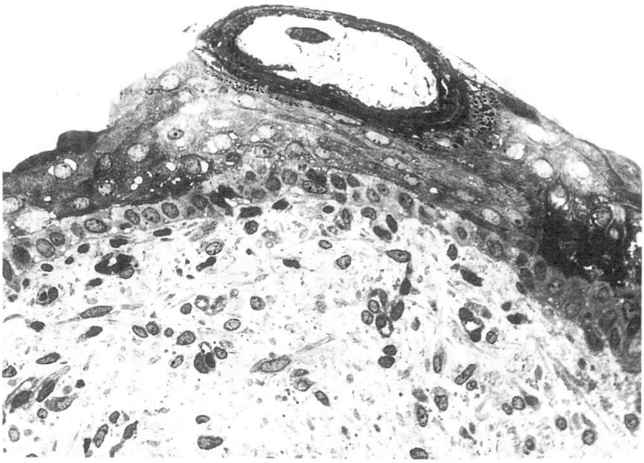

(b)

Figure 11 (a,b) Ichthyosis congenita type II, cholesterol type. The specific postnatal marker, islands of cholesterol crystals in the horny layer (a, affected newborn, postnatal skin) is not yet expressed in fetal skin. Fetal expression (see Fig. 11d) is restricted to the keratinizing distal portions of the hair canal (b, affected fetus at week 21 + 5, cf. Fig. 1d, normal skin, Fig. 9d, harlequin ichthyosis, and Fig. 10a, ichthyosis congenita type IV), with slight hyperkeratosis and irregular arrangement of horn lamellae, while the interfollicular epidermis is still unkeratinized.

Holbrook and coworkers in four consecutive pregnancies does not concern congenital ichthyosiform erythroderma (congenital ichthyosis), as diagnosed by the investigators (50,53) but rather ichthyosis congenita gravis of harlequin ichthyosis.

At present, PD is possible for this group of genodermatoses only by means of fetal skin biopsy and EM analysis. The time for PD is restricted to the end of the second trimester because of the late expression of keratinization markers: type II

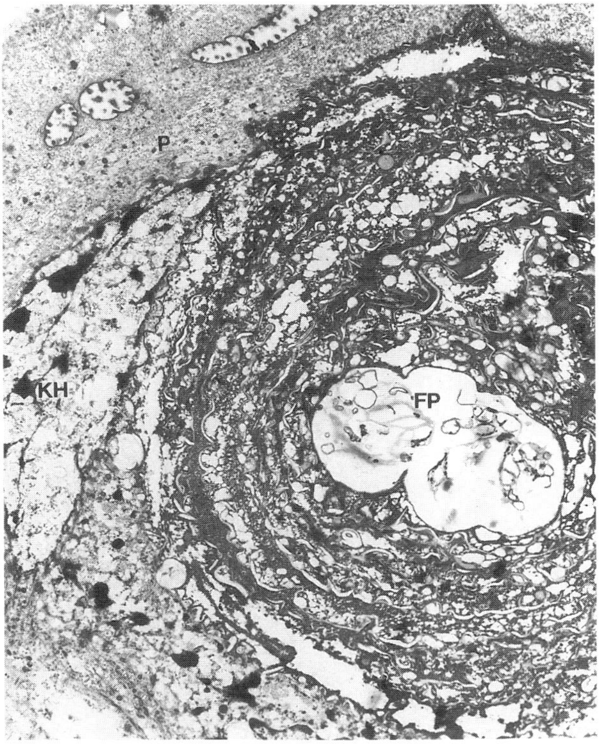

(c)

Figure 11 (c) Fetal expression of ichthyosis congenita type II. Ultrastructural appearance of hyperkeratotic distal hair canal in slightly tangential section (same fetus as in Fig. 11b at week 21 + 5), initial stage of plugged follicle (FP, cf. Fig. 9e, harlequin ichthyosis). KH, keratohyalin granules in surrounding granular cells; P, periderm cell at skin surface.

from week 20, better in weeks 21–22; type III probably not before the twenty-second week; type IV from weeks 19–20. (For further details, see Refs. 8–10.)

D. Sjögren-Larsson Syndrome

(SLS) is a severe neurocutaneous disorder characterized by the triad of congenital ichthyosis, spastic diplegia or tetraplegia, and mental retardation. The disorder has recently been ascribed to an enzyme deficiency of the lipid metabolism, fatty alcohol:NAD oxireductase (FAO) (67). Only two cases of positive PD of SLS have been reported (53,79). In the first case, positive PD of SLS was based on the light

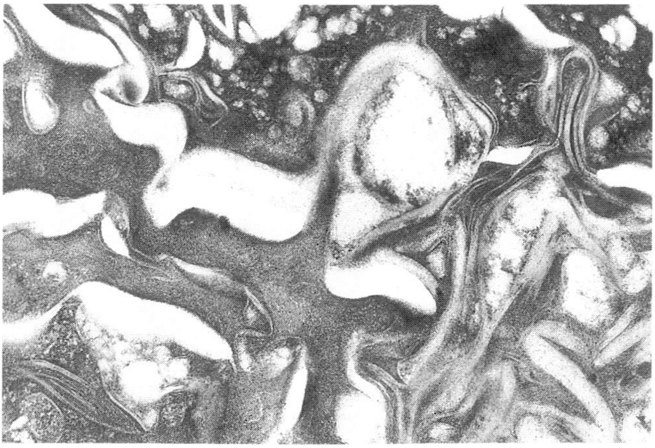

(d)

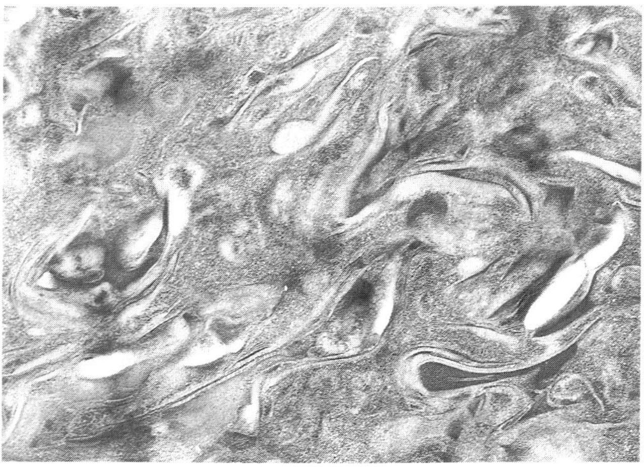

(e)

Figure 11 (d,e) Fetal expression of ichthyosis congenita type II. Membrane proliferation, deep membrane infoldings, and intercellular deposition of homogeneous (lipid?) material characterize the specific pattern of cornified cells in plugging follicles of affected fetuses (d, same fetus as in Figs. 11b and c at week 21 + 5). The same specific pattern may still be demonstrable in the uppermost layers of the collodion membrane and within plugged follicles of affected newborns (e, postnatal skin).

microscopic demonstration of hypergranulosis and hyperkeratosis, especially of hair canals in a fetus at week 23 (79). In the second case, the fetal skin samples obtained at 19 + 2 weeks appeared normal, whereas the FAO values from cultured amniotic fluid cells obtained at the same time were markedly decreased (53). Repeat of fetal biopsy at 23 + 5 weeks revealed marked hypergranulosis, hyperkeratosis, and acanthosis. Thus, the morphological features of SLS were only expressed with the late onset of keratinization. Biochemical analysis of FAO values from cultured amniotic fluid cells or fetal fibroblasts can be applied in the future when FAO deficiency is proven for the at-risk family (67).

IX. GENODERMATOSES THAT CANNOT BE DIAGNOSED AT PRESENT

Negative results have been experienced with PD in certain other genodermatoses:

Chondrodysplasia punctata of the rhizomelic type, presenting with an ichthyosis at birth, is not yet expressed before week 24 in affected fetuses (20).

Netherton syndrome: characterized by the triad of erythrodermic, sometimes ichthyosiform scaling, bamboo hairs (trichorrhexis invaginata), and atopy. It cannot be diagnosed prenatally from fetal skin samples of fetal hair as to our Heidelberg experience (10), and therefore also cannot be safely excluded.

Restrictive dermopathy: an always lethal disorder with recessive inheritance, this disorder belongs to those genodermatoses that are not manifest before week 24. The dramatic pathological process obviously starts only in the third trimester; before week 24, the fetal skin is developed completely normally and according to fetal age. The previous assumption of a primary arrest of the development of skin and appendages about weeks 12–15 thought to be suitable as criterion for PD does not hold true (10).

Connective tissue disorders: for example, Ehlers-Danlos syndrome, cutis laxa, Marfan syndrome, or pseudoxanthoma elasticum (70), also cannot be identified or excluded prenatally from fetal skin samples in the second trimester, as the matrix constituents of the dermal connective tissue are either synthesized only after the twenty-fourth week (elastin) or differ specifically from postnatal skin in the fetus (collagen) (77). (For details, see Refs. 28,29, and 70).

X. RESULTS OF PRENATAL DIAGNOSIS OF GENODERMATOSES

Results of PD performed in Heidelberg, predominantly in cooperation with the two gynecologists Prof. Dr. Rüdiger Rauskolb, Northeim, Germany, and Docent Björn Gustavii, Lund, Sweden, are summarized in Table 1. Table 2 presents the results

Table 2 Prenatal Diagnosis of Genodermatoses: Results of the International Centers 1979–1992 (18th World Congress of Dermatology, New York, 1992)[a]

Center	Total no. cases of PD	No. of fetuses affected
Heidelberg	149	45
London	116	26
Paris	128	43
Seattle	71	14
Tokyo	2	1
Nagoya	2	2
Total number of cases 1992	468	131
Results of Additional Centers (Dec. 1994)		
Milano[b]	14	6
Melbourne[c]	7	4
Adelaide[d]	1	1

[a]Modified from Ref. 34.
[b]Data summarized from Ref. 27 and Dr. Brusasco, personal communication, Milan.
[c]Data according to Dr. C. W. Chow and Dr. Dowling, Melbourne, personal communications.
[d]Data not complete, according to Ref. 78.

of PD of the international centers at the time of the last World Congress of Dermatology 1992 in New York City (34), including results from Milan, Italy, Melbourne, and Adelaide, Australia (December 1994).

XI. CONCLUSIONS AND FUTURE ASPECTS

With the advancing progress in the understanding and clarification of the basic abnormalities underlying genetic skin disorders on the DNA level, and with the identification of the specific mutations in individual patients and families, prenatal diagnosis will be shifted more and more to early pregnancy. This will make it a bit easier for the families to accept the considerable ethical problems related to the consequence of terminating a pregnancy.

As long as DNA-based PD in early pregnancy is, however, restricted to some few cases, fetal skin biopsy and subsequent ultrastructural evaluation of the respective target structures and ultrastructural markers of the genodermatosis at risk, as discussed in this chapter, offers a chance for prenatal diagnosis to many families with severe genodermatoses. More important than to identify affected fetuses prenatally is the chance safely to exclude a severe and often disabling genodermatosis at risk by means of PD, even if this is presently possible only in mid pregnancy, to overcome fear in the family and to save healthy children from unnecessary abortion merely because of the statistical risk of recurrence of a genodermatosis.

ACKNOWLEDGMENTS

I am most thankful to all my colleagues who took part in one or the other case of PD, especially to Prof. Dr. Rüdiger Rauskolb, Northeim, Germany, and to Docent Dr. Björn Gustavii, Lund, Sweden, for performing most of the fetal skin biopsies. Thanks are also due to all my coworkers who participated in this work over the years, to Wiebke Tubbesing for her invaluable help with the preparation of this manuscript, and to Birgit Kandt for preparing the accompanying figures.

I dedicate this chapter to the memory of my husband.

REFERENCES

1. D. Aberdam, M. F. Galliano, J. Vailly, et al. Herlitz's junctional epidermolysis bullosa is linked to mutations in the gene (LAMC2) for the γ2 subunit of nicein/kalinin (LAMININ-5), *Nature Genet. 6*:299–304 (1994).
2. I. Anton-Lamprecht. Electron microscopy in the early diagnosis of genetic disorders of the skin, *Dermatologica 157*:65–85 (1978).
3. I. Anton-Lamprecht. Prenatal diagnosis of genetic disorders of the skin by means of electron microscopy, *Hum. Genet. 59*:392–405 (1981).
4. I. Anton-Lamprecht. Genetically induced abnormalities of epidermal differentiation and ultrastructure in ichthyoses and epidermolyses: pathogenesis, heterogeneity, fetal manifestation, and prenatal diagnosis, *J. Invest. Dermatol. 81*:149s–156s (1983).
5. I. Anton-Lamprecht. Prenatal diagnosis of epidermolysis bullosa hereditaria: A review, *Semin. Dermatol. 3*:229–240 (1984).
6. I. Anton-Lamprecht. Pränatale Diagnostik von Genodermatosen, *Hautarzt 39*(Suppl. VIII):16–20 (1988).
7. I. Anton-Lamprecht. Pathomorphogenese von Genodermatosen. Möglichkeiten der Identifizierung und Charakterisierung von Genodermatosen mit Hilfe elektronenmikroskopischer Untersuchungen und deren praktische Anwendung in der frühen postnatalen sowie in der pränatalen Diagnostik schwerer erblicher Hautkrankheiten, *Ulmensien 2*:129–159 (1989).
8. I. Anton-Lamprecht. Heterogeneity and prenatal diagnosis of congenital ichthyosis, *Dermatologia Pediatrica*, 4th International Symposium on Pediatric Dermatology, (G. Fabrizi, F. Serri, and D. Cerimele, eds.), Selinunte (Trapani) 25–28, September 1991. Casa Editrice l'Antologia, Naples.
9. I. Anton-Lamprecht. The skin, *Diagnostic Ultrastructure of Non-neoplastic Diseases* (J. M. Papadimitriou, D. W. Henderson, and D. V. Spagnolo, eds.). Churchill Livingstone, Edinburgh, 1992, pp. 459–550.
10. I. Anton-Lamprecht. Prenatal diagnosis of genodermatoses, *La diagnosi fetale* (F.

Dagna Bricarelli, M. Casini Lemmi, G. Storti, eds.). Suppl Analysis No. 7, 1992, pp. 131–154.

11. I. Anton-Lamprecht. Ultrastructural identification of basic abnormalities as clues to genetic disorders of the epidermis, *J. Invest. Dermatol. 103*:6s–12s (1994).
12. I. Anton-Lamprecht and M.-L. Arnold. Pränatale Diagnostik von erblichen Hautkrankheiten, Murken J (ed) *Pränatale Diagnostik und Therapie.* (J. Murken, ed.). Enke, Stuttgart, 1987, pp. 187–214.
13. I. Anton-Lamprecht and M.-L. Arnold. Prenatal diagnosis of severe genetic disorders of the skin, *Pediatric Dermatology. Advances in Diagnosis and Treatment* (R. Happle and E. Grosshans, eds.). Springer, Berlin, 1987, pp. 3–22.
14. I. Anton-Lamprecht, M.-L. Arnold, and K. A. Holbrook. Methodology in sampling of fetal skin and pitfalls in the interpretation of fetal skin biopsy specimens, *Semin. Dermatol. 3*:203–215 (1984).
15. I. Anton-Lamprecht, M.-L. Arnold, R. Rauskolb. et al. Prenatal diagnosis of anhidrotic ectodermal dysplasis, *Hum. Genet. 62*:180 (1982).
16. I. Anton-Lamprecht, C. Blanchet-Bardon, and K. A. Holbrook. Prenatal diagnosis of genodermatoses, *Dermatology in Five Continents.* Proceedings of the XVII World Congress of Dermatology, Berlin, May 24–29, 1977. Springer, Berlin, pp. 838–843.
17. I. Anton-Lamprecht and I. Hashimoto. Epidermolysis bullosa dystrophica dominans (Pasini)—A primary structural defect of the anchoring fibrils, *Hum. Genet. 32*:69–76 (1976).
18. I. Anton-Lamprecht and R. Rauskolb. Pränatale Diagnostik von Genodermatosen, *Gynakologe 27*:296–308 (1994).
19. I. Anton-Lamprecht, R. Rauskolb, V. Jovanovic, et al. Prenatal diagnosis of epidermolysis bullosa dystrophica Hallopeau-Siemens with electron microscopy of fetal skin, *Lancet 14*:1077–1079 (1981).
20. M.-L. Arnold and I. Anton-Lamprecht. Problems in the prenatal diagnosis of the ichthyosis congenita group. *Hum. Genet. 71*:301–311 (1985).
21. M.-L. Arnold and I. Anton-Lamprecht. Prenatal diagnosis of epidermal disorders, *Curr. Prob. Dermatol. 16*:120–128 (1987).
22. M.-L. Arnold, I. Anton-Lamprecht, and R. Rauskolb. Prenatal diagnosis of ectodermal dysplasias, *Semin. Dermatol. 3*:247–252 (1984).
23. M.-L. Arnold, R. Rauskolb, I. Anton-Lamprecht, et al. Prenatal diagnosis of anhidrotic actodermal dysplasia, *Prenat. Diagn. 4*:85–98 (1984).
24. H. J. Bandmann and M. V. Ingersleben, eds. Die Dermatologische Indikation zur Interruptio. 105. Tagung der Vereinigung Südwestdeutscher Dermatologen, München 1978. *Hautarzt 31*(Suppl. IV): (1980).
25. C. Blanchet-Bardon and Y. Dumez. Prenatal diagnosis of a harlequin fetus, *Semin. Dermatol. 3*:225–228 (1984).
26. R. A. Briggaman and C. E. Wheeler. Epidermolysis bullosa dystrophica-recessive: A possible role of anchoring fibrils in the pathogenesis, *J. Invest. Dermatol. 65*:203–211 (1975).
27. A. Brusasco, U. Nicolini, R. Cavalli, et al. Diagnosi prenatale mediante biopsia cutanea fetale. Esperienza di 12 casi, *G. Ital. Dermatol. Venereol. 129*:135–142 (1994).
28. P. H. Byers and R. J. Wenstrup. Prenatal diagnosis of inherited connective tissue disorders, *Semin. Dermatol. 3*:257–264 (1984).

29. P. H. Byers, R. J. Wenstrup, J. E. Bonadio, et al. Molecular basis of inherited disorders of collagen biosynthesis: Implication for prenatal diagnosis, *Curr. Probl. Dermatol. 16*:158–174 (1987).
30. Y. Chan, I. Anton-Lamprecht, Q. C. Yu, et al. A human keratin 14 "knockout": The absence of K14 leads to severe epidermolysis bullosa simplex and a function for an intermediate filament protein, *Genes Dev. 8*:2574–2587 (1994).
31. J. Cheng, A. J. Syder, Q. C. Yu, et al. The genetic basis of epidermolytic hyperkeratosis: A disorder of differentiation-specific epidermal keratin genes, *Cell 70*:811–819 (1992).
32. B. A. Dale, K. A. Holbrook, P. Fleckman, et al. Heterogeneity in harlequin ichthyosis, an inborn error of epidermal keratinization: Variable morphology and structural protein expression and a defect in lamellar granules, *J. Invest. Dermatol. 94*:6–18 (1990).
33. R. A. J. Eady. Prenatal diagnosis of oculocutaneous albinism: Implications for other hereditary disorders of pigmentation, *Semin. Dermatol. 3*:241–246 (1984).
34. R. A. J. Eady, K. A. Holbrook, C. Blanchet-Bardon, and I. Anton-Lamprecht. Chair's summary: Prenatal diagnosis of skin diseases (Workshop), *Dermatology. Progress and Perspectives* (W. H. C. Burgdorf and S. I. Katz, eds.). Proceedings of the 18th World Congress of Dermatology. Parthenon Publishing Group, New York, Casterton, London, 1993, pp. 1159–1165.
35. S. Elias, M. Mazur, R. Sabaggha, et al. Prenatal diagnosis of harlequin ichthyosis, *Clin. Genet. 17*:275–280 (1980).
36. J. D. Fine, K. A. Holbrook, S. Elias, et al. Applicability of 19-DEJ-1 monoclonal antibody for the prenatal diagnosis or exclusion of junctional epidermolysis bullosa, *Prenat. Diagn. 10*:219–229 (1990).
37. E. Fuchs. Intermediate filaments and disease: Mutations that cripple cell strength. Mini-review on the cellular mechanisms of disease, *J. Cell. Biol. 125*:511–516 (1994).
38. W. Fuhrmann, R. Rauskolb, and V. Jovanovic. Pränatale Diagnostik. Aufgaben und Methoden, *Schwangerschaft* I. *Die normale Schwangerschaft*, Vol. 4 (W. Künzel and K.-H. Wulf, eds.). *Klinik der Frauenheilkunde und Geburtshilfe* (K.-H Wulf and H. Schmidt-Matthiesen, (eds.). Urban & Schwarzenberg, Munich, 1992, pp. 285–314.
39. T. Gedde-Dahl, Jr., and I. Anton-Lamprecht. Epidermolysis bullosa, *The Principles and Practice of Medical Genetics*, 2nd ed. (A. E. H. Emery and D. L. Rimoin, ed.). Churchill Livingstone, Edinburgh, 1990, pp. 855–876.
40. S. G. Gil, T. A. Brown, M. C. Ryan, and W. G. Carter. Junctional epidermolysis bullosis: Defects in expression of epiligrin/nicein/kalinin and integrin β4 that inhibit hemidesmosome formation, *J. Invest. Dermatol. 103*:31s–38s (1994).
41. M. S. Golbus, R. W. Sagebiel, R. A., et al. Prenatal diagnosis of bullous congenital ichthyosiform erythroderma (epidermolytic hyperkeratosis) by fetal skin biopsy, *N. Engl. J. Med. 302*:93–95 (1980).
42. D. A. Greenhalgh, J. A. Rothnagel, and D. R. Roop. Epidermis: An attractive target tissue for gene therapy, *J. Invest. Dermatol. 103*:63s–69s (1994).
43. E. Haneke and I. Anton-Lamprecht. Ultrastructure of blister formation in epidermolysis bullosa hereditaria: V. Epidermolyis bullosa simplex localisata type Weber-Cockayne, *J. Invest. Dermatol. 78*:219–223 (1982).
44. I. Haußer and I. Anton-Lamprecht. Ultrastructure of first trimester chorionic villi with regard to the prenatal diagnosis of genodermatoses, *Prenat. Diagn. 8*:511–524 (1988).

45. I. Hauβer and I. Anton-Lamprecht, and B. Gustavii. Prenatal diagnosis of junctional epidermolysis bullosa. Herlitz type, *Lancet O. 28*:1035–1036 (1989).
46. Hauβer and I. Anton-Lamprecht. Prenatal diagnosis of genodermatoses by ultrastructural diagnostic markers in extra-embryonic tissues: Defective hemidesmosomes in amnion epithelium of fetuses affected with epidermolysis bullosa Herlitz type (an alternative prenatal diagnosis in certain cases). *Hum. Genet. 85*:367–375 (1990).
47. A. H. Heagerty, R. A. J. Eady, A. R. Kennedy, et al. Rapid prenatal diagnosis of epidermolysis bullosa letalis using GB3 monoclonal antibody, *Br. J. Dermatol. 117*:271–275 (1987).
48. K. A. Holbrook. Progress in prenatal diagnosis of bullous congenital ichthyosiform erythroderma (epidermolytic hyperkeratosis), *Semin. Dermatol. 3*:216–220 (1984).
49. K. A. Holbrook, B. A. Dale, L. T. Smith, et al. Markers of adult skin expressed in the skin of the first trimester fetus, *Curr. Probl. Dermatol. 16*:94–108 (1987).
50. K. A. Holbrook, B. A. Dale, M. L. Williams, et al. The expression of congenital ichthyosiform erythroderma in second trimester fetuses of the same family: Morphologic and biochemical studies, *J. Invest. Dermatol. 91*:521–531 (1988).
51. K. A. Holbrook and M. S. Hoff. Structure of the developing human embryonic and fetal skin, *Semin. Dermatol. 3*:185–202 (1984).
52. K. A. Holbrook and L. I. T. Smith. Ultrastructural aspects of human skin during the embryonic, fetal, premature, neonatal, and adult periods of life. Birth defects: Original article series vol. 17, no 2. March of Dimes Birth Defects Foundation. Liss, New York, 1981, pp. 9–13.
53. K. A. Holbrook, L. T. Smith, and S. Elias. Prenatal diagnosis of genetic skin disease using fetal skin biopsy samples, *Arch. Dermatol. 129*:1437–1454 (1993).
54. A. Hovnanian, P. Duquesnoy, C. Blanchet-Bardon, et al. Genetic linkage of recessive dystrophic epidermolysis bullosa to the type VII collagen gene, *J. Clin. Invest. 90*:1032–1036 (1992).
55. A. Hovnanian, L. Hilal, C. Blanchet-Bardon, et al. DNA-based prenatal diagnosis of generalized recessive dystrophic epidermolysis bullosa in six pregnancies with risk of recurrence, *J. Invest Dermatol.* In press.
56. L. Löfberg, I. Anton-Lamprecht, G. Michaelsson, and B. Gustavii. Prenatal exclusion of Herlitz syndrome by electron microscopy of fetal skin biopsies obtained at fetoscopy, *Acta Derm. Venereol* (*Stockh.*) *63*:185–189 (1983).
57. M. P. Marinkovich. The molecular genetics of basement membrane diseases, *Arch. Dermatol 129*:1557–1565 (1993).
58. M. P. Marinkovich, R. E. Burgeson, G. Meneguzzi, et al. Prenatal diagnosis of Herlitz junctional epidermolysis bullosa by amniocentesis. Submitted.
59. G. Meneguzzi, M. P. Marinkovich, D. Aberdam, et al. Kalinin is abnormally expressed in epithelial basement membranes of Herlitz's junctional epidermolysis bullosa patients, *Exp. Dermatol. 1*:221–229 (1992).
60. C. Peracchia and B. S. Mittler. Fixation by means of glutaraldehyde-hydrogen peroxide reaction products, *J. Cell. Biol. 53*:234–238 (1972).
61. T. B. Perry. Clinical procedures for prenatal diagnosis of inherited skin disease: Amniocentesis, ultrasound, fetoscopy and fetal skin biopsy and blood sampling, chorionic villus sampling, *Semin. Dermatol. 3*:155–166 (1984).
62. L. Pulkkinen, A. M. Christiano, T. Airenne, et al. Mutations in the $\gamma 2$ chain gene

(LAMC2) of kalinin/laminin 5 in the junctional forms of epidermolysis bullosa, *Nature Genet.* *6*:293–298 (1994).

63. L. Pulkkinen, A. M. Christiano, D. Gerecke, et al. A homozygous nonsense mutation in the β3chain gene of laminin 5 (LAMB3) in Herlitz junctional epidermolysis bullosa. *Gernomics.* In press.
64. R. Rauskolb. *Fetoskopie. Eine klinische Methode zur pränatalen Diagnostik.* Thieme, Stuttgart, 1980.
65. R. Rauskolb. Fetoscopy, *J. Perinat. Med.* *11*:223–231 (1983).
66. R. Rauskolb and I. Anton-Lamprecht. Pränatale Diagnostik von erblichen Hautkrankheiten durch Fetoskopie und Elektronenmikroskopie, *Pränatale Medizin* (W. Holzgreve, ed.). Springer, Berlin, 1987, pp. 80–104.
67. W. B. Rizzo and D. A. Craft. Sjögren-Larsson syndrome: deficient activity of the fatty aldehyde dehydrogenase component of fatty alcohol: NAD* oxidoreductase in cultured fibroblasts, *J. Clin Invest.* *88*:1643–1648 (1991).
68. C. H. Rodeck, R. A. J. Eady, and C. M. Gosden. Prenatal diagnosis of epidermolysis bullosa letalis, *Lancet 1*: 949–952 (1980).
69. J. A. Rothnagel, M. P. Fisher, S. M. Axtell, et al. A mutational hot spot in keratin 10 (KRT 10) in patients with epidermolytic hyperkeratosis, *Hum. Mol. Genet.* 2:2147–2150 (1993).
70. P. M. Royce and B. Steinmann, eds. *Connective Tissue and Its Heritable Disorders. Molecular, Genetic and Medical Aspects.* Wiley-Liss, New York, 1992.
71. E. L. Rugg, W. H. I. McLean, E. B. Lane, et al. A functional "knockout" of human keratin 14, *Genes Dev.* *8*:2563–2573 (1994).
72. M. Ryynanen, R. G. Knowlton, M. G. Parente, et al. Human type VII collagen: genetic linkage to the gene (COL7A1) on chromosome 3 to dominant dystrophic epidermolysis bullosa, *Am. J. Hum. Genet.* *49*:797–803 (1991).
73. Schmidt. *Schmelzhypoplasien—Eine Manifestation des Gendefektes der Epidermolysis bullosa atrophicans? Vergleichende licht- und elektronenmikroskopische Untersuchung von Zahnkeimen bei Feten mit hereditären junktionalen Epidermolysen und Feten mit normaler Zahnentwicklung.* Dissertation, Heidelberg, 1987.
74. H. Shimizu, J. D. Fine, Suzumori, et al. Prenatal exclusion of pyloric atresia-junctional epidermolysis bullosa syndrome, *J. Am. Acad. Dermatol.* *31*:429–433 (1994).
75. H. Shimizu, A. Ishiko, A. Kikuchi, et al. Prenatal diagnosis of tyrosinase-negative oculocutaneous albinism. *Lancet* *340*:739–740 (1992).
76. H. Shimizu, H. Niizeki, K. Suzumori, et al. Prenatal diagnosis of oculocutaneous albinism by analysis of the fetal tyrosinase gene, *J. Invest. Dermatol.* *103*:104–106 (1994).
77. L. T. L. Smith, K. A. Holbrook, and P. H. Byers. Structure of the dermal matrix during development and in the adult, *J. Invest. Dermatol.* *79*(Suppl. 1):93s–104s (1982).
78. G. R. Sutherland and D. W. Henderson. Prenatal diagnosis of genetic disease by electron microscopy, *Diagnostic Ultrastructure of Non-neoplastic Diseases* (J. H. Papadimitriou, D. W. Henderson, and D. V. Spagnolo, eds.). Churchill Livingstone, Edinburgh, 1992, pp. 133–140.
79. R. Trepeta, K. S. Stenn, and M. J. Mahoney. Prenatal diagnosis of Sjögren-Larsson syndrome, *Semin. Dermatol.* *3*:221–224 (1984).
80. J. Uitto, L. Pulkkinen, and A. M. Christiano. Molecular basis of the dystrophic and

junctional forms of epidermolysis bullosa: Mutations in the type VII collagen and kalinin (laminin 5) genes, *J. Invest. Dermatol. 103*:39s–46s (1994).

81. J. Vailly, L. Pulkkinen, C. Miquel, et al. Identification of a homozygous one basepair deletion in exon 14 of the LAMB3 gene in a patient with Herlitz junctional epidermolysis bullosa for recurrence and prenatal diagnosis in a family at risk. Submitted.
82. C. Valenti. Endoamnioscopy and fetal biopsy: A new technique, *Am. J. Obstet. Gynecol 114*:561–564 (1972).
83. J. Zonana, A. Clarke, M. Sarfarazi, et al. PS X-linked hypohidrotic ectodermal dysplasia: Localization within the region Xq11-21.1 by linkage analysis and implications for carrier detection and prenatal diagnosis, *Am. J. Hum. Genet. 43*:75–85 (1988).
84. J. Zonana, A. Schinzel, M. Upadhyaya, et al. Prenatal diagnosis of X-linked hypohidrotic ectodermal dysplasia by linkage analysis, *Am. J. Med. Genet. 35*:132–135 (1990).

Index

About the Editors

MARWALI HARAHAP is Professor of Dermatology at the University of North Sumatra School of Medicine, Medan, Indonesia. The author of numerous professional publications and the editor or coeditor of six books, Dr. Harahap is a Fellow of the American Academy of Dermatology and a member of the Indonesian Society of Dermatology and Venereology; the International Society of Dermatology: Tropical, Geographic and Ecologic; the International Society of Dermatologic Surgery; and the Medical Society for the Study of Venereal Diseases; among others. He received the M.D. degree (1960) from the University of Indonesia, Jakarta.

ROBERT C. WALLACH is Professor of Clinical Obstetrics and Gynecology at New York University School of Medicine, New York, New York; Attending Obstetrician-Gynecologist at Bellevue Hospital, New York, New York; Professional Lecturer at the University of Puerto Rico School of Medicine, San Juan; and Director Emeritus of, and Consultant to, the Department of Obstetrics and Gynecology at Beth Israel Medical Center, New York, New York. A Fellow of the American College of Obstetricians and Gynecologists, the American College of Surgeons, and the New York Obstetrical Society, Dr. Wallach is a member of the Society of Gynecologic Oncologists, the American Association for the Advancement of Science, and the International Society of Gynecologic Pathologists, among others. He received the B.A. degree with honors (1956) in mathematics and the natural sciences from Swarthmore College, Pennsylvania, and the M.D. degree (1960) from Yale University School of Medicine, New Haven, Connecticut.